The Evidence
for Vascular
or Endovascular
Reconstruction

Commissioning Editor: Paul Fam
Project Development Manager: Sean Duggan
Project Manager: Jane Duncan
Project Controller: Hilary Hewitt
Designer: Andy Chapman
Cover illustration: Jenni Miller

The Evidence
for Vascular
or Endovascular
Reconstruction

Edited by

Roger M Greenhalgh MA, MD, MChir, FRCS

Jean–Pierre Becquemin MD
Alun Davies DM FRCS
Peter Gaines MRCP FRCR
Peter Harris MD FRCS
Krassi Ivancev MD PhD
Adam Mitchell MB BS FRCAS FRCR
Dieter Raithel MD PhD

W. B. SAUNDERS

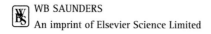
WB SAUNDERS
An imprint of Elsevier Science Limited

© 2002, Elsevier Science Limited. All rights reserved.

The right of Roger M Greenhalgh to be identified as author of this work has been asserted by him in accordance with the Copyright, Designs and Patents Act 1988

First published 2002

ISBN 0 7020 2675 1

British Library Cataloguing in Publication Data
A catalogue record for this book is available from the British Library

Library of Congress Cataloging in Publication Data
A catalog record for this book is available from the Library of Congress

Note
Medical knowledge is constantly changing. As new information becomes available, changes in treatment, procedures, equipment and the use of drugs become necessary. The editors, contributors and the publishers have taken care to ensure that the information given in this text is accurate and up to date. However, readers are strongly advised to confirm that the information, especially with regard to drug usage, complies with the latest legislation and standards of practice.

Existing UK nomenclature is changing to the system of Recommended International Nonproprietary Names (rINNs). Until the UK names are no longer in use, these more familiar names are used in this book in preference to rINNs, details of which may be obtained from the British National Formulary.

Typeset by Phoenix Photosetting, Chatham, Kent
Printed and bound in Great Britain at The Bath Press, Bath

The
Publisher's
policy is to use
paper manufactured
from sustainable forests

Contents

Contributors

Aadahl P, MD PhD
Associate Professor of Anaesthesiology
University Hospital of Trondheim
Trondheim, Norway

Aasland J, RN
Research Nurse
University Hospital of Trondheim
Trondheim, Norway

Ahmadi R, MD
Institute for Interdisciplinary Research
    in Clinical Vascular Medicine
Vienna, Austria

Arko FR, MD
Director of Endovascular Surgery
Assistant Professor of Surgery
Stanford University Hospital
Stanford, California, USA

Barjau E, MD
Servei d'Angiologia I Cirurgia Vascular
Hospital Universitari de Bellvitge
University of Barcelona
Barcelona, Spain

Bates Mc, , MD, FAAC
Instituto Cardiovascular de Buenos Aires
Buenos Aires, Argentina

Beattie DK, MD, FRCS (Gen Surg) FRCSI
Department of Surgery
Charing Cross Hospital
London, UK

Becquemin JP, MD
Professor of Vascular Surgery
Department of Vascular Surgery
Henri Mondor Hospital, AP/HP Paris
University of Paris XII
Creteil, France

Bell PRF, MBChB, MD, FRCS
Professor of Surgery
Robert Kilpatrick Building
Leicester Royal Infirmary
Leicester, UK

Bell RE, MBBS, FRCS
Clinical Research Fellow
Department of General and Vascular Surgery
Guy's and St Thomas' Hospital
London, UK

Bergeron P, MD
Chef de Service
Chirurgie Cardio-Thoracique et Vasculaire
Fondation Hôpital Saint Joseph
Marseille, France

Bergqvist D, MD, PhD
Professor, Department of Surgery
University Hospital
Uppsala, SwedEN

Bezzi M, MD
Assistant Professor of Radiology
Instituto di Radiologia
Universita "La Sapienza"
Policlinico Umberto I
Rome, Italy

Biasi GM, MD, FACS, FRCS
Professor of Vascular Surgery
Universita degli Studi di Milano-Bicocca
Bassini & San Gerardo Teaching Hospitals
Cinisello Balsamo, Milan, Italy

Blankensteijn J, MD
Chief Division of Vascular Surgery
University Medical Center,
Utrecht, The Netherlands

Boeckler D, MD
Clinical Research Fellow
Department of Surgery
Klinikum Nuernberg Sued
Nuernberg, Germany

Bolia A, MBCh, (Glasgow), DMRD, FRCR
Department of Radiology
The Leicester Royal Infirmary NHS Trust
Leicester, UK

Bradbury A, BSc, MD, FRCSEd
Professor, University Department of Vascular Surgery

Lincoln House (Research Institute)
Birmingham Heartlands Hospital
Bordesley Green East
Birmingham, UK

Burns P, BSc, FRCSEd
Research Fellow
University Department of Vascular Surgery
Lincoln House (Research Institute)
Birmingham Heartlands Hospital
Bordesley Green East
Birmingham, UK

Buth Jaap, MD, PhD
Consultant Vascular Surgeon
Catharina Hospital
Eindhoven, The Netherlands

Buth Jacob, MD
Regional Vascular Unit 8C Link
Royal Liverpool University Hospital
Liverpool, UK

Cairols MA, MD
Servei d'Angiologia I
Cirurgia Vascular
Hospital Universitari de Bellvitge
University of Barcelona
Barcelona, Spain

Campbell WB, MS, FRCP, FRCS
Professor and Consultant Surgeon
Royal Devon and Exeter Hospital
Exeter, UK

Cao P, MD
Unità Operativa di Chirurgia Vascolare
Policlinico Monteluce
Perugia, Italy

Celerien J
Assistant in Vascular Surgery
University Hospital
Strasbourg, France

Chakfe N
Professor of Vascular Surgery
University Hospital
Strasbourg, France

Clayton G, MBBS, MRCS
Clinical Research Fellow
Imperial College School of Medicine
Charing Cross Hospital
London, UK

Cleveland T, FRCS, FRCR
Consultant Vascular Radiologist
Sheffield Vascular Institute
Northern General Hospital
Sheffield, UK

Cuypers PWM, MD, PhD
Consultant Vascular Surgeon
Catharina Hospital
Eindhoven, The Netherlands

Daenens K, MD
Department of Vascular Surgery
University Clinic Gasthuisberg
Leuven, Belgium

Davies AH, MA, DM, FRCS
Reader in Surgery and Consultant Surgeon
Department of Surgery
Charing Cross Hospital
London, UK

Deleo G, MD
Universita degli Studi di Milano-Bicocca
Bassini & San Gerardo Teaching Hospitals
Cinisello Balsamo, Milan, Italy

Diethrich EB, MD
Professor, Medical Director
Arizona Heart Institute & Arizona Heart Hospital
Phoenix, AZ 85006, USA

Dix F, BSc, MBBS, FRCS
Venous Research Fellow
Vascular Research Department
University of Manchester
Wythenshawe Hospital
Manchester, UK

Domenig C, MD
Institute for Interdisciplinary Research
   in Clinical Vascular Medicine
Vienna, Austria

Duijm LEM, MD, PhD
Consultant Interventional Radiologist
Catharina Hospital
Eindhoven, The Netherlands

Fanelli F, MD
Junior Attendine in Vascular Radiology
Instituto di Radiologia
Universita "La Sapienza"
Policlinico Umberto I
Rome, Italy

Fogarty TJ, MD
Director of Endovascular Surgery
Assistant Professor of Surgery
Stanford University Hospital
Stanford
California, USA

Forneau I, MD
Department of Vascular Surgery
University Clinic Gasthuisberg
Leuven, Belgium

Gaines PA, MRCP, FRCP
Consultant Vascular Radiologist
Sheffield Vascular Institute
Sheffield, UK

Geissler C, MD
Kurhessisches Diakonissenhaus
Kassel, Germany

Gilling-Smith GL, MS, FRCS
Consultant Vascular Surgeon
Regional Vascular Unit
Royal Liverpool University Hospital
Liverpool UK

Gough MJ, ChM, FRCS
Consultant Vascular Surgeon
The General Infirmary at Leeds
Leeds LS1 3EX, UK

Greenhalgh RM, MA, MD, MChir, FRCS
Professor of Surgery
Imperial College School of Medicine
Charing Cross Hospital
London, UK

Grønholdt MLM, MD, PhD
Research Fellow
Department of Vascular Surgery,
Rigshospitale
Copenhagen, Denmark

Gruss J-D, MD
Kurhessisches Diakonissenhaus
Kassel, Germany

Guerrero F
Servei d'Angiologia I
Cirurgia Vascular
Hospital Universitari de Bellvitge
University of Barcelona
Barcelona, Spain

Gunther G, MD
Department of Vascular and Thoracic Surgery
Krankenhaus Nordwest
Frankfurt, Germany

Hamilton G, MBChB, FRCS
Consultant Vascular Surgeon
University Department of Surgery
Royal Free Hospital
London, UK

Hanschke D, MD
Kurhessisches Diakonissenhaus
Kassel, Germany

Harris JP, MS FRACS, FRCS, FACS, DDU
Department of Surgery
University of Sydney DO6
New South Wales, Australia

Harris PL, MD,FRCS
Regional Vascular Unit 8C Link
Royal Liverpool Hopsital
Liverpool, UK

Hassani O
Assistant in Vascular Surgery
University Hospital
Strasbourg, France

Hatlinghus S, MD
Consultant Radiologist
University Hospital of Trondheim
Trondheim, Norway

Hawdon A, PhD
Department of Surgery
Charing Cross Hospital
London, UK

Heilbron M Jr, MD
Staff Vascular Surgeon
Harbor-UCLA Medical Center
Torrance, California, USA

Hill BB, MD
Assistant Professor of Surgery
Stanford University Medical Center
Stanford, California, USA

Hinchliffe RJ, MRCS
Research Fellow Vascular Surgery
Department of Vascular and Endovascular Surgery
University Hospital, Nottingham, UK

Hölzenbein T, MD
Institute for Interdisciplinary Research
    in Clinical Vascular Medicine
Vienna, Austria

Hopkinson BR, ChM, FRCS
Professor of Vascular Surgery
Department of Vascular and Endovascular Surgery
University Hospital, Nottingham, UK

Iborra E, MD
Servei d'Angiologia I Cirurgia Vascular
Hospital Universitari de Bellvitge
University of Barcelona, Barcelona, Spain

Ince H, MD
Abteilung fur Kardiologie
Universitatsklinikum Rostock
Rostock, Germany

Ivancev K, MD, PhD
Head of Endovascular Centre
Department of Radiology
Malmo University Hospital
Malmo, Sweden

Kakisis JD, MD
Clinical Research Fellow
Athens, Greece

Kirch M, MD
Department of Surgery
University of Duesseldorf Medical School
Augusta Hospital
Duesseldorf, Germany

Kolvenbach R, PhD
Professor, Department of Vascular Surgery and
Plebology
Augusta Hospital
Duesseldorf, Germany

Kretschmer G, MD
Institute for Interdisciplinary Research
in Clinical Vascular Medicine
Vienna, Austria

Kretz J–G
Professor of Cardiovascular Surgery
University Hospital
Strasbourg, France

Lacroix H, MD
Department of Vascular Surgery
Universsity Clinic Gasthuisberg
Leuven, Belgium

Laheij R, MD
Regional Vascular Unit 8C Link
Royal Liverpool University Hospital
Liverpool, UK

Lammer J, MD
Institute for Interdisciplinary Research in Clinical
Vascular Medicine
Vienna, Austria

Lee JT, MD
Fellow, Vascular Surgery
Harbor–UCLA Medical Center
Torrance, California, USA

Liapis CD, MD, FACS
Associate Professor of Vascular Surgery
Athens, Greece

Lindblad B, MD, PhD
Department of Radiology
Malmo University Hospital
Malmo, Sweden

Lundbom J, MD, PhD
Consultant Vascular Surgeon
University Hospital of Trondheim
Trondheim, Norway

Malina M, MD, PhD
Department of Radiology
Malmo University Hospital
Malmo, Sweden

May J, AC, MD, MS, FRACS, FACS
Department of Surgery
University of Sydney DO6
New South Wales, Australia

McCollum CN, MBChB, MD, FRCS
Professor of Surgery
Vascular Research Department
University of Manchester
Wythenshawe Hospital
Manchester,UK

Minar E, MD
Professor of Internal Medicine
Department of Angiology
University of Vienna
General Hospital Vienna
Vienna, Austria

Moss JG, MBChB, FRCS, FRCR
North Glasgow Hospitals NHS Trust
Gartnavel Hospital
Glasgow, UK

Myhre HO, MD, PhD
Professor of Surgery
University Hospital of Trondheim
Trondheim, Norway

Nevelsteen A, MD
Professor, Head of Department of Vascular Surgery
University Clinic Gasthuisberg
Leuven, Belgium

Nicholas T, MS, FRCS,
Specialist Registrar
Regional Vascular Unit
Royal Liverpool University Hospital
Liverpool, UK

Nicholson T, FRCR
Consultant Cardiovascular Radiologist
Hull & East Yorkshire Hospitals Trust
Hull, UK

Nienaber CA, MD
Abteilung fur Kardiologie
Universitatsklinikum Rostock
Rostock, Germany

Ohki T, MD
Chief, Vascular and Endovascular Surgery
Montefiore Medical Center
Associate Professor of Surgery
Albert Einstein College of Medicine
New York, New York, USA

Ouriel K, MD, FACS, FACC
Chairman Department of Vascular Surgery
The Cleveland Clinic Foundation
Cleveland, Ohio, USA

Paaske W, MD, DMSc, FRCS, FACS
Professor, Department of Cardiothoracic & Vascular
    Surgery
Aarhus University Hospital
Skejby Sygehus
Aarhus N, Denmark

Parodi JC, MD
Professor, Director, Instituto Cardiovascular de
    Buenos Aires
Buenos Aires, Argentina

Peloschek P, MD
Institute for Interdisciplinary Research
    in Clinical Vascular Medicine
Vienna, Austria

Pfeiffer T, MD
Attending Vascular Surgeon
Department of Vascular Surgery
    and Kidney Transplantation
Heinrich-Heine-University of Dusseldorf
Dusseldorf, Germany

Pinter L, MD
Department of Surgery
University of Duesseldorf Medical School
Augusta Hospital
Duesseldorf, Germany

Poetter R, MD
Professor of Radiotherapy
University of Vienna
General Hospital Vienna
Vienna, Austria

Pokrajac B, MD
Professor of Radiotherapy
University of Vienna
General Hospital Vienna
Vienna, Austria

Polterauer P, MD
Institute for Interdisciplinary Research
    in Clinical Vascular Medicine
Vienna, Austria

Poussier B, MD
Department of Vascular Surgery
Henri Mondor Hospital, AP/HP Paris
University of Paris XII
Creteil, France

Prescher H, MD
Kurhessisches Diakonissenhaus
Kassel, Germany

Puech–Leao P, MD
Instituto Cardiovascular de Buenos Aires
Buenos Aires, Argentina

Raithel D, MD, PhD
Professor and Head
Department of Surgery
Klinikum Nuernberg Sued
Nuernberg, Germany

Reekers JA, MD, PhD
Professor of Radiology
Academic Medical Centre
Amsterdam, The Netherlands

Rehders TC, MD
Abteilung fur Kardiologie
Universitatsklinikum Rostock
Rostock, Germany

Resch T, MD, PhD
Department of Radiology
Malmo University Hospital
Malmo, Sweden

Rinckenbach S
Resident in Vascular Surgery
University Hospital
Strasbourg, France

Rossi M, MD
Assistant Professor of Radiology
Instituto di Radiologia
Universita "La Sapienza"
Policlinico Umberto I
Rome, Italy

Rossi P, MD
Professor of Radiology,
Instituto di Radiologia
Universita "La Sapienza"
Policlinico Umberto I
Rome, Italy

Salvatori FM, MD
Interventional Radiologist
Instituto di Radiologia
Universita "La Sapienza"
Policlinico Umberto I
Rome, Italy

Sandmann W, MD
Professor and Chairman
Department of Vascular Surgery
    and Kidney Transplantation
Heinrich-Heine-University of Dusseldorf
Dusseldorf, Germany

Sautner T, MD
Institute for Interdisciplinary Research
    in Clinical Vascular Medicine
Vienna, Austria

Schillinger M, MD
Institute for Interdisciplinary Research
    in Clinical Vascular Medicine
Vienna, Austria

Schroeder TV, MD, DMSc
Professor, Department of Vascular Surgery
Rigshospitalet
Blegdamsvej
Copenhagen, Denmark

Sillesen HH, MD, DMSc
Chief Vascular Surgeon
Department of Vascular Surgery
Rigshospitalet
Blegdamsvej
Copenhagen, Denmark

Simeon JM, MD
Servei d'Angiologia I Cirurgia Vascular
Hospital Universitari de Bellvitge
University of Barcelona
Barcelona, Spain

Sonesson B, MD, PhD
Department of Radiology
Malmo University Hospital
Malmo, Sweden

Taylor PR, MA, MChir, FRCS
Consultant Vascular Surgeon
Department of General and Vascular Surgery
Guy's and St Thomas' Hospital
London, UK

Tielbeek AV, MD, PhD
Consultant Interventional Radiologist
Catharina Hospital
Eindhoven, The Netherlands

Towne JB, MD
Medical College of Winsconsin
Milwaukee, Wisconsin, USA

Tshomba Y, MD
Universita degli Studi di Milano-Bicocca
Bassini & San Gerardo Teaching Hospitals
Cinisello Balsamo, Milan, Italy

van Marrewijk C, MD
Regional Vascular Unit 8C Link
Royal Liverpool University Hospital
Liverpool, UK

van Urk H, MD, PhD, FRCS(Ed)
Professor of Vascular Surgery
University Hospital Rotterdam
Rotterdam, The Netherlands

Veith FJ, MD
Albert Einstein College of Medicine
New York, New York, USA

Verzini F, MD
Unità Operativa di Chirurgia Vascolare
Policlinico Monteluce
Perugia, Italy

Vorwerk D, MD
Professor and Chairman
Department of Radiology
Klinikum Ingolstadt
Ingolstadt, Germany

Wahba A, MD, PhD
Consultant Cardiac Surgeon
University Hospital of Trondheim
Trondheim, Norway

White GH, MB BS FRACS
Department of Surgery
University of Sydney DO6,
New South Wales, Australia

White RA, MD, FACS
Professor of Surgery
Harbor-UCLA Medical Center
Torrance, California, USA

Wolfram R, MD
Clinical Research Fellow
University of Vienna
General Hospital Vienna
Vienna, Austria

Yilmaz N, MD
Clinical Fellow in Vascular Surgery
Catharina Hospital
Eindhoven, The Netherlands

Zannetti S, MD
Clinical Study Manager
Peripheral Vascular Division
Medtronic Europe SA
Tolochenaz, Switzerland

Zegelman M, MD
Head, Department of Vascular and Thoracic Surgery
Krankenhaus Nordwest
Frankfurt, Germany

Preface

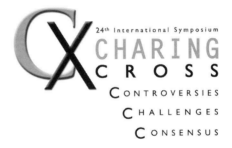

24th International Symposium

CHARING
CROSS

CONTROVERSIES
CHALLENGES
CONSENSUS

This is a novel book. It is in a series of volumes, each published at the time of the Charing Cross Symposium – an annual event since 1978. Technologies and techniques have changed in the communication world. Books are part of that change. The Charing Cross Symposium is an international event and has a most distinguished following of registrants who come from all over the world. The outstanding feature of the meeting is that it is compact and relates to a single topic in general and World Class speakers contribute to it.

Over the years the book has been designed first – not as a conference summary but as a book in its own right. The chapters have been written in advance, edited, and the book produced so that it has been ready for the participants at the time of the meeting. It has always been on time.

In the year 2001 Symposium we enjoyed two days of the latest techniques and the 4th edition of the Atlas was produced. Last year we had the techniques, this year the evidence! A hallmark of the Charing Cross Symposium is to look for the evidence for interventions. Those who met in 2001 screamed out for evidence of interventions but the speakers were detailed not to give any more than technique in that year and the evidence had to wait.

This is the moment when we look at evidence. The titles in recent years have been vascular and endovascular. The endovascular revolution has been the dominant issue of the 1990s in the subject, perhaps triggered by the endovascular aneurysm repair early in the decade. Now there are options of management and this year the programme directors decided to set up the whole of the book and meeting in terms of gentle confrontation and a series of debates. These days a performance can be recorded and televised. The book is a companion to other forms of communication. Readers have found that this series of books is valuable for a number of reasons but mainly for the referencing and up-to-date aspects of the rapidly changing subject. So often textbooks are out of date before they reach the shelves but this series is bang up to date and summarizes the key points of each topic with 'bullet points'. This time the book represents a series of controversies which are challenged as a debate. At the time of writing no author had seen what another author had stated – and each was asked to concentrate on their argument and not to give a balanced approach. At the end of every combination of arguments a short editorial piece is included. At the meeting in April 2002 surgeons and radiologists will debate the rights and the wrongs and it is hoped that a consensus will prevail. The editorial comments are therefore imaginary comments ahead of the argument. Readers can see that the cast-list of authors is highly distinguished. What better than to get the world's experts to hit the high spots and challenge a controversy?

R M Greenhalgh

February 2002

Plaque type can determine the need for asymptomatic carotid intervention

For the motion

Giorgio M Biasi, Yamume Tshomba, Gaetano Deleo

Introduction

The results of the NASCET and ECST studies, which were published at the beginning of the 1990s[1,2] consecrated for posterity carotid endarterectomy as the treatment of choice in the prevention of stroke from symptomatic tight stenoses of the carotid bifurcation. The efficacy of carotid endarterectomy was further defined and confirmed a few years later[3] also for asymptomatic patients presenting with the same conditions, when performed by surgeons with low complication rates.

It is worth noticing that for all these studies, indication for carotid endarterectomy was essentially based on the presence or absence of neurological symptoms and the rate of carotid stenosis. More recently, carotid stenting has appeared on the international scene and has been proposed as a less invasive and more attractive alternative to carotid endarterectomy for symptomatic and asymptomatic patients affected by tight carotid stenosis, with a rate of neurological complications comparable and sometimes even better, than that reported with carotid endarterectomy. In addition, recent publications[4] including the Carotid and Vertebral Artery Transluminal Angioplasty Study (CAVATAS)[5] seem to confute the extremely good results following carotid endarterectomy, as appeared from the NASCET and ECST studies. Furthermore, even though there is no demonstration that there is a difference in terms of neurological complications between brain protection and non-protection in the course of carotid stenting, it is quite evident that so-called 'high risk' patients, may benefit from a capturing device in preventing an intraprocedural brain embolization.[6,7] Apart from the fact that there is no definition of what is a high risk patient for carotid stenting, it should be remarked once more that as for the carotid endarterectomy, also for the stenting procedure, indication is based on the percentage of carotid stenosis and presence or absence of neurological symptoms.

Technique

This consideration led to a series of recent reports[8-10] and discussions, which tend to question the validity of these two parameters: rate of stenosis and neurological

1

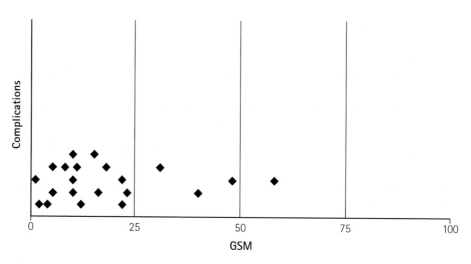

Figure 1. Concentration of neurological complications in cases of carotid stenting. The majority of complications occurred in patients with very soft, echolucent plaques with a grey scale median (GSM)<25.

symptoms, as reliable criteria for indicating conventional or endoluminal repair of the carotid stenosis, in the prevention of brain ischaemia. Those who have been treating carotid bifurcation lesions for years, have certainly experienced situations where symptomatic patients with a similar rate of carotid stenoses, but having completely different plaques, may intuitively be categorized as at low, intermediate or high risk for brain embolization, in relation to the features of the plaque (Fig. 1). The question of the potential risk of embolization of some plaques compared with others, has long been discussed and several publications have pointed to the need for analysing the plaque before any procedure on the carotid bifurcation is undertaken.[11–13] In an experimental study published in 1998, Ohki et al. could demonstrate that echolucent plaques produce more embolic particles.[14] The extreme accuracy in the manipulation during isolation of the carotid bifurcation during the course of carotid endarterectomy, or when crossing a lesion with a wire during carotid stenting, are recognized as mandatory to prevent plaque debris from embolizing to the brain. The potential risk of embolization is high during carotid endarterectomy, but it is even higher during carotid stenting where the plaque is not removed but remodelled, which may represent a source of embolization during the procedure, since whatever brain protection device is used, no protection is provided throughout the entire procedure, nor during the post-procedural hours and days. Even though these facts are well-known and acknowledged, indication for any procedures (conventional or endoluminal) on the carotid bifurcation, still relies on rate of stenosis and neurological symptoms.

Evidence

These considerations brought us initially to the perception, and finally to the conclusion, that these two parameters: percentage of carotid stenosis and presence or absence of neurological symptoms, are quite obsolete and no longer adequate for a correct indication to any carotid procedure and that other criteria, i.e. plaque characteristics, should be exploited and their clinical application consequently recognized and implemented.

Symptomatology is a vexed question. The issue of neurological symptoms in fact, involves two different aspects. One is a moral aspect, the other is purely clinical. The first poses the problem of whether it is ethical to perform any interventional act which implies a risk of permanent injury or even death in a symptom-free patient. The question can be puzzling and carry many moral as well as medico-legal, but not clinical implications. The other aspect is a false problem, since symptoms are often just the epiphenomenon of an underlying carotid lesion. The latter has to be the real concern of the physician and not the presence or absence of symptoms. If an asymptomatic malignancy is identified in a patient, it would be a nonsense or even criminal to wait for symptoms to become evident, before it is removed or in any case treated. It could be objected that the substantial difference between the two cases, is that malignancies usually have a progressively negative evolution, whilst it is not necessarily so for a carotid stenosis. Nevertheless, if a carotid plaque progresses to produce stroke or death, this is more a consequence of the characteristics of the plaque, rather than the presence or absence of symptoms.

The ICAROS study was designed and proposed for participation to a number of Centres practising carotid stenting worldwide, with the aim of correlating the risk of embolization during carotid stenting with the echographic characteristics of the plaque.

The rationale of the study was to demonstrate that an accurate selection of the patients, candidates for carotid stenting on the basis of the plaque characteristics, could improve the post-procedural results. The study utilizes a computer elaboration of the echographic image of the carotid plaque, which gives an index of echogenicity (grey scale median: GSM) that can be correlated with the outcome of the procedure.[15] The study will be concluded in January 2002, but with the data collected so far, we can anticipate that ICAROS is feasible, reliable since it provides a quantifiable number (the GSM), and reproducible through the standardization of the images collected from different centres, with different machines, by different technicians.[15]

From July 2000 to July 2001, 409 cases were reported from 12 different centres worldwide; 334 patients were entered in the study, while 75 were excluded because of: 1) low quality of the images; 2) incomplete information on data forms or 3) lost to follow-up. There were 237 male and 97 female patients. In 112 cases the underlying pathology was restenosis (33.5%) and a primary lesion in 222 cases (66.5%). In all cases a stent procedure was applied (100%). A brain protection device was applied in 177 cases (53%). The overall neurological complications were 21 (6.3%): ten transient ischaemic attacks (3%), seven minor strokes (2.1%) and four major strokes (1.2%). Two of the ten transient ischaemic attacks, two of the seven minor strokes and one of the four major strokes, occurred during the course of brain-protected procedures.

Seventeen of the 21 complications (81%) occurred in cases with a GSM<25 (very soft, echolucent plaques), three (14.3%) with a GSM between 25 and 50, and one (4.7%) with a GSM>50 (Fig. 2). It is worth noticing that, of the total of the 334 cases observed, the incidence of the GSM<25 is 21%, GSM>50 is 14% and the majority of cases have a 25<GSM <50. On the basis of these preliminary data of the ICAROS study, we concluded that any indication to carotid endarterectomy or carotid stenting should not prescind from:

1. rate of carotid stenosis,
2. neurological symptoms,
3. echogenicity of the plaque.

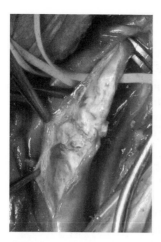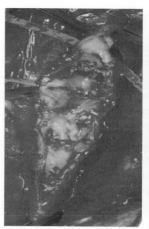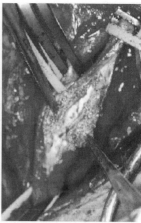

Figure 2. Intraoperative images of three different patients operated on for symptomatic tight stenosis, of similar rate, of the internal carotid artery. The discriminating factors in these three patients for the indications for any procedure, should not be based on the presence or absence of neurological symptoms, nor the percentage of stenosis but rather the characteristics of the plaque.

In addition:

1. carotid stenting should be contraindicated when the pre-procedural GSM is less than 25,
2. carotid stenting could safely be performed with the mandatory application of a capturing device with a GSM of between 25 and 50.
3. Finally, carotid stenting could be indicated also when the GSM is over 50. Nevertheless, in these cases, the application of a brain-protection device may be optional or even contraindicated

Summary

- Carotid endarterectomy remains the gold standard for the prevention of brain ischaemia consequent to embolization from carotid bifurcation plaque.

- Carotid stenting seems to be an appealing procedure providing encouraging and comparable results.

- Indication for both procedures is mostly based on 1: Rate of carotid stenosis and 2: Presence or absence of neurological symptoms.

- The validity of these two parameters, as sufficient and reliable for a safe indication, is questioned.

- The parameters and algorithms to identify the grade of potential risk intrinsic in a plaque to embolize to the brain are numerous, but, on the basis of the preliminary results of the ICAROS study, we can conclude that the pre-procedural identification of the grey scale median of the plaque, is a reliable, quantifiable and reproducible method to determine the need for a safe carotid intervention in symptomatic and asymptomatic patients.

References

1. North American Symptomatic Carotid Endarterectomy Trial Collaborators. Beneficial effect of carotid endarterectomy in symptomatic patients with high-grade carotid stenosis. *N Engl J Med* 1991; **325**: 445–453.
2. European Carotid Surgery Trialists Collaborative Group. MCR European carotid surgery trial: Interim results for symptomatic patients with severe (70–99%) or with mild (0–29%) carotid stenosis. *Lancet* 1991; **337**: 1235–1243.
3. Executive Committee for the Asymptomatic Carotid Atherosclerosis Study. Endarterectomy for asymptomatic carotid artery stenosis. *JAMA* 1995; **73**: 1421–1428.
4. Wennberg DE, Lucas FL, Birkmeyer JD *et al.* Variations in carotid endarterectomy mortality in the Medicare population: Trial hospitals, volume, and patient characteristics. *JAMA* 1998; **279**: 1278–1281.
5. CAVATAS Investigators. Endovascular versus surgical treatment in patients with carotid stenosis in the Carotid and Vertebral Artery Transluminal Angioplasty Study (CAVATAS); A randomized trial. *Lancet* 2001; **357**: 1729–1737.
6. Henry M, Amor M, Henry I *et al.* Carotid stenting with cerebral protection: First clinical experience using the PercuSurge GuardWire system. *J Endovasc Surg* 1999; **6**: 321–331.
7. Parodi JC. Initial evaluation of carotid angioplasty and stenting using three different cerebral protection devices (Abstract). *J Endovasc Ther* 2000; **7** (suppl.): I30–I31.
8. Dangas G, Laird JR, Mehran R *et al.* Carotid artery stenting in patients with high risk anatomy for carotid endarterectomy. *J Endovasc Ther* 2001; **8**: 39–43.
9. Diethrich EB. Characterizing the carotid revascularization candidate: Will plaque morphology be important? (Editorial) *J Endovasc Ther* 2001; **8**: 44–45.
10. Biasi GM. Is it time to reconsider the selection criteria for conventional or endovascular repair of carotid artery stenosis in the prevention of cerebral ischemia? *J Endovasc Ther* 2001; **8**: 339–340.
11. Biasi GM, Mingazzini P, Sampaolo A, Ferrari S. Echographic characterization of the carotid plaque and risk for cerebral ischemia. In *Progress in Angiology and Vascular Surgery*. Minerva Medica Eds. 1995: 59–65.
12. Nicolaides AN. Asymptomatic carotid stenosis and risk of stroke. Identification of a high risk (ACSRS) group. A natural history study. *Int Angiol* 1995; **14**: 21–23.
13. Biasi GM, Sampaolo A, Mingazzini PM *et al.* Computer analysis of ultrasonic plaque echolocency in identifying high risk carotid bifurcation lesions. *Eur J Vasc Endovasc Surg* 1999; **17**: 476–479.
14. Ohki T, Marin ML, Lyon RT *et al.* *Ex vivo* human carotid artery bifurcation stenting: Correlation of lesion characteristics with embolic potential. *J Vasc Surg* 1998; **27**: 463–471.
15. Biasi GM, Ferrari SA, Nicolaides AN, Mingazzini PM, Reid D. The ICAROS Registry of Carotid Artery Stenting. *J Endovasc Ther* 2001; **8**: 46–52.

Plaque type can determine the need for asymptomatic carotid intervention

Against the motion
Torben V Schroeder,
Marie Louise Moes Grønholdt,
Henrik H Sillesen

Introduction

Stroke is one of the leading causes of death worldwide with the consequence that huge resources are spent on rehabilitation. Approximately 20% of ischaemic strokes are associated with carotid artery disease, mainly due to embolization from degenerative breakdown of complex plaques. Carotid endarterectomy is effective in reducing the risk of ipsilateral stroke in patients with symptomatic high-grade carotid artery stenosis in the European Carotid Surgery Trial (ECST) as well as in the North American Symptomatic Carotid Endarterectomy Trial (NASCET).[1,2]

Evidence

Stenosis severity and asymptomatic carotid surgery

The substantial number of strokes in patients with carotid artery disease occurring without warning, suggests, that carotid surgery could also reduce the risk of stroke in asymptomatic patients with severe carotid stenosis. The largest and most recent randomized trial, the Asymptomatic Carotid Atherosclerosis Study (ACAS) indicated a substantial relative risk reduction in patients with carotid stenosis of 60% or more.[3] In absolute terms the 5-year risk reduction was cut from 11% to 5%. Two systematic reviews and meta-analyses pooling the ACAS data with three smaller trials have confirmed the evidence favouring endarterectomy for asymptomatic carotid stenosis, but the effect is at best barely significant.[4,5]

The absolute risk reduction may only be 3–4% over 3–5 years, and it is necessary to operate on about 50 patients to prevent one stroke in the next 3 years – or even more to prevent just disabling and fatal strokes.[6]

Recent NASCET data also question the justification for endarterectomy in patients with asymptomatic stenosis.[7] Counting only large-artery strokes as the outcome of interest, rather than strokes from any cause, halves the risk reduction. The remaining

Table 1. Carotid endarterectomy for asymptomatic carotid stenosis. Any stroke or perioperative death[5]

Study (year)	Surgical group	Medical group	Mean follow-up (years)	Peto odds ratio (95% CI)
AURC (1989)[8]	10/128	16/109	5	0.5 (0.2–1.1)
MACE (1992)[9]	3/36	0/35	2	7.6 (0.8–75)
VA (1993)[10]	25/211	30/233	4	0.9 (0.5–1.6)
ACAS (1995)[3]	60/825	86/834	2.7	0.68 (0.48–0.96)
TOTAL	98/1215	132/1225		0.73 (0.56–0.96)

strokes had a lacunar or cardioembolic cause, and were therefore not attributable to carotid artery disease. Applying these results to the ACAS data[3] diminishes the absolute risk reduction from 5.9 to 3.5% at 5 years. In consequence, the number needed to treat rises to 111 patients to prevent a single large-artery stroke within 2 years. ACAS reported a low 2.3% rate of perioperative stroke and death associated with endarterectomy. In contrast, recent large multicentre studies on asymptomatic patients[11-13] report rates between 4 and 5%, whereby endarterectomy causes more strokes than it prevents. As these morbidity figures are more appropriate to apply, when endarterectomy for asymptomatic disease is performed in the general community outside of the ACAS trial the benefit is hard to visualize. With occlusion of the contralateral carotid artery the risk of perioperative stroke and death may even be as high as 12% in asymptomatic patients.[11]

Thus transatlantic data are in accord: the absolute benefit of carotid surgery in asymptomatic patients is extremely small in terms of absolute risk reduction – in fact so small that medical management remains the sensible alternative; unless high risk subgroups can be readily identified on other grounds than the degree of stenosis.[4]

The atherosclerotic plaque

From studies on coronary atherosclerosis it is known that only a minority of plaques protrude into and compromise the lumen because of compensatory remodelling during plaque growth.[14] Thus, the lumen may remain normal, despite a build-up of a large volume of atherosclerotic plaque in the vessel wall. Atherosclerosis is a diffuse disease with superimposed focal luminal narrowing. The vulnerability and thrombogenicity of atherosclerotic plaques rather than their stenosis severity, together with the status of the collateral circulation, are the most important determinants for the outcome.[15] Thus, angiography may not be the best method to identify high-risk thrombosis-prone lesions.[16] Although the stroke-risk increases with stenosis severity, it is suggestive that the great majority of ischaemic strokes occur distal to low degree steno-

Table 2. Asymptomatic carotid stenosis: progression to stroke

Angiography in 2240 patients

Stenosis at baseline	n	Ipsilateral stroke	
		%, 3-years	n, 4.5-years
0–29%	1270	1.8	28 ⎫ 54
30–69%	843	2.1	26 ⎭
70–99%	127	5.7	13
All	2240		67

sis. Asymptomatic plaques at the carotid bifurcation, contralateral to symptomatic lesions, were evaluated and followed in the European Carotid Surgery Trial (n=2240).[17]

Only one-fifth of new strokes were judged to originate from initially asymptomatic lesions that at baseline caused more than 70% angiographic stenosis, because lower grade stenotic lesions plaques outnumbered by far the high grade stenotic ones.

Plaque morphology and asymptomatic carotid surgery

Many studies have addressed carotid plaque morphology and symptomatology and/or structural brain damage. Applying subjective criteria cerebrovascular symptoms and brain infarction are more frequent with echolucent than hyperechoic plaques. More recent studies have applied computer assessment of plaque echogenicity, i.e. the grey scale median, and found low values to be associated with a higher prevalence of symptomatology and cerebral infarction on computed tomography images, compared with high grey scale median values.[18,19-24] Validation against histology, has consistently reported that an echolucent plaque was associated with a high content of lipid and haemorrhage, whereas the echorich plaque contained more calcification and fibrous tissue.[25-27] The surface characteristics of the plaque, i.e. ulcerations, once believed to be of importance, are not easy to detect reliably, either using ultrasound[28-30] or angiography.[31]

Using computer-assisted ultrasound imaging we have showed that plaque morphology is an independent predictor of ipsilateral ischaemic stroke when adjusting for age in a cohort of 246 patients.[21] In the 135 symptomatic patients echolucency and high degree of stenosis were independent risk factors for stroke, whereas no such increased risk could be shown in the 111 asymptomatic patients followed for 4.4 years (Table 3). In this context it is noteworthy that the group of asymptomatic patients actually had an incidence of ipsilateral stroke resembling the 11% 5-year cumulative risk found in ACAS.[3]

Table 3. Relative risk of ipsilateral ischaemic stroke as a function of carotid plaque echogenicity and severity of stenosis.[21]

Echogenicity	Stenosis	Number of patients	Relative risk (95% CI)	Absolute risk at 4.4 years	Absolute risk increase
All patients (n = 246)					
Echorich	50–79%	77	1	12%	
Echorich	80–99%	31	1.1 (0.3–3.6)	13%	1%
Echolucent	50–79%	96	1.7 (0.8–3.8)	20%	8%
Echolucent	80–99%	42	3.1 (1.3–7.4)	29%	17%
Asymptomatic patients (n = 111)					
Echorich	50–79%	38	1	16%	
Echorich	80–99%	10	0	0%	−16%
Echolucent	50–79%	43	0.6 (0.2–1.8)	12%	−4%
Echolucent	80–99%	20	1.4 (0.4–4.9)	20%	4%
Symptomatic patients (n = 135)					
Echorich	50–79%	39	1	8%	
Echorich	80–99%	21	3.1 (0.7–14)	19%	11%
Echolucent	50–79%	53	4.2 (1.2–15)	26%	18%
Echolucent	80–99%	22	7.9 (2.1–30)	36%	28%

Relative risks are based on Cox regression analysis adjusted for age. Echolucent = grey scale median <74. Echorich = grey scale median ≥74.

The only other follow-up study using stroke as the primary endpoint investigated 4886 asymptomatic individuals, and found that echolucent plaques – subjectively evaluated – had an increased risk ratio for incident stroke.[20] However, adjusted for confounders in a Cox regression model, the degree of stenosis over 50% had a more prominent relative risk than echolucency. Finally the study by Holdsworth et al.[32] concluded that plaque morphology and degree of carotid stenosis were mutually dependent factors, whereas morphology did not add to the sensitivity of stenosis in predicting the presence of symptoms.

Conclusion

Other measures of carotid atherosclerosis than the degree of asymptomatic stenosis put the patients at increased risk, but it is impossible to identify carotid plaque types with sufficiently high risk, to determine the need for carotid endarterectomy.

Epilogue

Some clinicians are still in doubt, as to whether surgery or best medical treatment is better in subgroups of patients. These patients in the 'grey area', are currently randomized in the ongoing Asymptomatic Carotid Surgery Trial (ACST) which together with the ongoing Asymptomatic Carotid Stenosis and Risk of Stroke Study will add to our knowledge about the medical and surgical prevention of stroke in patients with asymptomatic carotid-artery disease.[33,34]

Summary

- Though the risk of stroke rises with increasing degrees of asymptomatic carotid stenosis, it remains low – and much lower than in patients with symptomatic stenosis.

- Plaque echolucency, evaluated by ultrasound B-mode, also increases stroke risk in asymptomatic patients, but not beyond that of severe stenoses.

- The benefit of carotid surgery in patients with asymptomatic atherosclerotic lesions – whether severely stenotic or hypoechoic – is extremely small in terms of absolute risk reduction.

References

1. Randomised trial of endarterectomy for recently symptomatic carotid stenosis: final results of the MRC European Carotid Surgery Trial (ECST). *Lancet* 1998; **351**: 1379–3887.
2. Barnett HJ, Taylor DW, Eliasziw M *et al.* Benefit of carotid endarterectomy in patients with symptomatic moderate or severe stenosis. North American Symptomatic Carotid Endarterectomy Trial Collaborators. *N Engl J Med* 1998; **339**: 1415–1425.
3. Executive Committee for the Asymptomatic Carotid Atherosclerosis Study. Endarterectomy for asymptomatic carotid artery stenosis. *JAMA* 1995; **273**: 1421–1428.
4. Benavente O, Moher D, Pham B. Carotid endarterectomy for asymptomatic carotid stenosis: a meta-analysis. *BMJ* 1998; **317**: 1477–1480.

5. Chambers BR, You RX, Donnan GA. Carotid endarterectomy for asymptomatic carotid stenosis. *Cochrane Database Syst Rev* 2000; CD001923.

6. Warlow C. Carotid endarterectomy for asymptomatic carotid stenosis. Better data, but the case is still not convincing. *BMJ* 1998; 317: 1468.

7. Inzitari D, Eliasziw M, Gates P *et al.* The causes and risk of stroke in patients with asymptomatic internal-carotid-artery stenosis. North American Symptomatic Carotid Endarterectomy Trial Collaborators. *N Engl J Med* 2000; 342: 1693–1700.

8. Lagneau P. [Asymptomatic carotid stenoses. Analysis of randomized studies] Stenoses carotidiennes asymptomatiques. Analyse des études randomisées. *J Mal Vasc* 1993; 18: 209–212.

9. Mayo Asymptomatic Carotid Endarterectomy Study Group. Results of a randomized controlled trial of carotid endarterectomy for asymptomatic carotid stenosis. *Mayo Clin Proc* 1992; 67: 513–518.

10. Hobson RW, Weiss DG, Fields WS *et al.* Efficacy of carotid endarterectomy for asymptomatic carotid stenosis. The Veterans Affairs Cooperative Study Group. *N Engl J Med* 1993; 328: 221–227.

11. Taylor DW, Barnett HJ, Haynes RB *et al.* Low-dose and high-dose acetylsalicylic acid for patients undergoing carotid endarterectomy: a randomised controlled trial. ASA and Carotid Endarterectomy (ACE) Trial Collaborators. *Lancet* 1999; 353: 2179–2184.

12. Hertzer NR, O'Hara PJ, Mascha EJ, Krajewski LP, Sullivan TM, Beven EG. Early outcome assessment for 2228 consecutive carotid endarterectomy procedures: the Cleveland Clinic experience from 1989 to 1995. *J Vasc Surg* 1997; 26: 1–10.

13. Kucey DS, Bowyer B, Iron K, Austin P, Anderson G, Tu JV. Determinants of outcome after carotid endarterectomy. *J Vasc Surg* 1998; 28: 1051–1058.

14. Glagov S, Weisenberg E, Zarins CK, Stankunavicius R, Kolettis GJ. Compensatory enlargement of human atherosclerotic coronary arteries. *N Engl J Med* 1987; 316: 1371–1375.

15. Falk E, Shah PK, Fuster V. Coronary plaque disruption. *Circulation* 1995; 92: 657–671.

16. Falk E, Fuster V. Atherogenesis and its determinants. In *Hurst's the Heart.* Fuster V, Alexander RW, O'Rourke RA, Roberts R KS, Wellens HJJ (eds). New York: McGraw-Hill, 2001.

17. The European Carotid Surgery Trialists Collaborative Group. Risk of stroke in the distribution of an asymptomatic carotid artery. *Lancet* 1995; 345: 209–212.

18. Langsfeld M, Gray-Weale AC, Lusby RJ. The role of plaque morphology and diameter reduction in the development of new symptoms in asymptomatic carotid arteries. *J Vasc Surg* 1989; 9: 548–557.

19. Giannoni MF, Speziale F, Faraglia V *et al.* Minor asymptomatic carotid stenosis contralateral to carotid endarterectomy (CEA): our experience. *Eur J Vasc Surg* 1991; 5: 237–245.

20. Polak JF, Shemanski L, O'Leary DH *et al.* Hypoechoic plaque at US of the carotid artery: an independent risk factor for incident stroke in adults aged 65 years or older. Cardiovascular Health Study. *Radiology* 1998; 208: 649–654.

21. Gronholdt ML, Nordestgaard BG, Schroeder TV, Vorstrup S, Sillesen H. Ultrasonic echolucent carotid plaques predict future strokes. *Circulation* 2001; 104: 68–73.

22. Mathiesen EB, Bonaa KH, Joakimsen O. Echolucent plaques are associated with high risk of ischemic cerebrovascular events in carotid stenosis : the tromso study. *Circulation* 2001; 103: 2171–2175.

23. El Barghouty N, Nicolaides A, Bahal V, Geroulakos G, Androulakis A. The identification of the high risk carotid plaque. *Eur J Vasc Endovasc Surg* 1996; 11: 470–478.

24. Sabetai MM, Tegos TJ, Nicolaides AN *et al.* Hemispheric symptoms and carotid plaque echomorphology. *J Vasc Surg* 2000; 31: 39–49.

25. Montauban van Swijndregt AD, Elbers HR, Moll FL, de Letter J, Ackerstaff RG. Ultrasonographic characterization of carotid plaques. *Ultrasound Med Biol* 1998; 24: 489–493.

26. Gronholdt ML, Wiebe BM, Laursen H, Nielsen TG, Schroeder TV, Sillesen H. Lipid-rich carotid artery plaques appear echolucent on ultrasound B- mode images and may be associated with intraplaque haemorrhage. *Eur J Vasc Endovasc Surg* 1997; 14: 439–445.

27. European Carotid Plaque Study Group. Carotid artery plaque composition—relationship to clinical presentation and ultrasound B-mode imaging. *Eur J Vasc Endovasc Surg* 1995; 10: 23–30.

28. Ratliff DA, Gallagher PJ, Hames TK, Humphries KN, Webster JH, Chant AD. Characterisation of carotid artery disease: comparison of duplex scanning with histology. *Ultrasound Med Biol* 1985; 11: 835–840.

29. Ricotta JJ, Bryan FA, Bond MG *et al.* Multicenter validation study of real-time (B-mode) ultrasound, arteriography, and pathologic examination. *J Vasc Surg* 1987; 6: 512–520.

30. O'Leary DH, Holen J, Ricotta JJ, Roe S, Schenk EA. Carotid bifurcation disease: prediction of ulceration with B-mode US. *Radiology* 1987; 162: 523–525.

31. Streifler JY, Eliasziw M, Fox AJ *et al.* Angiographic detection of carotid plaque ulceration. Comparison with surgical observations in a multicenter study. North American Symptomatic Carotid Endarterectomy Trial. *Stroke* 1994; 25: 1130–1132.

32. Holdsworth RJ, McCollum PT, Bryce JS, Harrison DK. Symptoms, stenosis and carotid plaque morphology. Is plaque morphology relevant? *Eur J Vasc Endovasc Surg* 1995; 9: 80–85.

33. Nicolaides AN. Asymptomatic carotid stenosis and risk of stroke. Identification of a high risk group (ACSRS). A natural history study. *Int Angiol* 1995; 14: 21–23.

34. Halliday AW, Thomas D, Mansfield A. The Asymptomatic Carotid Surgery Trial (ACST). Rationale and design. Steering Committee. *Eur J Vasc Surg* 2001; 8: 703–710.

Plaque type can determine the need for asymptomatic carotid intervention

Charing Cross Editorial Comments towards Consensus

It would be a major step forward if plaque type was proved to point to an increased risk of stroke. It is plain that asymptomatic carotid stenoses of high grade do not relate to stroke nearly as much as symptomatic carotid stenoses. Therefore a degree of stenosis alone is not the only factor. It is entirely reasonable to search for differences in the plaque to point to a relationship with stroke risk. The problem is that this has been investigated now for some 30 years and a breakthrough has been imminent throughout all that time. Haemorrhages into plaques were seen 30 years ago. We were told that the use of aspirin would increase haemorrhage into plaques and that this could cause sudden occlusions and would be contraindicated. Then the beneficial affects of aspirin were argued and on went the discussion.

The fact that it has taken so long for plaque type to be shown to relate to stroke risk in the asymptomatic severely stenosed carotid artery can mean one of two things. It can mean a plaque type never has and never will, relate to stroke risk – and second it can mean that the precise combination of findings has not been clearly recognized. The authors have argued their corners extremely well and at the time of writing I believe that it is fair to say that the jury has been out for a long time and is still out.

Roger M Greenhalgh
Editor

Carotid endarterectomy under general anaesthesia is the treatment of choice

For the motion

Jonathan B Towne

Introduction

Over the past two decades, there have been significant advances in the treatment of extracranial cerebral vascular disease, the most significant of which was the publication of several co-operative randomized prospective studies which demonstrated the efficacy of the treatment of carotid bifurcation disease for the prevention of stroke in patients with both symptomatic and asymptomatic lesions.[1-4]

The focus has now shifted to try to minimize neurological and non-neurological morbidity and mortality following carotid artery surgery. Increasingly, over the past ten years, it has been proposed that the type of anaesthetic technique used has a great effect on the outcome of carotid artery surgery.

This chapter will outline the advantages of general anaesthesia for the performance of carotid endarterectomy, and compare and contrast this technique with regional anaesthesia. The analysis of the type of anaesthetic agent can be divided into three categories. The first is the effect, if any, on neurological morbidity – principally temporary and permanent neurological deficit. The second is the effect on non-neurological adverse events – most importantly the morbidity and mortality related to coronary artery disease. The third is the examination of fiscal efficacy, namely which technique allows for a shorter stay in hospital, therefore making it more cost-effective.

Evidence

The literature on anaesthetic technique for carotid artery surgery reveals many studies with a variety of flaws. The most profound flaw is the lack of truly prospective randomized studies. The second is the increasing tendency of many authors to use historical controls; for example early in their experience they did the procedure using one technique, later they used another. Assuming all else had remained equal, these studies have a limited ability to discriminate the differences in treatment, particularly if the differences are not large. Several studies use a control group of patients not selected for regional anaesthesia because of the stated bias of the surgeon. An important caveat is that any study that compares two techniques

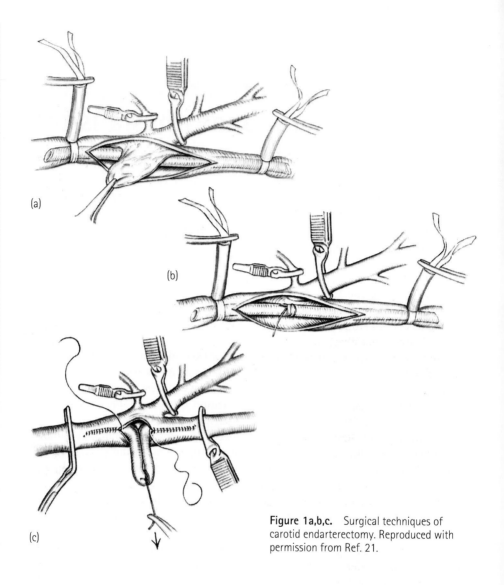

(a)

(b)

(c)

Figure 1a,b,c. Surgical techniques of carotid endarterectomy. Reproduced with permission from Ref. 21.

whether they be surgical or anaesthetic, makes the presumption that the physician performing these techniques is equally skilled at both alternatives and that the enthusiasm for one technique or the other has not biased their opinion. The shortcomings of using historical controls is best illustrated by using length-of-stay data to demonstrate the superiority of an anaesthetic technique. Over the past decade, the length of stay for carotid endarterectomy on our vascular surgery service has decreased from over 5 days to currently an average of 2 days. We did not vary our anaesthesia technique during this period. Had we done so, it might be assumed that indeed the change in technique had affected the length of stay. In fact the change was due to other factors such as hospital reimbursement and the desire of insurance companies to decrease costs.

Effect of type of anaesthesia on neurological outcome following carotid endarterectomy

When one reviews the current literature, several facts become quite obvious. The principal of these is that the surgeon's preferred surgical technique affects the anaesthetic technique. Surgeons who prefer patching tend to use regional anaesthesia less often. The incidence of patching in series using regional anaesthesia is much lower than in many reported series where general anaesthesia is employed. The average duration of the procedure is significantly shorter for regional anaesthesia. Similarly, those who prefer to use regional anaesthesia are less inclined to perform intraoperative assessment of the vascular repair.

Intraoperative evaluation is the best way to determine the haemodynamic status of the repair because immediate operative revision is possible when technical defect is identified. Our average time for performing intraoperative evaluation was 10.6 minutes ($\pm$1 min).[5] Since a technically precise repair is the most important determinant of success of carotid endarterectomy, this becomes a major point of difference when evaluating anaesthesia techniques. Several studies have demonstrated a significant correlation between technical errors of the carotid repair, and the development of perioperative neurological deficits.[6-8] Hand in glove with the intraoperative assessment of the vascular repair has come an increased incidence of patching of the artery because of the demonstrated improvement in heamodynamics, clearly seen on intraoperative assessment.[5,9,10]

Currently, we patch 70% of the carotid reconstructions. Since regional anaesthesia tends to place a premium on the temporal efficacy of the procedure, there is an inherent disinclination on the part of the surgeon to do anything that would extend that procedure. In the reported series that compare the duration of the procedure and the incidence of carotid patching and/or intraoperative assessment, the operative times are shorter in the regional group, the incidence of carotid patching is decreased, and intraoperative assessment is rarely done.[11,12]

The reported temporary and permanent neurological deficit rates are similar for procedures done under regional and general anaesthesia. There have been no prospective randomized trials to evaluate adequately the effect of anaesthesia techniques on neurological outcomes. Also there are no studies evaluating the status of the repair either in the perioperative period or long-term. Studies that evaluate the status of the operative repair are important to determine if the relatively infrequent use of carotid patching and absence of intraoperative assessment affects the short- and long-term patency and neurological outcome of the carotid repair.

Non-neurological morbidity

Coronary artery disease is the most important non-neurological factor affecting morbidity and mortality of carotid endarterectomy. In multiple studies it has been the aetiological factor in 60–100% of cases.[13-15] In these studies the neurological contribution to mortality ranged from 17 to 33%. The goal is to perform carotid endarterectomy for the least cost in terms of myocardial complications. The choice of anaesthetics provides an interesting contrast.

The use of general anaesthetic allows precise control of blood pressure, and certainly avoids any episode of hypoxia. Perhaps most critically, general anaesthetic allows the anaesthesiologist effectively to avoid tachycardia which is the most important factor affecting myocardial function and outcome. McCann and Clements, in an evaluation of 50 consecutive patients who underwent continuous perioperative electrocardiographic monitoring during vascular surgery procedures, found that tachycardia was often associated with myocardial ischaemia.[16] On the other hand, these positive effects must be balanced by the depressive effect that inhalation of anaesthetics have on myocardial function. Several studies have addressed the fact that regional anaesthetics result in fewer perioperative myocardial complications.[17, 18]

In a randomized prospective study, Sbarigia and colleagues compared regional and general anaesthetics in groups of patients with and without myocardial disease.[17] Mean pressure in patients with local anaesthesia was higher and the accumulated number of haemodynamic events was not statistically different between the two groups, but the prevalence of hyperdynamic events was higher in the group receiving local anaesthesia. In contrast, hypodynamic events were more frequent in those receiving general anaesthesia. Of note, is that the use of electrocardiogram monitored episodes of myocardial ischaemia was slightly more frequent and longer in the postoperative period than in the intraoperative period. Under general anaesthesia only patients with ischaemic heart disease exhibited myocardial ischaemia, whereas for the group of patients operated on under local anaesthesia, the prevalence of myocardial ischaemia was equally distributed between those with and without myocardial ischaemia. They noted a significant trend towards higher rate of myocardial ischaemia in patients allocated to the general anaesthesia group who had known ischaemic heart disease. Because of the small number of patients in this study, no definitive conclusion on the impact of early cardiac morbidity could be determined. Similar findings were noted by Allen *et al.* in a non-randomized study.[11] General anaesthesia for carotid endarterectomy needs to avoid myocardial ischaemia by keeping haemodynamic variables, especially heart rate, at normal levels and maintaining high normal blood pressures to aid in the collateral flow to the operative side.[6] In the absence of crescendo transient ischaemic attacks, which mandate urgent operative intervention, patients with uncontrolled hypertension should have procedures delayed because of the haemodynamic lability which can result in myocardial ischaemic events. Also, surgical reconstruction should be avoided in patients who have had a myocardial infarction more recently than 3 months because of an increase in myocardial ischaemia.[16]

Fiscal efficacy of the procedure

There are really no definitive data that favour either technique in terms of overall cost. The studies that do suggest that regional anaesthesia results in shorter lengths of stay in hospital tend to be sequential rather than randomized or concurrent. As anaesthesia techniques are refined, the general anaesthetic is not a factor in the patient's length of stay. Currently on our service, it is other factors such as myocardial ischaemia that are the primary determinant of length of stay.

Discussion

The advantages of general anaesthesia are an unhurried approach which allow for a technically precise repair permitting the surgeon to use his technique of choice for cerebral protection. The advantage that the patient does not move during the procedure cannot be understated. In patients who have difficult dissections because of high bifurcations or disease extending into the internal carotid artery, there is more flexibility with general anaesthesia. Because the approach is unhurried, it allows for intraoperative evaluation of the repair, which in the long-term provides better results. Contraindications to regional anaesthetic are patients who are confused, apprehensive or are hard of hearing.

With the increasing experience of regional anaesthesia, unique complications are being reported.[19] In patients with contralateral phrenic nerve paralysis, the local anaesthesia from the regional block will affect the phrenic nerve, which arises from cervical levels three, four and five. Emery and associates have demonstrated that 55% of patients undergoing regional block for carotid endarterectomy developed a phrenic nerve block.[19] In addition, because the patient tolerates test clamping does not mean they will not have trouble later during a period of internal carotid clamping. Lawrence and his group noted that in five of nine patients cerebral ischaemia occurred between 20 and 30 minutes after cross-clamping – all occurring during relative intraoperative hypotension (average reduction of 35 mmHg in systolic pressure).[20] This emphasizes the need for the anaesthesiologist to maintain continuous, meticulous evaluation of the patient's neurological status.

If the patient is given general anaesthesia, thiopental can be used to protect the brain. For some patients, carotid anatomy precludes shunting. In these situations the patient is better protected by having general anaesthesia.

In the final analysis, results are the most important aspect when evaluating anaesthesia technique. The skill administering each technique can be variable. Each surgeon should do the procedure the way they do it best. The main trade-off between the two techniques is a more precise repair under general anaesthesia versus the decreased incidence of myocardial ischaemic events with regional anaesthesia. Carotid artery surgery is unforgiving of a lack of technical skill in both doing the procedure or administering the anaesthesia.

Summary

- Results are the most important aspect when evaluating anaesthesia technique.

- Both anaesthesia skill and surgical skill can vary widely and are the primary determinants of outcome.

- General anaesthesia allows a technically more precise repair.

- Carotid artery surgery is unforgiving of a lack of technical skill in both doing the procedure or administering the anaesthesia.

References

1. North American Symptomatic Carotid Endarterectomy Trial Callaborators. Beneficial effect of carotid endarterectomy in symptomatic patients with high- grade stenosis. *N Engl J Med* 1991; **325**: 445–453.
2. Executive Committee for Asymptomatic Carotid Atherosclerosis Study. Endarterectomy for asymptomatic carotid stenosis. *JAMA* 1995; **273**: 1421–1428.

3. European Carotid Study Trialists' Collaborating Group. MCR European Carotid Surgery Trial: Interim results for symptomatic patients with severe (70–90%) or mild (0–29%) carotid stenosis. *Lancet* 1991; **337**: 1235–1243.

4. Hobson RW II, Weiss DG, Fields W *et al*. Efficacy of carotid endarterectomy for asymptomatic carotid stenosis. *N Engl J Med* 1993; **328**: 221–227.

5. Mays BW, Towne JB, Seabrook GR, Cambria RA, Jean-Claude J. Intraoperative carotid evaluation. *Arch Surg* 2000; **135**: 525–528.

6. Towne JB, Weiss DG, Hobson RW II. First phase report of cooperative Veteran's Administration Asymptomatic Carotid Stenosis Study – Operative morbidity and mortality. *J Vasc Surg* 1990; **12**: 252–259.

7. Riles TS, Imparato AM, Jacobowitz GR *et al*. The cause of perioperative stroke after carotid endarterectomy. *J Vasc Surg* 1994; **19**: 206–216.

8. Kinney EV, Seabrook GR, Kinney LY, Bandyk DF, Towne JB. The importance of intraoperative detection of residual flow abnormalities after carotid artery endarterectomy. *J Vasc Surg* 1993; **113**: 580–586.

9. Dykes JR, Bergamini TM, Lipski DA, Fulton RL, Garrison RN. Intraoperative duplex scanning reduces both residual stenosis and postoperative morbidity of carotid endarterectomy. *Am Surg* 1997; **63**: 50–54.

10. Baker WH, Koustas G, Burks K, Littooy FN, Grenske HP. Intraoperative duplex scanning and late carotid stenosis. *J Vasc Surg* 1994; **19**: 829–833.

11. Allen BT, Anderson CB, Rubin BG *et al*. The influence of anesthetic techniques on perioperative complication after carotid endarterectomy. *J Vasc Surg* 1994; **19**: 834–843.

12. Bowyer MW, Zierold D, Loftus JP *et al*. Carotid endarterectomy: A comparison of regional versus general anesthesia in 500 operations. *Ann Vasc Surg* 2000; **14**: 145–151.

13. Sundt FM Jr, Sharbough FW, Piepgras DG *et al*. Correlation of cerebral blood flow and electroencephalographic changes during carotid endarterectomy. *Mayo Clin Proc* 1981; **56**: 533–543.

14. Hartzer NR, Lees CD. Fatal myocardial infarction following carotid endarterectomy. Three hundred thirty-five patients followed 6-11 years after operation. *Ann Surg* 1981; **194**: 212–218.

15. Ennix CL Jr, Lawrie GM, Morris GC Jr *et al*. Improved results of carotid endarterectomy in patients with symptomatic disease; and analysis of 1,546 consecutive carotid operations. *Stroke* 1979; **10**: 122–125.

16. McCann RL, Clements FM. Silent myocardial ischemia in patients undergoing peripheral vascular surgery: Incidence and association with perioperative cardiac morbidity and mortality. *J Vasc Surg* 1989; **9**: 583–587.

17. Sbarigia E, DarioVizza C, Antonini M *et al*. *J Vasc Surg* 1999; **30**: 131–138.

18. Shah DM, Darling RC III, Chang BB *et al*. Carotid endarterectomy in awake patients: Its safety, acceptability and outcome. *J Vasc Surg* 1994; **19**: 1015–1020.

19. Emery G, Handley G, Davies MJ, Mooney PH. Incidence of phrenic nerve block and hypercapnia in patients undergoing carotid endarterectomy under cervical plexus block. *Anaesth Intens Care* 1998; **26**: 377–381.

20. Lawrence PF, Alves JC, Jicha D, Bihrangi K, Dobrin PB. Incidence, timing and causes of cerebral ischemia during carotid endarterectomy with regional anesthesia. *J Vasc Surg* 1998; **27**: 329–337.

21. Thompson JE. Carotid endarterectomy. In *Vascular and Endovascular Surgical Techniques* 4th edn. Greenhalgh RM (ed). London: WB Saunders, 2001; 29–33.

Carotid endarterectomy under general anaesthesia is the treatment of choice

Against the motion
Michael J Gough

Introduction

Proof that carotid endarterectomy is superior to best medical therapy, both in the short and long-term, in patients with a significant carotid stenosis was confirmed by the ECST[1] and NASCET[2] trials. Despite this, the 30-day stroke/death rates were 7.5% and 5.8% respectively. A number of techniques have been explored with a view to making carotid endarterectomy safer. Whilst there seems to be no advantage associated with either eversion or conventional endarterectomy techniques,[3] and the role of post-carotid endarterectomy quality control is unproven, there is strong evidence that routine patching of the internal carotid artery is beneficial.[4,5]

Of the other techniques employed during carotid endarterectomy the use of a shunt has caused the most debate. Vascular surgeons have adopted three approaches to shunting: routine use in all patients, no routine shunting and selective shunt insertion. Although a systematic review suggests that routine shunting may confer a small advantage[6] this has not been assessed in a large randomized controlled trial. Clearly the most sensible approach would be that of selective shunting but this has been thwarted by difficulties in accurately identifying those patients who develop post-clamping cerebral ischaemia.

This difficulty can be overcome by performing carotid endarterectomy under local anaesthetic. This allows awake neurological testing that accurately predicts the patients who require a shunt for cerebral hypoperfusion following carotid clamp application. Thus patients who do not need a shunt avoid the potential complications associated with its use. Furthermore, evidence is accumulating to indicate that carotid endarterectomy performed under local anaesthetic is associated with a reduction in stroke and death rates.[7] This is consistent with the findings of a recent systematic review that demonstrates a reduction in morbidity and mortality for a wide variety of surgical procedures performed under local or regional anaesthesia.[8] Such a finding is not suprising given the co-existent cardiac, respiratory and other co-morbidities that are often present in elderly patients requiring surgery although previous authors have questioned its benefit for carotid endarterectomy.

This chapter considers the theoretical, practical and clinical benefits of local anaesthetic carotid endarterectomy and makes a strong case to suggest that it offers considerable advantages over carotid endarterectomy performed under general anaesthesia.

Technique

Table 1 outlines the techniques for both general and local anaesthesia. Although it is feasible for the surgeon to administer the local anaesthetic it is strongly advised that an anaesthetist is present for the purposes of monitoring and blood pressure control although the need for the latter is uncommon (unlike with general anaesthetic). Additionally, on rare occasions conversion to general anaesthetic may be required.

Table 1. Suggested format for administering general and local anaesthesia for carotid endarterectomy

General anaesthesia	Local anaesthesia
Premedication: benzodiazepine or none	Premedication: benzodiazepine or none
IV access + arterial line under LA	IV access + arterial line under LA
IV induction + opiate analgesia	Judicious sedation: benzodiazepine/opiate
Muscle relaxant	Deep and superficial cervical plexus block: 20ml bupivacaine 0.25% + 20ml prilocaine 1%
Tracheal intubation	Local infiltration of incision: 20ml bupivacaine 0.25%
Ventilation to normocapnia	Intraoperative LA if required: 1% lignocaine
Maintain systemic BP to preoperative levels:	Maintain systemic BP to preoperative levels:
IV fluids/cardioactive drugs if required	IV fluids/cardioactive drugs if required
Reversal of anaesthetic and extubation	O$_2$ by nasal cannulae/mask during cross-clamping of carotid vessels
O$_2$ overnight by nasal cannulae/mask	

IV: intravenous; LA: local anaesthetic; BP: blood pressure; O$_2$ oxygen.

Two techniques have been suggested for local anaesthesia carotid endarterectomy. The simplest is direct infiltration of the proposed incision and deeper tissues although a combination of superficial and deep cervical plexus blocks produces superior anaesthesia with smaller doses of anaesthetic. Improved postoperative analgesia is also provided by the deep cervical plexus block. Prior to administering the block the anterior and posterior borders of the sternocleidomastoid are marked. The superficial cervical plexus emerges at the mid-point of the latter and is anaesthetized by fan-wise infiltration of the local anaesthetic. The former marks the line of the incision and this is infiltrated using a long spinal needle. Finally, the deep cervical plexus is blocked by insertion of local anaesthetic adjacent to the transverse processes of C$_{2-4}$.

The set-up in theatre is important to allow maximum comfort for patients undergoing local anaesthetic carotid endarterectomy. After routine preparation, and draping of the surgical site, a translucent orthopaedic hip drape is used to create a 'tent' for the patient. This avoids darkness and allows a nurse or the anaesthetist to talk to the patient. If required, small sips of water can be administered via a straw and an electric fan can be used to provide cool air (Fig. 1). Small doses of a short-acting benzodiazepine or opiate may also be given if the patient becomes anxious or uncomfortable. During general anaesthetic carotid endarterectomy inotropic support to maintain blood pressure at or above preoperative levels may be required but this is unusual with local anaesthetic carotid endarterectomy.

The surgical techniques employed during carotid endarterectomy are the same

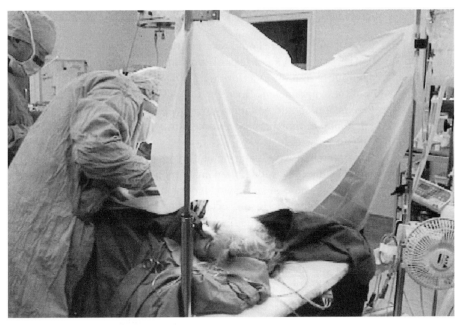

Figure 1. Set-up in operating theatre.

regardless of the method of anaesthesia. The use of a patch and the type of patch material, there being no obvious advantage to either synthetic or vein patches, are dependent upon individual surgeon choice. Similarly the use of a shunt and selection of monitoring techniques during general anaesthetic procedures are dictated by surgical policy. In contrast the indication for using a shunt during local anaesthetic carotid endarterectomy are dictated by the results of awake testing. Following carotid clamp application patients are quizzed to ensure that they are orientated in time and place, that they can perform relatively simple mental tests (count from 1–10), can answer a number of general knowledge questions, and can move both limbs contralateral to the side of surgery. Failure to complete all of these simple tasks is an indication that cerebral perfusion may be inadequate, as is increasing confusion or the development of severe hypertension. Under these circumstances a shunt should be inserted.

Evidence

The aim of anaesthesia for carotid endarterectomy is to maintain normal PaO_2, $PaCO_2$ and blood pressure and to preserve cerebral autoregulation. Furthermore, the anaesthetic technique should allow accurate monitoring of cerebral oxygenation or function, particularly when a policy of selective shunting is adopted. Finally, the method of anaesthesia should be safe, be associated with a good clinical outcome, be cost-effective, and be acceptable to the patient.

The evidence to support the hypothesis that these aims are best met by local anaesthetic techniques for carotid endarterectomy will now be considered.

Maintenance of normal PaO$_2$ and PaCO$_2$

Both local and general anaesthesia should result in the maintenance of normal PaO$_2$ and PaCO$_2$ levels. The potential drawbacks of local anaesthetic are that injudicious sedation may compromise respiratory effort and the technique does not easily allow for manipulation of these parameters. However, provided oxygen is administered via nasal cannulae blood gases should remain normal and the benefit of manipulation of PaO$_2$ and PaCO$_2$, that may be more easily achieved during general anaesthetic carotid endarterectomy requires discussion.

Hypercarbia causes cerebral vasodilatation and hypoventilation increases cerebral blood flow. However, induced vasodilatation in normal cerebral tissue may divert blood away from an ischaemic area despite increasing total cerebral blood flow. Furthermore if significant hypoperfusion occurs after carotid clamping the intra-cerebral vessels will already be maximally dilated. Thus there is no evidence to suggest that manipulation of PaCO$_2$ under general anaesthetic is of benefit. Conversely, experimental data suggest that *hypocarbia* may increase flow to an area of ischaemic cerebral tissue despite a reduction in total cerebral blood flow, a phenomenon known as reverse steal.

In summary there is no clinical evidence to indicate that manipulating pCO$_2$ is of benefit and current anaesthetic practice is to maintain normal pCO$_2$ levels. It follows therefore that there is no proven or theoretical benefit from general anaesthesia, as opposed to loco-regional anaesthesia, in this regard.

Maintenance of blood pressure

Since the intracerebral vessels in the relevant territory become maximally dilated after carotid clamping cerebral blood flow will be dependent upon the perfusion pressure. Local anaesthetic carotid endarterectomy is associated with a significant rise in mean arterial pressure during surgery, both prior to and following carotid clamping. These changes do not occur during general anaesthetic surgery. That this rise in blood pressure may be beneficial is suggested by animal work that indicates a reduction in neurological events with moderate hypertension that also causes a rise in stump pressure. Similarly, if neurological function deteriorates after carotid clamping during local anaesthetic, carotid endarterectomy pharmacologically induced hypertension may reverse this.

It has been suggested that the rise in systemic blood pressure during local anaesthetic carotid endarterectomy, whilst enhancing cerebral perfusion, may increase cardiac morbidity as a result of increased myocardial oxygen requirements. Equally, periods of hypotension during general anaesthesia are common and these may reduce both cerebral and myocardial perfusion. As a result there might be a need to administer pressor agents that increase myocardial work and the risk of infarction. In ESCT and NASCET, where the majority of surgery was performed under general anaesthetic, perioperative cardiac events were almost as common as neurological deficits.[1,2] Thus there is no evidence that general anaesthetic is essential to optimize blood pressure control or that it reduces cardiac morbidity or mortality.

Intraoperative cerebral protection

General anaesthesia

Proponents of both general and local anaesthesia for carotid endarterectomy suggest that the respective techniques offer a degree of cerebral protection during carotid

Table 2. Cerebral protection by anaesthetic agents

	Cerebral protection mode of action	Supporting evidence	Disadvantages	Clinical use
Barbiturates	Electrical activity $\downarrow \rightarrow \downarrow$ CMRO$_2$ $\rightarrow \downarrow$ O$_2$ demand Redistribution of CBF Intracranial pressure $\downarrow$ Ca^{++} influx $\downarrow$	Single clinical trial of protection during cardiopulmonary bypass Animal studies – high doses that would cause unacceptable cardiac and respiratory compromise in man	$\downarrow$ Electrical activity does not protect against severe ischaemia Large doses required producing: i. Cardiovascular depression ii. Respiratory depression	Often used in small doses during neurosurgery, CEA and cardiopulmonary bypass (one study indicating protection)
Volatile anaesthetics	Electrical activity $\downarrow$ CMRO$_2\downarrow$ Sympathetic activity $\downarrow$ (nitrous oxide has opposite effect) $\downarrow$ Glutamate receptors $\rightarrow \downarrow$ Ca^{++} influx (cytotoxic)	Animal studies Isoflurane reduces critical CBF at which EEG changes occur during CEA (compared with enflurane and halothane). No evidence of clinical benefit	Hypotension	Isoflurane agent of choice in most centres – probably $\downarrow$ CMRO$_2$ at doses that do not cause $\downarrow$ blood pressure
Propofol	Electrical activity $\downarrow$ CMRO$_2\downarrow$	Conflicting animal studies No clinical studies Effective dose does not cause cardiac/respiratory depression	Theoretical risk: Seizures Myoclonus Opisthotonus	In common use
Etomidate	Electrical activity $\downarrow$ CMRO$_2\downarrow$ Redistribution of CBF Free fatty acid release $\downarrow$	Animal studies No clinical studies Effective dose does not cause cardiac/respiratory depression	Must be used as continuous infusion Potential for: i. Adrenocortical suppression ii. Myoclonic movements	Infusion used in research only
Nitrous oxide			$\uparrow$ sympathetic activity $\rightarrow \uparrow$ CMRO$_2$ $\uparrow$ ICP	Not apparently detrimental Commonly used as 'carrier gas'

CMRO$_2$: cerebral metabolic rate for oxygen; CBF: cerebral blood flow; O$_2$: oxygen; EEG: electroencephalography; CEA: carotid endarterectomy; ICP: intracranial pressure clamping. For general anaesthesia it is claimed that the pharmacological properties of various anaesthetic agents afford protection against cerebral ischaemia whilst there is increasing evidence that local anaesthesia preserves cerebrovascular autoregulation.

The putative actions of common general anaesthetic agents are summarized in Table 2 and these have been discussed in detail elsewhere.[9] Most of the work supporting a role in cerebral protection for these drugs has been obtained from animal studies that may not be clinically relevant. Furthermore, some agents, such as nitrous oxide, may have detrimental effects upon cerebral physiology (increased cerebral metabolic rate for oxygen ($CMRO_2$), rise in intracranial pressure). Interestingly nitrous oxide does not appear to have a detrimental effect upon neurological outcome. Thus despite considerable experimental data suggesting that various general anaesthetic agents offer some degree of cerebral protection there are no trials to prove any clinical benefit.

Local anaesthesia

There is good evidence that physiological protective mechanisms are preserved when local anaesthesia is used. Thus near infrared spectroscopy demonstrates that cerebral oxygenation is initially reduced following carotid clamp application during loco-regional anaesthesia but recovers spontaneously over the next 2 minutes (Fig. 2a). When general anaesthesia is used cerebral oxygenation does not recover until a shunt is inserted (Fig. 2b).[10] This phenomenon (autoregulation) appears to be the result of a reflex rise in blood pressure that is not seen in general anaesthetic patients (Fig. 3). Further, changes in cytochrome oxidase levels (caa_3) seem to mirror those of blood pressure (Fig. 4). Cytochrome oxidase is the terminal link in oxidative phosphorylation and a reduction in its concentration is a sensitive marker of intracellular cerebral ischaemia. The mechanism by which reflex hypertension occurs is unknown although it does not appear to be mediated by the carotid sinus nerve and baroreceptors as the former was blocked by local anaesthetic infiltration in these studies. This would be an attractive hypothesis, however, since volatile anaesthetic agents impair the baroreflex.

A transient rise in blood pressure is often observed in acute stroke and appears to be mediated by the sympathetic nervous system. Again volatile anaesthetic agents such as isoflurane depress the latter although this effect seems to be 'dose-dependent'. Thus it is possible that the reflex may be preserved by a 'light general anaesthesia' as advocated by Roizen.[11] This could explain McCleary's finding that cerebral autoregulation was present in a few general anaesthetic patients although it occurred significantly less often than in local anaesthetic patients (Fig. 5).[10] The concept that local anaesthesia preserves cerebral oxygenation is also supported by data from Wellman[12] who showed that ischaemic electroencephalography (EEG) changes were less common with local anaesthesia (6.3% vs 15.7%).

Finally, a portion of the reticular activating system in the medulla appears to be sensitive to hypoxia, especially in the presence of hypotension, stimulating an increase in systemic blood pressure. Of course the posterior cerebral artery supplies the medulla but other similar centres may exist within the internal carotid artery territory.

If autoregulation is preserved during local anaesthetic carotid endarterectomy then it might be expected that cerebral injury is reduced during surgery. Evidence that this may be the case is supported by significantly higher neuron-specific enolase levels, an enzyme released from damaged cells, in the jugular venous blood of general anaesthetic patients during reperfusion.[13] Similarly it appears that postoperative cognitive performance is worse after general anaesthetic carotid endarterectomy than following local anaesthetic surgery.[14]

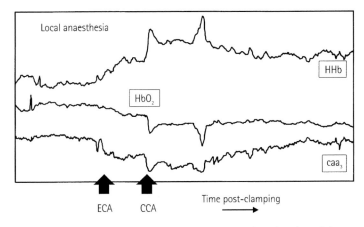

Figure 2a. Changes in parameters of cerebral oxygenation following clamping of the external carotid artery and then the common carotid artery during local anaesthetic carotid endarterectomy.

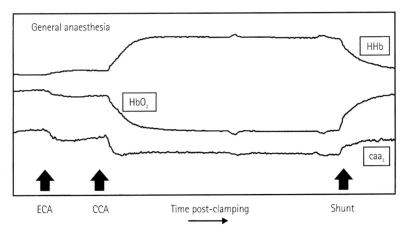

Figure 2b. Changes in parameters of cerebral oxygenation following clamping of the external carotid artery and then the common carotid artery during general anaesthetic carotid endarterectomy. Further changes occur following insertion of a carotid shunt.

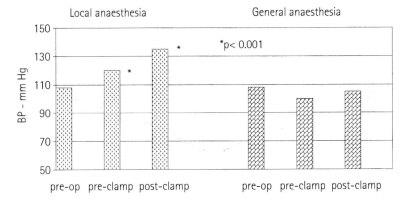

Figure 3. Mean arterial blood pressure (BP) prior to surgery (pre-op), post-induction of anaesthesia (pre-X) and after application of carotid clamps (post-x) in patients undergoing carotid endarterectomy under local or general anaesthesia.

25

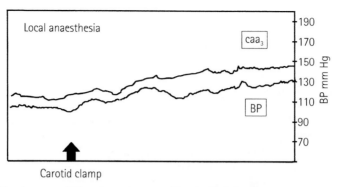

Figure 4. Blood pressure (BP) and cytochrome oxidase levels following application of carotid clamps during local anaesthetic carotid endarterectomy.

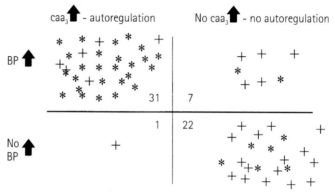

Figure 5. Blood pressure (BP) and caa_3 changes in patients undergoing carotid endarterectomy local (*) or general (+) anaesthetic; r = 0.75.

Clinical outcome

Although research data indicate potentially beneficial differences in cerebrovascular physiology and surrogate markers of cerebral injury these are only relevant if they are mirrored by a clinical benefit. The evidence that exists strongly supports the concept that local anaesthetic carotid endarterectomy is safer and is associated with a 50% reduction in 30-day stroke and death rates compared with general anaesthetic procedures. This was first suggested by a systematic review of both randomized and non-randomized studies involving >6000 patients.[7] Since this original analysis by the Cochrane Stroke Review Group[6] further non-randomized studies have been published and the potential benefit for local anaesthetic persists (30-day stroke/death rate: 66/3221 (2.05%) for local anaesthetic vs 218/5120 for general anaesthetic (4.26%); OR 0.5, 95% CI 0.4–0.7). Our own results are also consistent with this data. In 200 consecutive endarterectomies performed by one surgeon where the patient was given a free choice as to the type of anaesthesia (local anaesthetic: n = 97, general anaesthetic: n = 103) the 30-day stroke rates were 0% (local anaesthetic) vs 3.9% (general anaesthetic), myocardial infarction rates 1.1% (local anaesthetic) vs 2.9% (general anaesthetic) and combined 30-day stroke and death rates 1.1% (local anaesthetic) vs 5.8% (general anaesthetic). Although non-randomized, the indications for surgery and risk factors were the same in both groups. Although these data strongly support the hypothesis that local anaesthesia is safer the usual potential for bias to which all non-randomized series are susceptible exists and this issue can only be resolved by an appropriately designed randomized controlled trial.

Cardiac morbidity and mortality

Patients with carotid disease have a high incidence of ischaemic heart disease. The possibility that the higher systemic blood pressures during local anaesthetic carotid endarterectomy might increase the risk of myocardial ischaemia and infarction has been considered earlier. Despite these concerns there is no evidence that this is the case. Indeed the available literature would suggest the opposite, including data from the Cochrane Stroke Review Group systematic review which demonstrates a significantly lower incidence of myocardial events in local anaesthetic patients (0.6% vs 1.3%, OR 0.34, 95% CI 0.18-0.63, p<0.001).[7]

The reasons for an apparent reduction in cardiac morbidity with local anaesthesia are unclear. The respective roles of local anaesthetic-induced hypertension and hypotension during general anaesthetic have been considered above. An alternative possibility is that myocardial ischaemia is precipitated by the use of volatile anaesthetic agents which may produce a steal phenomenon in patients with ischaemic heart disease.[15]

Carotid shunts and intraoperative monitoring of cerebral function

Although preservation of normal cerebrovascular reflexes are an attractive hypothesis for the apparent superiority of local anaesthetic carotid endarterectomy the use of a carotid shunt might also be important. Shunts are used less frequently during local anaesthetic surgery which reflects both the rise in blood pressure with local anaesthetic and the unreliability of monitoring techniques to determine the need for a shunt in general anaesthetic patients.

Although it is difficult to determine the cause of an intraoperative neurological deficit with certainty it is estimated that 80% are embolic in nature and 20% are due to hypoperfusion.[16] In addition an embolus on a background of hypoperfusion may be more significant than an embolus to well perfused brain.[17]

Not suprisingly the majority of surgeons attempt to avoid hypoperfusion by using a carotid shunt. The benefit from shunt insertion is not proven, however, and many series in which shunts were used routinely report similar results to those in which shunts are used selectively or not at all. Whilst two randomized trials and a systematic review of obligatory shunting vs non-shunting have shown a non-significant trend suggesting a benefit from routine shunting[6,18,19] other authors have suggested that the use of a shunt increases the risk of complications.[19-21] These are attributed to intimal damage that may promote early thrombosis or late stenosis, the risk of platelet and air emboli from the shunt, or embolization of atheromatous debris from the common carotid artery. Further, the shunt may compromise surgical exposure and the need for more extensive dissection may increase the risk of cranial nerve injury.[23] In view of these potential hazards the benefit of shunt insertion might be cancelled out by complications resulting from their use and logically a policy of selective shunting would be more appropriate. That this may be the case is supported by one study that reported a 4.4% major stroke rate in routinely shunted patients compared with 0.5% in the selectively shunted group.[24] The main challenge of a policy of selective shunting policy is to ensure that patients at risk of hypoperfusion are shunted whilst those with an adequate collateral circulation are not.

A variety of techniques have been proposed for detecting post-clamping cerebral ischaemia and these fall into three categories. They are based on direct or indirect measures of cerebral blood flow and assessment of either cerebral oxygenation or cerebral function. The criteria for inserting a shunt, the false positive and false negative rates for each technique, and comments on their value are shown in Table 3.

Cerebral blood flow

Internal carotid artery stump pressure measurement is arguably the most widely used technique for assessing the need for a shunt. Sensitivity and specificity are low and it only provides information at a single instant in time, taking no account of changes in perfusion during the period of cross-clamping. Although measurement of middle cerebral artery velocity by transcranial Doppler ultrasound allows continuous monitoring of blood flow the technique requires considerable expertise to obtain a reliable signal and 10–15% of patients do not the required acoustic window. However transcranial Doppler ultrasound will also detect intraoperative emboli which may be valuable during carotid dissection.

Cerebral oxygenation

Measurements of cerebral blood flow rely upon the assumption that this reflects the adequacy of cerebral oxygenation. Indirect information about this is also provided by continuous jugular venous oximetry that determines the oxygen content ($SjvO_2$) of jugular bulb venous blood. Although this technique is commonly used to monitor patients with severe head injuries or patients undergoing cerebral aneurysm surgery its value during carotid endarterectomy is not established.

Near infrared spectroscopy (niroscopy) directly assesses cerebral oxygenation but only samples a small volume of brain. Furthermore, the contribution by the extracranial circulation to measurements of oxyhaemogobin, deoxyhaemoglobin and cytochrome oxidase (caa_3) is difficult to quantify.

Cerebral function

Since neurological function deteriorates before irreversible neuronal damage occurs both EEG and somatosensory evoked potentials have been proposed as tools for identifying those patients in whom a shunt is required. However, interpretation is difficult and requires a neurophysiologist. In addition, hypotension, arterial $PaCO_2$, anaesthetic agents, a previous stroke and diathermy may influence the data. Thus sensitivity and specificity are relatively low.

The most reliable method of assessing neurological function during carotid endarterectomy is awake neurological testing although this is only applicable when local anaesthetic surgery is performed. It provides a continuous assessment of cerebral function throughout the period of carotid cross-clamping, does not require expensive equipment and is wholly reliable. Awake testing should include tests of higher function (orientation in time and place, simple general knowledge questions, mental mathematics) together with test of motor function in the contralateral limbs (e.g. squeaky toy in the contralateral hand). Whilst the majority of patients requiring a shunt loose consciousness immediately after clamping the common carotid artery hesitancy in the performance of the tests of higher function or confusion, often

Table 3. Cerebral monitoring and criteria for shunting. False positives and negatives are derived from studies in which monitoring has been compared with awake testing.

Parameter assessed	Technique	Criteria for shunting	Shunting rates	False +ve	False -ve	Comments
Cerebral blood flow – direct	Cerebral blood flow (Xe^{133} washout)	< 18ml/100g/min	50%	Unknown	Unknown	Limited availability , research tool Radiation hazard, technician required Measures CBF in superficial cortex
Cerebral blood flow – indirect	Stump pressure	<50 mmHg	Up to 60%	20–40%	0–23%	Cheap, universally available Single measurement ∴ non-continuous High false +ve rates Compensates for variations in BP
	Stump pressure index (SPx100/systemic BP	<33		40%	0	
	Transcranial doppler (TCD)	MCAV fall by 60–70%	20%	4–45%	Up to 17% if >70% fall used	10% of patients have no acoustic window, technician required
Cerebral function	Awake testing	Contralateral neurological signs, impaired higher function/conscious level	5–21%	Gold standard	Gold standard	Only applicable to LA CEA Requires good patient communication Shunt needed if very high BP/confusion
	EEG	>50% ↓ α or β activity ↑ in δ activity Asymmetry	15–30%	5–13%	5–25%	Requires expert interpretation – processed EEG not validated Variable influences of anaesthetic agents Only assesses superficial cortex Influenced by previous CVA
	Somatosensory evoked potentials	> 1ms prolongation of conduction time >50% ↓ amplitude		Unknown	Unknown	Requires expert interpretation Variable influences of anaesthetic agents Influenced by previous CVA
Cerebral oxygenation	Near infrared spectroscopy	> 5% ↓ cerebral O$_2$ saturation ↓ caa$_3$ concentration (no criteria established)		Unknown	Unknown	Influenced by scalp and skull perfusion Difficulties in quantification Research tool
	Continuous jugular venous oximetry	SJvO$_2$ < 50 %		Unknown	Unknown	Catheter position needs determining and maintaining – research tool

SP: stump pressure; BP: blood pressure; EEG: electroencephalography; CBF: cerebral blood flow.

accompanied by a marked rise in systemic blood pressure are more subtle signs of the need for a shunt. If this is not inserted delayed loss of consciousness may occur 10–45 minutes later. Similarly if blood pressure (perfusion pressure) falls during surgery late shunt insertion may be needed. Thus the ability of awake testing to continuously monitor cerebral function throughout the procedure is extremely valuable.

Not all patients are able to co-operate with awake testing (prior cerebrovascular accident with residual motor weakness, dysarthria, receptive or expressive dysphasia, deafness, language problems) and for these either local anaesthetic with routine shunting or general anaesthetic carotid endarterectomy are indicated.

During local anaesthetic carotid endarterectomy shunts are required less often than with any of the monitoring techniques used during general anaesthetic surgery (Table 3) and this may be beneficial for the reasons outlined earlier. Furthermore, all general anaesthetic monitoring techniques have a false negative rate and all studies report patients who develop a deficit despite normal monitoring.[25-27] In summary therefore local anaesthetic and awake testing ensures that all patients with significant hypoperfusion are shunted and that the potential risks of a shunt are avoided in all patients with satisfactory cerebral perfusion.

Cost–effectiveness

Although not proven it is our experience that patients undergoing local anaesthetic carotid endarterectomy are normally discharged from hospital 24 hours earlier than patients undergoing general anaesthetic surgery. In addition they are less likely to require admission to either a high dependency or intensive care unit postoperatively. These end-points together with a comparison of 30-day stroke and death rates for carotid endarterectomy performed using either local anaesthetic or general anaesthetic are currently being assessed in a randomized study, The GALA (general anaesthetic vs local anaesthetic) Trial. That there is no requirement for expensive monitoring equipment nor a technologist are further cost savings associated with local anaesthetic carotid endarterectomy.

Of course if the trial confirms that local anaesthetic carotid endarterectomy is associated with fewer neurological complications, as suggested by the data from non-randomized studies this will have a major impact on the relative cost-effectiveness of local anaesthetic.

Patient and surgeon acceptability

It often suggested that both surgeon and patient anxiety are increased by the use of local anaesthetic. However, surgeons who use local anaesthetic techniques are reassured by the knowledge that a patient is neurologically intact both during surgery and immediately postoperatively. This facility also allows unhurried and careful surgery, usually without the added difficulties associated with shunt deployment. The ability to fully expose the carotid vessels is not affected by local anaesthetic even in obese patients, and worries about the need to convert to general anaesthetic are unfounded, this being required in 1–3% of patients at most. Further, the advent of the laryngeal mask has made this both easy and safe.

It is not disputed that some patients find local anaesthetic carotid endarterectomy rather tedious, particularly if prolonged. Patient comfort is enhanced by the methods described in the **Techniques** section at the beginning of this chapter. We have assessed patient satisfaction with either general or local anaesthesia in 144 patients randomized to either local anaesthetic or general anaesthetic. There was no difference in pre-operative anxiety or peroperative satisfaction with the two techniques although there were significant advantages to local anaesthetic in terms of postoperative nausea, discomfort, and the time taken to return to normal activity. A reduction in postoperative pain after local anaesthetic carotid endarterectomy has also been shown in another study and appears to be greater when a deep cervical plexus block is performed.[28]

Summary

Local anaesthesia for carotid endarterectomy does the following.

- Preserves cerebrovascular reflexes.

- Results in less cerebral injury than general anaesthesia.

- Accurately identifies patients requiring a shunt.

- Allows continuous, cheap and accurate monitoring of neurological function during carotid clamping.

- Is associated with a reduction in the frequency of shunt deployment.

- Reduces the risk of shunt-related complications.

- Appears to be associated with a lower 30-day stroke and death rate.

- Is likely to be more cost-effective than general anaesthetic surgery.

- Allows careful, precise and unhurried surgery.

- Is associated with high levels of surgeon and patient acceptability.

References

1. European Carotid Surgery Trialists Group. MRC European Carotid Surgery Trial. Interim results for symptomatic patients with severe (70–99%) or with mild (0–29%) carotid stenosis. *Lancet* 1991; **337**: 1235–1243.

2. North American Symptomatic Carotid Endarterectomy Trial Collaborators. Beneficial effect of carotid endarterectomy in symptomatic patients with high-grade stenosis. *N Eng J Med* 1991; **325**: 445–453.

3. Cao P, Giordano G, De Rango P *et al.* Collaborators of the EVEREST study group. A randomised study on eversion versus standard carotid endarterectomy: study design and preliminary results. *J Vasc Surg* 1998; **27**: 595–605.

4. Counsell C, Salinas R, Naylor AR, Warlow CP. A systematic review of the randomised trials of carotid patch angioplasty in carotid endarterectomy. *Eur J Vasc Surg* 1997; **13**: 345–354.

5. Aburhama AF, Khan JH, Robinson PA *et al.* Prospective randomised trial of carotid endarterectomy with primary closure and patch angioplasty with saphenous vein, jugular vein and polyte-traflouroethylene: perioperative (30 day) results. *J Vasc Surg* 1996; **24**: 998–1007.

6. Counsell C, Salinas R, Naylor R, Warlow C. Routine or selective shunting during carotid endarterectomy and the different methods of monitoring in selective shunting (Cochrane Review). *The Cochrane Library* 1998; Issue 3: 1–12.

7. Tangkanakul C, Counsell C, Warlow C. Local versus general anaesthesia in carotid endarterectomy: a systematic review of the evidence. *Eur J Vasc Surg* 1997; **13**: 491–499.

8. Rodgers A, Walker N, Schug S *et al.* Reduction in postoperative mortality and morbidity with epidural or spinal anaesthesia: results from overview of randomised trials. *BMJ* 2000; **321**: 1493–1497.

9. McCleary AJ, Maritati G, Gough MJ. Carotid endarterectomy; local or general anaesthesia? *Eur J Vasc Endovasc Surg* 2001; **22**: 1–12.

10. McCleary AJ, Dearden NM, Dickson DH, Watson A, Gough MJ. The differing effects of regional and general anaesthesia on cerebral metabolism during carotid endarterectomy. *Eur J Vasc Endovasc Surg* 1996; **12**: 173–181.

11. Roizen MF. Anaesthesia goals for operations to relieve or prevent cerebrovascular insufficiency. In *Clinical Neuroanaesthesia* 2nd edn. RF Cucchiara, S Black, JD Michenfelder (eds). New York: Churchill Livingstone, 1998: 103–122.

12. Wellman BJ, Loftus CM, Kresowik TF, Todd M, Granner MA. The differences in electroencephalographic changes in patients undergoing carotid endarterectomy while under local versus general anaesthesia. *Neurosurgery* 1998; **43**: 769–773.

13. Wijeyaratne SM, Cruickshank J, Collins M *et al*. Jugular venous neurone-specific enolase and s-100 levels after carotid endarterectomy under local or general anaesthesia. *Br J Surg* 2001, **88**: 600.

14. Calvey TAJ, Bollom P, Cruickshank J *et al*. Differences in cognitive function and s-100 production after carotid endarterectomy under local or general anaesthetic. *Br J Surg* 2000, **87**: 493.

15. Sbarigia E, Dario Vizza C, Antonini M *et al*. Locoregional versus general anaesthesia in carotid surgery: is there an impact on perioperative myocardial ischaemia? Results of a prospective monocentric randomised trial. *J Vasc Surg* 1999; **30**: 131–138.

16. Spencer M. Transcranial Doppler monitoring and causes of stroke from carotid endarterectomy. *Stroke* 1997; **28**: 1845–1846.

17. Krul JMJ, van Gijn J, Ackerstaff RJA *et al*. Site and pathogenesis of cerebral infarction associated with carotid endarterectomy *Stroke* 1989; **20**: 324–328.

18. Gummerlock MK, Neuwelt EA. Carotid endarterectomy: to shunt or not to shunt. *Stroke* 1988; **19**: 1485–1490.

19. Sandmann W, Willeke F, Kovenbach R, Godehardt E. To shunt or not to shunt: the definite answer with a randomised study. In *Current Clinical Problems in Vascular Surgery* Vol 5. Veith FJ (ed). St Louis, Missouri: Quality Medical Publishing Inc, 1993: 434–440.

20. Spencer MP, Thomas GI, Nicholls SC *et al*. Detection of middle cerebral artery emboli during carotid endarterectomy using transcranial Doppler ultrasonography. *Stroke* 1990; **21**: 415–423.

21. Fode NC, Sundt TM, Robertson JT, Peerless SJ, Shields CB. Multicentre retrospective review of results and complications of carotid endarterectomy in 1981. *Stroke* 1986; **17**: 370–376.

22. Halsey JH for The International Transcranial Doppler Collaborators. Risks and benefits of shunting in carotid endarterectomy. *Stroke* 1992; **23**: 1583–1587.

23. Forrsell C, Kitzing P, Bergqvist D. Cranial nerve injuries after carotid surgery. A prospective study of 663 operations. *Eur J Vasc Surg* 1995; **10**: 445–449.

24. Salvian AJ, Taylor DC, Hsiang YN *et al*. Selective shunting with EEG monitoring is safer than routine shunting for carotid endarterectomy. *Cardiovasc Surg* 1997; **5**: 481–485.

25. Cao P, Giordano G, Zanetti S *et al*. Transcranial Doppler monitoring during carotid endarterectomy: is it appropriate for selecting patients in need of a shunt? *J Vasc Surg* 1997; **26**: 973–979.

26. Connolly JE. Carotid endarterectomy in the awake patient. *Am J Surg* 1985; **150**: 159–165.

27. Bornstein NM, Rossi GB, Treves TA, Shifrin EG. Is transcranial Doppler effective in avoiding the hazards of carotid surgery. *Cardiovasc Surg* 1996; **4**: 335–377.

28. Stoneham MD, Doyle AR, Knighton JD, Dorje P, Stanley JC. Prospective, randomised comparison of deep or superficial cervical plexus block for carotid endarterectomy surgery. *Anesthesiology* 1998; **89**: 907–912.

Carotid endarterectomy under general anaesthesia is the treatment of choice

Charing Cross Editorial Comments towards Consensus

Carotid endarterectomy has been with us now since 1953 and extremely fine results have been achieved under general anaesthetic in some single centres. The operation is an unforgiving operation if techniques are not perfect and in the early days there were some awful results, but in time some excellent practitioners showed us that good results were possible. There are those who claim that general anaesthetic confers a type of protection but from time to time there has been a call for patients to be allowed to stay awake by either using a local infiltration or a regional block of anaesthesia. With the patient awake it is possible to get him/her to move the contralateral limb and then to check the cerebral function during the procedure; this gives a sense of reassurance to supporters of this method.

At the time of writing it would be fair to say that there is considerable dispute concerning the benefits of general or local anaesthesia and a random controlled trial, the general anaesthetic vs local anaesthetic (GALA) trial, is underway which could contribute to the argument. Whatever happens there can be no doubt that the election of patients for carotid surgery and the performance of the procedure will contribute greatly to the outcome which will certainly not just depend upon whether a patient is managed with general or local anaesthesia.

Roger M Greenhalgh
Editor

Carotid stenting will become the gold standard

For the motion
Thomas J Fogarty, Frank R Arko

Introduction

Stroke is the third most common cause of death in North America, and approximately 500 000 new strokes are reported annually in the USA. Of these, 75% of strokes occur in the distribution of the carotid arteries. Carotid occlusive disease is the most common cause of thromboembolic strokes. The 30-day and 5-year mortality rates for stroke that occur in the carotid distribution are 17% and 40%, respectively.[1-2]

Carotid endarterectomy reduces the reported incidence of stroke alone and stroke and death in symptomatic patients with high-grade ≥70% stenosis. In addition, the North American Symptomatic Carotid Endarterectomy Trial (NASCET) investigators have confirmed the efficacy of carotid endarterectomy for ≥50% stenosis.[3-4]

However, this surgical procedure is not without risk. Rates of stroke or death within 30 days of surgery have ranged from 2.3% to 6.7% in well-controlled randomized trials. In 1995, the American Heart Association Council on Stroke established surgical guidelines identifying upper limits of acceptable perioperative (30-day) stroke and death rates for carotid endarterectomy, with updated recommendations in 1998 (Table 1).

Table 1. American Heart Association Council on Stroke surgical guidelines

Patient	Stenosis (%)	Upper limits of acceptable perioperative death and stroke rates (%)
Symptomatic	≥70	5.8
Asymptomatic	≥60	2.3
History of		
Transient ischaemic attack		5.0
Prior cerebrovascular accident		7.0
Restenosis after carotid endarterectomy		10.0
Contralateral occlusion with ipsilateral stenosis		14.0

In the last decade there has been an increasing interest in less invasive means to treat carotid artery occlusive disease with carotid angioplasty and stenting. Numerous case reports and clinical series have been published regarding carotid artery angioplasty and stenting. The first report of a multicentre prospective protocol-based study of carotid angioplasty was the North American Percutaneous Transluminal Angioplasty Register in 1993. In this study the 30-day combined rate of death and stroke from all causes was 9%. This early study reported a restenosis rate of 22% (8/37).[5] This data after angioplasty alone stimulated clinicians to perform stenting after angioplasty as a routine practice. The widespread application of these techniques has been limited by a significant incidence of perioperative neurological complications ranging between 5.2% and 9.3%.[6-7] However, as technology improves and experience accumulates results will continue to improve.

The standard with which carotid artery angioplasty and stenting is compared is the result of conventional carotid endarterectomy for symptomatic patients (NASCET total neurological event rate 5.8%) and for asymptomatic patients (ACAS total neurological event rate of 2.65%).[3,8] In order for carotid angioplasty and stenting to become an acceptable alternative to conventional surgery for carotid occlusive disease the procedure-related neuroembolism complications need only to be equivalent to those of carotid endarterectomy.

Evidence

On the basis of the conclusions of a multidisciplinary panel at the recent Montefiore Vascular symposium,[9] subgroups of patients should currently be considered for carotid artery angioplasty and stenting. These groups include high-risk patients with significant medical co-morbidities and patients with carotid restenosis after previous carotid endarterectomy, anatomically inaccessible lesions above C2, and radiation-induced stenoses.

Technique of carotid stenting

Arterial access is obtained with a 5-French sheath, a pigtail flush catheter is passed into the ascending aorta and a 30-degree left anterior oblique view is obtained of the arch anatomy. The patient is systemically heparinized to a target activated clotting time of 225–250 seconds. Gaining access to the carotid arteries is dependent on using the correct catheter for the anatomy. An angled catheter is used to access the origins of the innominate and left carotid arteries. The VTK catheter (Cook Inc, Bloomington, Ind) possesses an angle that makes it well suited to gain access to the arch vasculature.

Once the vessel is cannulated, a 0.035-inch angled glidewire (Boston Scientific, Natick, Mass) is advanced staying below the lesion. Once the wire is positioned the catheter is advanced into the common carotid artery. The position of the catheter is confirmed with contrast injection under fluoroscopy. The angled glidewire is then advanced into the external carotid artery. The catheter is advanced into the external carotid artery over the wire. The glidewire is is then exchanged for an exchanged length 0.035-inch Amplatz super stiff wire (Cook) with a 1-cm flexible tip. This wire will allow the sheath to access the common carotid artery.

A 7-French, 90-cm Shuttle (Cook) sheath is then advanced into the common carotid artery over the Amplatz wire. Once the sheath is positioned, a 0.018-inch wire is advanced across the lesion. The wire is positioned at the base of the skull. Predilation of the lesion is then performed with a 4-mm low profile balloon for pre-stent dilation. For most lesions, a self-expanding stent appropriately sized to the artery should be chosen. Stent length should be chosen such that there will be adequate length of the stent above and below the lesion to stabilize the stent. The stent is then post-dilated with either a 5-mm or 6-mm diameter balloon. Completion arteriography of the target lesion and intracranial circulation should be performed to assess stent placement.

The patient should be carefully observed during all inflations to assess neurological status and to ensure that the typical bradycardia response to carotid dilatation can be recognized and treated appropriately.

Outcome of carotid stenting

Although the precise outcome of carotid stenting is unknown, the technique continues to evolve and outcomes will continue to improve. Recent individual published series are presented in Table 2.

Table 2. Results of carotid stenting

Authors	Year	Patients	Lesions	Success (%)	Major stroke (%)	Minor stroke (%)	Death (%)	30-day combined stroke mortality (%)
Mathias et al.[10]	1999	633	799	99	1.1	1.6	0.3	3
Bergeron et al.[11]	1999	99	99	97	0	1	0	1
Wholey et al.[12]	2000	4757	5210	98.4	1.49	2.72	0.86	5.07
Dangas[13]	2000	133	140	99.3	0.9	5.3	0.7	6.9
Roubin et al.[14]	2001	528	604	98	1	4.8	1.6	7.4

These results are based on data from the most experienced centres in the world. Wholey et al. reviewed data from a registry incorporating worldwide data from Europe, North and South America, and Asia.[12] Most of these operations have been performed without the use of distal protection devices or improved technology that could enhance the outcome of carotid stenting. Various distal protection systems have been developed and are under investigation. These include the Angioguard (Angioguard Inc, Plymouth, Minn), Percusurge (Medtronic, Santa Rosa, CA), and Parodi Antiembolism System (Arteria) (Figs 1 and 2).

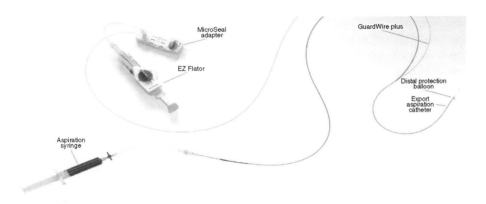

Figure 1. Percusurge device.

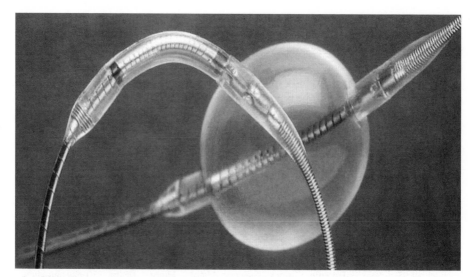

Figure 2. Atraumatic distal balloon from Percusurge device. Facilitates distal protection by completely occluding the vessel and preventing any particulate debris from moving distally.

Recently, the use of distal protection devices has been shown to reduce microemboli during critical phases of carotid stenting compared with controls (no protection). Microemboli signals were significantly decreased in patients with distal protection devices in place.[15] Microemboli were decreased during predilation, stent deployment, and post-dilation (Table 3).

Table 3. Microembolic signal counts in control vs distal protection groups

Procedural phase	Control group	Protection group	p-Value
Pre-dilatation	32 ± 36	12 ± 31	0.001
Stent deployment	75 ± 57	17 ± 22	0.004
Post-dilation	27 ± 25	5 ± 9	0.002
Total	164 ± 108	68 ± 83	0.002

The only available study comparing stenting with surgery is the CAVATAS study. The two procedures were similar in outcomes. The combined stroke/mortality rate was excessively high (10.3%) in the surgery group. However, the same can be said of the interventional results, with a combined stroke/mortality rate of 10.4%. Many of the interventional patients were treated with angioplasty alone with stenting reserved. Experience has shown that this form of therapy will increase the stroke risk.[16]

Alberts *et al.* described the methods of another randomized clinical trial that compared carotid stenting with endarterectomy in symptomatic patients (stenosis, 50–99%) that was sponsored by the Schneider Corporation. However, this trial has been discontinued because of procedural and recruitment difficulties.[17]

Although the final outcome of trials will determine how patients will be treated in the future it is clear that patients will ultimately help determine which procedure, carotid angioplasty and stenting or carotid endarterectomy, most benefits them. Certainly, there are patients for whom the morbidity of carotid endarterectomy is high and the small increased risk of stroke for carotid angioplasty and stenting is offset by risk of general anaesthesia. In addition, the technological development of low-profile stents and protection devices will allow even less morbid interventions for the treatment of carotid artery occlusive disease. Even without these technological advances it appears that in selected patients carotid artery angioplasty and stenting can be used to treat extracranial carotid stenosis in NASCET-eligible patients with periprocedural complications similar to those of carotid endarterectomy.

Summary

- The results of carotid angioplasty and stenting continue to improve in experienced hands.

- Currently, selected patients can be treated with carotid angioplasty and stenting with periprocedural complications similar to carotid endarterectomy.

- Technology for carotid angioplasty and stenting continues to improve.

- Distal protection devices will decrease the number of microemboli following carotid angioplasty and stenting.

- Patients will demand a less invasive procedure with equivalent results to treat extracranial carotid artery occlusive disease.

References

1. Chambers BR, Norris JW, Shurvell BL, Hachinski V. Prognosis of acute stroke. *Neurology* 1987; **37**: 221–225.
2. Wolf PA, Kannel WB, McGee DL. Epidemiology of strokes in North America. In *Stroke: Pathophysiology, Diagnosis, and Management*. Barnett HJM, Stein BM, Mohr JP, Yatsu FM (eds). New York: Churchill Livingstone, 1986: 19–29.
3. North American Symptomatic Carotid Endarterectomy Trial Collaborators. Beneficial effect of carotid endarterectomy in symptomatic patients with high-grade carotid stenosis. *N Engl J Med* 1991; **325**: 445–453.
4. Barnett HJM, Taylor DW, Eliasziw M *et al*. Benefit of carotid endarterectomy in patients with symptomatic moderate or severe stenosis. *N Engl J Med* 1998; **339**: 1415–1425.
5. NACPTAR Investigators: Ferguson R, Schwarten D, Purd P *et al*. Restenosis following cerebral percutaneous transluminal angioplasty [abstract]. *Stroke* 1995; **26**: 186.
6. Deitrich EB, Ndiye M, Reid DB. Stenting in the carotid artery: Initial experience in 110 patients. *J Endovasc Surg* 1996; **3**: 42–62.
7. Mathur A, Roubin GS, Piamsomboom C *et al*. Predictors of stroke following carotid stenting: univariate and multivariate analysis [abstract]. *Circulation* 1997; **96**: A1710.
8. Executive committee for the Asymptomatic Carotid Atherosclerosis Study. Endarterectomy for asymptomatic carotid stenosis. *JAMA* 1995; **273**: 1421–1428.
9. Veith FJ, Amor M, Ohki T *et al*. Current status of carotid bifurcation angioplasty and stenting based on a consensus of opinion leaders. *J Vasc Surg* 2001; **33**: S111–S116.
10. Mathias K, Jager H, Sahl H *et al*. Interventional treatment of arteriosclerotic carotid stenosis. *Radiology* 1999; **39**: 125–134.
11. Bergeron P, Becquemin JP, Jausseran JM *et al*. Percutaneous stenting of the internal carotid artery: The European CAST I Study. Carotid Artery Stent Trial. *J Endovasc Surg* 1999; **6**: 155–159.
12. Wholey MH, Wholey M, Mathias K *et al*. Global experience in cervical carotid artery stent placement. *Cathet Cardiovasc Interv* 2000; **50**: 160–167.
13. Dangas G, Laird JR Jr., Satler LF *et al*. Postprocedural hypotension after carotid artery stent placement: Predictors and short- and long-term clinical outcomes. *Radiology* 2000; **215**: 677–683.

14. Roubin GS, New G, Iyer S *et al*. Immediate and late clinical outcomes of carotid artery stenting in patients with symptomatic and asymptomatic carotid artery stenosis: A 5-year prospective analysis. *Circulation* 2001; 103: 532–537.

15. Al-Mubarek N, Roubin G S, Vitek JL *et al*. Effect of the distal-balloon protection system on microembolization during carotid stenting. *Circulation* 2001; 104: 1999.

16. Major ongoing stroke trials: carotid and vertebral artery transluminal angioplasty study (CAVATAS) [abstract]. *Stroke* 1996; 27: 358.

17. Alberts MJ, McCann R, Smith TP *et al*. A randomized trial: carotid stenting versus endarterectomy in patients with symptomatic carotid stenosis, study designs. *J Neurovasc Dis* 1997; November–December: 228–234.

Carotid stenting will become the gold standard

Against the motion
Roger Greenhalgh, Gill Clayton, Alun H Davies, Peter R F Bell

Introduction

The European Carotid Surgery Trial (ECST) and North American Symptomatic Carotid Endarterectomy (NASCET) multicentre randomized trials have demonstrated the value of carotid endarterectomy in patients with symptomatic severe carotid artery stenosis. The reduction in stroke risk as a result of endarterectomy is approximately 5% per annum, with a reduction in the risk of major stroke or death by two-fold compared with medical treatment alone.[1,2]

Patient-related factors have been shown to influence outcome following carotid endarterectomy. A single centre series of 460 patients following carotid endarterectomy by the senior author for symptomatic carotid artery stenosis of >70% illustrates that stroke rates vary according to presenting symptom. Stroke was significantly more common in patients with crescendo transient ischaemic attacks (TIA) than those with amaurosis fugax (p< 0.001), established stroke (p= 0.02), and TIA (p= 0.02).[3]

Also in terms of mortality there is a similar correlation with respect to presenting symptoms (Fig. 2). Patients with crescendo TIAs had the worst outcome and those with amaurosis fugax the best. Log rank analysis confirmed the significantly better survival following carotid endarterectomy for amaurosis fugax than for

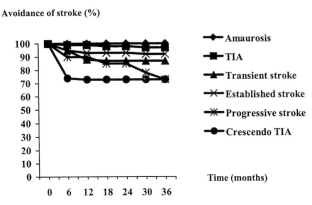

Figure 1. Life-table analysis of stroke related to presenting symptom.

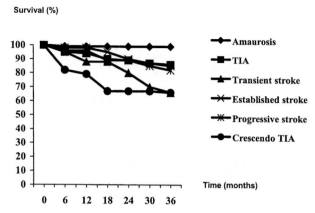

Figure 2. Life-table analysis of survival related to presenting symptom.

crescendo TIA (p< 0.001), TIA (p< 0.01), Transient stroke (p< 0.01) and progressive stroke (p< 0.05).[3]

Thus when carotid stenting and surgery are compared presentation is important.

Asymptomatic carotid artery stenosis can be detected by duplex ultrasound in approximately 25% of patients with peripheral vascular disease.[4] The natural history of asymptomatic carotid artery disease is dependent on the degree of internal carotid artery stenosis. Patients with <75% stenosis have an annual stroke rate of 1.3% whereas those with stenosis of >75% have an annual stroke rate of 3.3%.[5] This establishes clear guidelines for acceptable rates of postoperative stroke and death rates together with long-term outcome.

The Cochrane review of randomized controlled trials comparing carotid endarterectomy with medical management concluded that there is little benefit in terms of surgery for asymptomatic carotid artery stenosis[6] (Fig. 3).

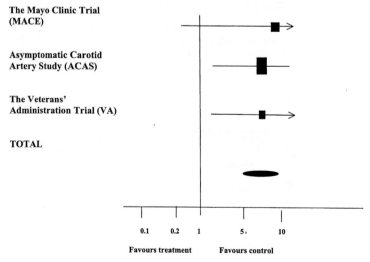

Figure 3. Odds ratio comparing 30-day combined stroke and death rates following carotid endarterectomy or medical therapy for aysmptomatic carotid artery stenosis.[6] The results of the Asymptomatic Carotid Artery Surgery Trial (ACST) are cautiously awaited.

Evidence

Operative technique is fairly well established. Surgeons vary in their choice of use of shunt (Fig. 4). There is also a variation of preference with respect to general anaesthetic or local anaesthetic and use of patch.

Whatever the method, it is regarded as crucially important that arterial blood pressure is maintained throughout the procedure and immediately before and after the procedure. Results have improved in two major British units in the last decade. Figure 5 shows combined 30-day stroke mortality figures following endarterectomy at Charing Cross Hospital and the Leicester Royal Infirmary. During the period 1980–1995, Charing Cross reported 460 symptomatic patients. Mortality is 2.4%, a stroke rate of 1.7% and total combined stroke mortality rate 4.1%.[3] The Leicester 1992–1996 results are 494 consecutive patients showed a 30-day death and stroke rate of 4.2%.[7]

Since 1996 the audited Charing Cross results of 291 patients showed a 30-day combined stroke and death rate of 2.4% and are similar to the Leicester published results of 500 consecutive patients 2.2%[8] (Fig. 5).

There can be no certainty why this improvement has occurred but the period does coincide with the use of transcranial Doppler which may have altered the indications for the use of shunt and also led to improved surgical techniques.

Follow-up of contralateral stenosis by duplex have been shown to be of little benefit.[9]

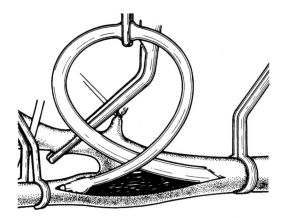

Figure 4. Open carotid surgery. Reproduced with permission from Ref. 14.

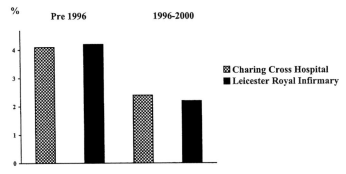

Figure 5. 30-Day stroke and death rates following carotid endarterectomy at Charing Cross and Leicester Royal Infirmary.

The patient is monitored in a high dependency unit for 24 hours. Attention is paid to controlling the arterial blood pressure, with glyceryl trinitrate infusion if necessary. An intensive care bed is not required. Discharge is routinely by the third postoperative day. Mortality and stroke rates following surgical carotid endarterectomy have improved over the last decade. An audit of postoperative complications using published data from two specialist centres, Charing Cross Hospital and Leicester Royal Infirmary in the United Kingdom confirm this.

A systematic comparison of the 30-day outcome following angioplasty and endarterectomy for symptomatic carotid artery disease reviewed the literature on 33 single centre studies published between 1990 and 1999; 13 angioplasty studies with 714 arteries and 20 surgical studies with 6970 arteries were analysed. The 30-day mortality following angioplasty was 0.8% compared with 1.2% following endarterectomy (p=0.6) and the risk of stroke or death was 7.8% for the angioplasty group and 4% following surgery (p<0.001)[10] (Fig. 6).

The results of the Carotid and Vertebral Artery Transluminal Angioplasty Study (CAVATAS) have recently been published in which 504 patients were randomized to surgery (253 patients) or endovascular treatment (251 patients). The rate of any stroke lasting more than 7 days, or death were 9.9% and 10% respectively.[11]

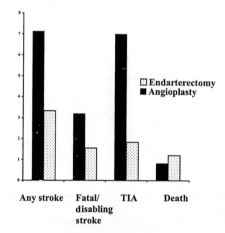

Figure 6.   Systematic comparison of the early outcome of angioplasty and endarterectomy for symptomatic carotid artery disease – 30-day stroke rate.

Carotid stenting: a minority option

The European Vascular and Endovascular Monitoring Panel (an initiative by *Vascular News*) consists of 250 expert centres across Europe. The EVEM data have been analysed for the fourth quarter of the year 2000 and the annual carotid angioplasty numbers have been estimated across Europe from the EVEM panel based on data from the third and fourth quarters of the year. These data include an estimated 103 520 carotid procedures during the calendar year, 8303 (8%) carotid angioplasties and 95 217 carotid endarterectomies.[12]

This puts into perspective the situation across Europe where carotid angioplasty is being used for a small minority of the total number of carotid procedures.

Random controlled trial?

Only if stenting results approach these levels should such a trial be undertaken. Complications in CAVATAS are too high.

Summary

- EVEM data illustrate how few carotid angioplasties are performed.

- Published 30-day stoke and mortality results are superior following carotid endarterectomy.

- Randomized controlled trials are needed, but only if endovascular results improve.

- Endovascular stenting is improving.

- There is no certainty at all that stenting results will ever approach best surgery.

- There is no place for endovascular intervention in asymptomatic carotid artery stenosis.

References

1. Anonymous. Randomised trial of endarterectomy for recently symptomatic carotid stenosis: Final results of the MRC European Carotid Surgery Trial (ECST). *Lancet* 1998; **351**: 1379–1387.
2. Anonymous. North American Symptomatic Carotid Endarterectomy Trial Collaborators (NASCET). Beneficial effect of carotid endarterectomy in symptomatic patients with high-grade carotid stenosis. *N Engl J Med* 1991; **325**: 445–453.
3. Golledge J, Cuming R, Beattie DK, Davies AH, Greenhalgh RM. Influence of patient-related variables on the outcome of carotid endarterectomy. *J Vasc Surg* 1996; **24**: 120–126.
4. Alexandrova NA, Gibson WC, Norris JW. Carotid artery stenosis in peripheral artery disease. *J Vasc Surg* 1996; **23**: 645–649.
5. Norris JW, Zhu CZ, Bornstein NM, Chambers BR. Vascular risks of asymptomatic carotid stenosis. *Stroke* 1991; **22**: 1485–1490.
6. Chambers BR, You RX, Donnan GA. Carotid endarterectomy for asymptomatic carotid stenosis (Cochrane review). The Cochrane Library 2001; 3.
7. Loftus IM, McCarthy MJ, Pau H *et al*. Carotid endarterectomy without angiography does not compromise operative outcome. *Eur J Vasc Endovasc Surg* 1998; **16**: 189–193.
8. Naylor AR, Hayes PD, Alroggen H *et al*. Reducing the risk of carotid surgery: a seven year audit of the role of monitoring and quality control assessment. *J Vasc Surg* 2000; **32**: 750–759.
9. Golledge J, Cuming R, Ellis M. Clinical follow-up rather than duplex surveillance after carotid endarterectomy. *J Vasc Surg* 1997 25, 53–55.
10. Golledge J, Mitchell A, Greenhalgh RM, Davies AH. Systematic comparison of the early outcome of angioplasty and endarterectomy for symptomatic carotid artery disease. *Stroke* 2000; **31**: 1439–1443.
11. CAVATAS investigators. Endovascular versus surgical treatment in patients with carotid stenosis in the Carotid and Vertebral Artery Transluminal Angioplasty Study (CAVATAS); a randomised trial. *Lancet* 2001; **357**: 1729–1737.
12. EVEM Newsflash 2001: 4.
13. Cuming R, Blair SD, Powell JT, Greenhalgh RM. The use of duplex scanning to diagnose perioperative carotid occlusions. *Eur J Vasc Surg* 1994; **8**: 143–147.
14. Greenhalgh RM. Selective shunting during carotid endarterectomy. In *Vascular and Endovascular Surgical Techniques* 4th edn. Greenhalgh RM (ed). London: WB Saunders, 2001: 35–38.

Carotid stenting will become the gold standard

For the motion
Peter A Gaines

Introduction

Intervention upon the carotid artery is usually performed as a prophylactic procedure to prevent stroke and carotid endarterectomy in combination with best medical treatment is currently the accepted treatment to manage high-grade symptomatic carotid disease. Surgery is not without problems but the truth about complication rates is difficult to find. Even with a highly selected group of surgeons operating on a highly selected group of patients there is a 5.8% perioperative stroke and any death rate and a 2.1% death and disabling stroke rate.[1] Within a trial that is less tightly proscribed the equivalent rates were 7.1% and 3.7% respectively.[2]

Treatment away from tightly structured trials is usually less good and carotid endarterectomy is no exception. The American Heart Association recognized a surgical death and major stroke rate of 4.8–9% outside major trial centres.

Care should also be taken when critically reviewing data, as authorship of the article appears to play a major factor in the reported stroke and death rate. Rothwell reviewed 50 published studies and reported a perioperative mortality and stroke rate of 7.7% (95% CI 5–10.2%) when patients were assessed by a Neurologist and a 2.3% rate (95% CI 1.8–2.7%) when the author was a surgeon.[3] Two recent reports of carotid endarterectomy from Germany and the USA where the patients were evaluated by an unbiased observer (a neurologist) detail a stroke and death rate of 11.1% and 11.4%.[4,5] The NASCET trial also detailed the non-neuroembolic complications of surgery, in particular cranial nerve damage in 7.6% of patients, wound complications in 8.9%, myocardial infarction in 0.9% and other cardiovascular complications in 1.2%.

Clearly carotid surgery is far from a benign procedure and the efficacy demonstrated by the tightly controlled surgical trials has not translated into effectiveness in the real world. In addition there is no un-biased evidence to suggest that the complication rate of carotid endarterectomy is reducing. It is time to look to carotid stenting as an alternative strategy.

Level 1 Evidence

For carotid stenting to be recognized as a useful prophylactic procedure it should have short- and long-term results comparable with or better than carotid endarterectomy. In the light of the vagaries of the outcome reporting detailed above it would

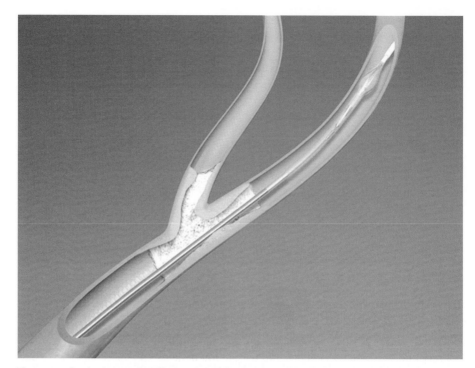

Figure 1. Cerebral protection filter deployed. Reproduced with permission from Ref. 9.

seem pertinent to review the available data from the three randomized trials comparing carotid stenting with carotid endarterectomy.

Table 1. Immediate outcome of randomized trials

		No. patients	Peri-procedural any stroke and/or death (%)	Peri-procedural disabling stroke and/or death (%)	Comments
CAVATAS	Surgery	253	9.9	5.9	Completed trial
	Endovascular	251	10.0	6.4	
WALLSTENT	Surgery	112	4.5		Stopped trial
	Stent	107	12.1		
LEICESTER	Surgery	10	0	0	Stopped trial
	Stent	7	71	43	

The CAVATAS Trial[6]

In all, 504 patients with carotid stenosis were randomized to carotid endarterectomy or endovascular treatment. In the endovascular group, stents were only used in 26% and there was no cerebral protection. A neurologist followed up the patients and was the principal author. The rates of major outcome events did not differ significantly between the endovascular treatment and surgery (disabling stroke or death: 6.4% vs 5.9% respectively, and any stroke lasting >7 days or death 10% vs 9.9%). The results were remarkably consistent with other outcome data when presented by an independent observer.[4,5] Not surprisingly there were more major non-neuroembolic complications in the surgery group. The data also demonstrated that in the long-term carotid stenting was as efficacious as carotid endarterectomy at preventing stroke.

These results were achieved without either dedicated devices, routine use of stents, contemporary pharmacological support and cerebral protection systems.

The Wallstent Trial[7]

Only 219 patients of the proposed 700 were recruited to this study comparing carotid stenting with carotid endarterectomy in patients with high-grade symptomatic carotid disease. The results in the stenting group were poor with an ipsilateral stroke, procedure-related death or vascular death rate at 1 year of 12.1% vs 3.6% for carotid endarterectomy (p=0.022). Cerebral protection was not used and the Wallstent was not a dedicated carotid device. In addition it is unclear whether the study was stopped because of the results or poor recruitment.

The Leicester Trial[8]

This trial, which randomized symptomatic patients with high-grade disease between surgery and stenting, was expected to recruit 300 patients but was stopped after only 17 had been treated because of an unacceptable complication rate in the stenting limb. Ten carotid endarterectomy operations had no complication but five of the seven patients who underwent carotid stenting had a stroke, three of which were disabling at 30 days. These results are so disparate compared with other centres that the structure of the study deserves consideration.

1. No prior imaging of the origin of the major vessels was undertaken to exclude disease that would be a contraindication to an endovascular procedure by most experienced interventionalists.
2. The interventionalist had only performed eight prior carotid procedures, most of these not in an experienced unit, whereas the surgeons had long expressed their wide experience and expertise at carotid endarterectomy.
3. Only a single anti-platelet agent was employed prior to carotid stenting, whereas major units were already recommending combining aspirin with clopidogrel or ticlopidine.[8]
4. The protocol required an attempt at passage of the stent before pre-dilatation. It has long been recognized that it is not possible to pass a 7F (2.3mm diameter) device across a >70% stenosis of a vessel with a normal lumen of 6mm or less (i.e. best residual lumen of only 1.8mm) without 'Dotterizing' the plaque. It is observed from their published data that of the five patients in whom failed passage of the stent was followed by balloon pre-dilatation and subsequent stent placement, four had a stroke (80%).

Unfortunately cerebral protection was not available at the time of the study.

Other data

The UK National Carotid Register has recently released its first report. In all, 147 patients (85.7% symptomatic) were treated by placement of a stent. There was a 4.1%

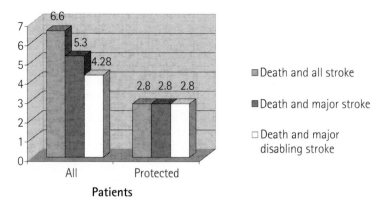

Figure 2. Sheffield 30-day outcomes (%). Total: 304 patients. Protected: 71 patients.

death and all stroke rate, and a 2.7% death and disabling stroke rate. The patients treated with cerebral protection had half the complication rate of those treated without protection.

The endovascular management of carotid disease is a recent innovation and a learning curve is to be expected. Unpublished data from the CAVATAS trial shows that there is a dramatic improvement in the peri-procedural complication rate with experience. The combined stroke and death rate for the first 30 patients treated in each centre was 11.1%. The stroke and death rate for the 51st to the 100th patient treated in the only centre to achieve that level of recruitment was 4.0%. The respective rates for surgery were less dramatic with a reduction from 10.8% to 6.4%.

The data from our own unit also demonstrate improvement in 30-day outcome with time and change in technique. All data were collected by neurologists. Overall we have a 6.6% death and any stroke rate, 5.35% death and major stroke rate, and 4.3% death and major disabling stroke rate. Our last 71 patients have all been treated with cerebral protection following which there were only two deaths (one ruptured right ventricle from a pacing wire, one cerebral haemorrhage) and no neuroembolic complications. The corresponding death and any stroke rate is therefore 2.8%, comparable with even the best surgical data.

Discussion

The motion to be debated is 'carotid stenting will become the gold standard'. Carotid stenting is a new technique in evolution and yet, already, the only level 1 data from a completed trial indicates that the endovascular management of carotid disease is at least as safe as carotid surgery and is equally efficacious at preventing stroke. Two other studies that were stopped suggest that the treatment has a higher peri-procedural risk. In addition there are data to suggest that the results are improving. Practitioners are learning to utilize adjunctive drug therapy, dedicated devices and cerebral protection. The indications are that this minimally invasive approach will supplant surgery as the treatment of choice for stenotic carotid disease and we welcome the new generation of randomized trials.

Summary

- The only completed randomized trial indicates that endovascular treatment of carotid stenosis is as efficacious as surgery.

- The results of endovascular therapy are improving.

- Carotid stenting will become the gold standard.

References

1. Beneficial effect of carotid endarterectomy in symptomatic patients with high-grade carotid stenosis. North American Symptomatic Carotid Endarterectomy Trial Collaborators. *N Engl J Med* 1991; 325: 445–453.
2. MRC European Carotid Surgery Trial: interim results for symptomatic patients with severe (70–99%) or with mild (0–29%) carotid stenosis. European Carotid Surgery Trialists' Collaborative Group. *Lancet* 1991; 337(8752): 1235–1243.
3. Rothwell PM, Warlow C. Is self-audit reliable? *Lancet* 1995; 346: 1623.
4. Chaturvedi S, Aggarwal R, Murugappan A. Results of carotid endarterectomy with prospective neurologist follow-up. *Neurology* 2000; 55: 769–772.
5. Hartmann A, Hupp T, Koch H *et al.* Prospective study on the complication rate of carotid surgery. *Cerebrovasc Dis* 1999; 9: 152–156.
6. Endovascular versus surgical treatment in patients with carotid stenosis in the Carotid and Vertebral Artery Transluminal Angioplasty Study (CAVATAS): a randomised trial. *Lancet* 2001; 357(9270): 1729–1737.
7. Alberts MJ. Results of a multicenter prospective randomised trial of carotid artery stenting vs carotid endarterectomy. *Stroke* 2001; 32: 325 (abs).
8. Yadav JS, Roubin GS, Iyer S *et al.* Elective Stenting of the Extracranial Carotid Arteries. *Circulation* 1996; 95: 376–381.
9. Gaines PA. The MedNova NeuroShield cerebral protection system. In *Vascular and Endovascular Surgical Technique* 4th edn. Greenhalgh RM (ed). London: WB Saunders, 2001: 57–62.

Carotid stenting will become the gold standard

Against the motion
Peter RF Bell

Introduction

Carotid endarterectomy has been an effective treatment for carotid stenosis for many years. The ECST and NASCET trials[1,2] demonstrated clearly that for symptomatic lesions the risk of stroke and death in the first 3 years for surgery was around 7% and for medical treatment close to 30%. These data represented what was the standard almost 10 years ago from a multicentre trial. Single centres with validation of results by neurologists can achieve results today which are much better than this at around 2–3% stroke and death rate for symptomatic patients on any presentation.[3] The causes of stroke and death during surgery are now well known and the risks at operation can be well controlled. Routine shunting, although controversial, now prevents many of the complications that were seen without shunts. The routine use of transcranial Doppler monitoring[4] allows intraoperative emboli to be easily detected (Fig. 1) and measures taken to stop them occurring immediately.[5] Assessment of the operation by angioscopy or duplex[6] also reduces the chances of stroke making control of the perioperative period almost complete. Mortality can be virtually eliminated by either using local anaesthesia[7] or investigating the patient prior to surgery where necessary and carrying out prior or synchronous coronary artery bypass grafting. In this way the death and stroke rate can be reduced to very low levels. The cost of the procedure used to be quoted as a reason for doing an angioplasty but this has now been reduced to levels comparable with or below

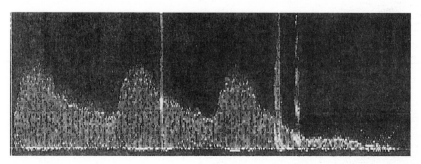

Figure 1. Emboli detected by transcranial Doppler during dissection at carotid endarterectomy.

those of angioplasty[8] with patients staying in hospital for 24 hours. The only down-side to the operation is the scar which nearly always heals very well and usually recoverable cranial nerve damage of around 1–2%.[9] Restenosis of the lesion can be reduced to 5% with routine patching[10] using vein or artificial material. Routine monitoring for 3 hours after surgery using transcranial Doppler has also largely abolished the thromboembolic events that occur in the immediate postoperative period.[11] We therefore have a situation where, at the appropriate centre, death and stroke rates of around 2% for symptomatic patients without exclusions can be routinely achieved with good long-term results. Quality carotid measures such as transcranial Doppler monitoring and some method of assessing the procedure such as angioscopy (Figs 2,3) are important.

For patients who are asymptomatic the surgical death and complication rates are even lower than that quoted for the symptomatic patients. In our own series we have had no strokes or deaths in the last 100 asymptomatic patients on whom we have operated.

With these results one has to ask the question, what can angioplasty with or without stenting do to improve matters, particularly when attempts are made to angioplasty lesions containing echogenic or soft plaques (Fig. 4). There are many non-randomized, non-validated series where selected patients, many of them

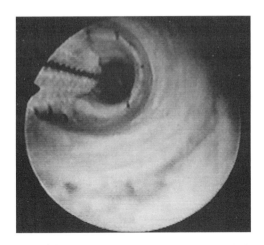

Figure 2. A view of a satisfactory technical procedure at angioscopy.

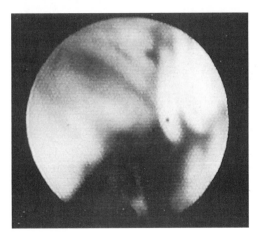

Figure 3. Thrombus can be seen at the endarterectomy site at angioscopy.

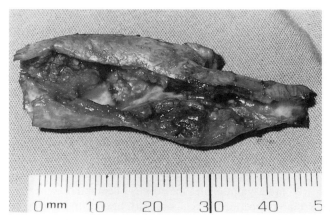

Figure 4. A plaque removed at endarterectomy showing soft material and possible thrombus which can easily embolize.

asymptomatic, are said to have complication rates of between 3 and 6%, often unverified by a neurologist.[12,13] Of the randomized studies, there are three, the first done in Leicester, which showed extensive embolization (Fig. 5) and an unacceptable complication rate in patients who were dealt with on an intention-to-treat basis without selection.[14] In other words no patients were excluded from surgical treatment or angioplasty and all were symptomatic. This study has been criticized because the numbers were too small, predilatation was not used and the radiologist who did the procedure was inexperienced. The trial was rightly stopped by the monitoring committee which is why the numbers were small. The radiologist had been mentored for the procedure and was an extremely experienced operator. Finally predilatation was used where necessary and this trial remains the only one where no patient was excluded. It showed quite clearly that angioplasty was dangerous and emboli are common and numerous (Table 1). After this study was published we were told that emboli to the brain did not matter. This soon changed when it was realized that they did matter and protection is now thought to be necessary.

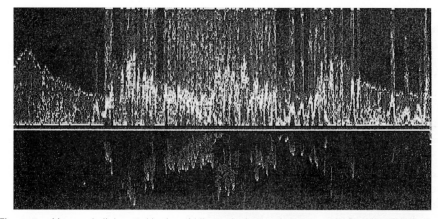

Figure 5. Many emboli detected in the middle cerebral artery by transcranial Doppler during angioplasty.

Table 1. Embolus count in seven patients at various stages of carotid angioplasty detected by transcranial Doppler.

Patient no.	Wire manipulation	Stent deployment	Balloon inflate	Balloon deflate
1	29	125	1	26
2	20	90	28	81
3	115	110	23	101
4	158	76	0	86
5	71	159	29	60
6	115	115	0	53
7	50	65	14	22

The second study[15] recently showed a complication rate in the angioplasty group of around 10% and about 1% for surgery. This study was multidisciplinary and stopped by the monitoring committee because of the very inferior results produced by angioplasty.

In the third study, the CAVATAS Study,[16] patients were excluded from angioplasty for ill-defined reasons on the basis that surgeons also chose which patients to operate on. Details of why exclusion took place were not mentioned. In this study the surgery and angioplasty group had a complication rate of around 10%. The surgical stroke and death rate is greatly in excess of what one would expect today and one must be concerned about the track record of the surgeons involved. The complications of angioplasty are also higher than other studies and may be a reflection of the experience of those taking part.

These studies have shown that angioplasty with or without stenting has a high complication rate and is an unacceptable treatment at the present time outside a properly controlled trial with well-defined aims. At present, even that would be difficult as informed consent is something which is not at all easy to obtain.

Equipoise is not present when comparing surgery with angioplasty and the only way it might be ethical do carry out a trial would be to use cerebral protection devices which have now become popular. These devices have been invented to prevent embolization which we were told was not important when they were reported after the Leicester trial. A recent consensus statement agreed in New York[17] clearly states that angioplasty and stenting should not be used except in a trial situation and should not be used to treat routine patients with carotid bifurcation disease. Protection devices may make a difference and feasibility studies have shown that they can be used effectively. The devices available use a balloon or filter placed above the stenosis to trap debris that would otherwise embolize. One device relies upon creating reversed flow to avoid embolization.[18] Even with these devices strokes still occur but the incidence may be lower than without them. Their availability and the knowledge that emboli are a major risk factor in causing strokes means that a trial to compare them with surgical treatment might be considered ethical. It is essential that if a trial is done, the same type of patient is treated by both methods, i.e. all symptomatic or non-symptomatic and equal degrees of stenoses are dealt with. It is impossible at present to pick out a dangerous lesion so we can reliably exclude these.

We know that most symptomatic patients do not require any form of treatment, only about 30% in fact would have a stroke if nothing was done. What we should be doing is trying to find out who these patients are and then treating them with the safest possible method available. It is not necessary to invent new treatments until they have been shown to be better or more efficient. It would be very difficult for angioplasty and stenting to be shown in a proper randomized scientific fashion to be better than surgery. Only when it is, should it be used routinely and not put forward as the primary treatment, which it is being done in many centres where ethics appear to have flown out of the window to be replaced by vested self-interest. Carotid stenting is a new treatment which remains unproven and can only become the gold standard for treatment of carotid stenosis if it is properly tested against the very effective and safe gold standard of carotid endarterectomy.

Summary

- Specialist centre stroke and death rates less than 2% for symptomatic patients after carotid endarterectomy.

- For asymptomatic patients results are even better than this.

- In two-thirds of randomized trials the stroke and death rate for carotid endarterectomy are much better than for angioplasty.

- Serious embolism occurs during angioplasty and stenting and it should not be used routinely.

- Emboli may be avoidable if protection is used.

References

1. Anonymous. Randomised trial of endarterectomy for recently symptomatic carotid stenosis: Final results of the European Carotid Surgery Trial (ECST) *Lancet* 1991; 351: 445–453.
2. Anonymous. North American symptomatic carotid endarterectomy trial collaborators (NASCET) Benefit of carotid endarterectomy in symptomatic patients with high grade carotid stenosis. *N Engl J Med* 1991; 325: 445–453.
3. Naylor AR, Gaunt ME. Quality control during carotid endarterectomy. *Vasc Med* 1996; 1: 125–132.
4. Naylor AR, Hayes PD, Alroggen H *et al*. Reducing the risk of carotid surgery: a seven year audit of the role of monitoring and quality control assessment. *J Vasc Surg* 2000; 32: 750–759.
5. Gaunt ME, Martin PJ, Smith JL. Clinical relevance of intraoperative embolisation detected by transcranial Doppler ultrasound during carotid endarterectomy. A prospective study of 100 patients. *Br J Surg* 1994; 81: 1345–1439.
6. Gaunt ME, Smith JL, Martin PJ *et al*. A comparison of quality control methods applied to carotid endarterectomy. *Eur J Vasc Endovasc Surg* 1996; 11: 4–11.
7. Shah DM, Darling C III, Cheng BB *et al*. Carotid endarterectomy awake patients, its safety, acceptability and outcome. *J Vasc Surg* 1994; 19: 1015–1020.
8. Back MR, Haward TB, Huber TS *et al*. Improving the cost effectiveness of carotid endarterectomy. *J Vasc Surg* 1997; 26: 456–465.
9. Schauber M, Fontenelle LJ, Solomon JW *et al*. Cranial/cervical nerve dysfunction after carotid endarterectomy. *J Vasc Surg* 1997; 25: 481–487.
10. Counsell C, Salinas R, Naylor AR *et al*. A systematic review of randomised trials of carotid patch angioplasty in carotid endarterectomy. *Eur J Vasc Endovasc Surg* 1997; 13: 345–354.
11. Dietrich EB, Ndiaye M, Reid DM. Stenting in the carotid artery. Initial experience in 110 patients. *J Endovasc Surg* 1996; 3: 42–62.
12. Theron J, Curthenex P, Alachkav F *et al*. A new triple catheter system for carotid angioplasty with cerebral protection. *Am J Neuroradiol* 1990; 11: 69–74.
13. Yadav JS, Roubin GS, Sriram I *et al*. Elective stenting of extra cranial carotid arteries. *Circulation* 1995; 2: 376–381.
14. Naylor AR, Bolia A, Abbott R *et al*. Randomised study of carotid angioplasty and stenting versus carotid endarterectomy. A stopped trial. *J Vasc Surg* 1998; 28: 326–334.

15. Alberti MJ. For the publications committee of the Wall stent. Results of a multicentre prospective randomised trial of carotid artery stenting versus carotid endarterectomy. *Stroke* 2001; **32**: 325 (abstracts).
16. Endovascular versus surgical treatment in patients with carotid stenosis in the carotid and vertebral artery. Transluminal angioplasty study (CAVATAS) a randomised trial. *Lancet* 2001; **357**: 1729–1737.
17. Veith FJ. In *Current Status of Carotid Bifurcation. Angioplasty Stenting.* Veith FJ, Amor M (eds). New York, Basel: Marcel Dekker Inc. 2001: pp 267–271.
18. Parodi JC, La Mura R, Marian Fexreera L *et al.* Initial evaluation of carotid angioplasty and stenting with three different cerebral protection devices. *J Vasc Surg* 2000; **6**: 1127–1137.

Carotid stenting will become the gold standard

For the motion

Plinio Rossi, Mario Bezzi, Fabrizio Fanelli, Michele Rossi, Filippo Maria Salvatori

With the collaboration of
Alberto Cremonesi, Fausto Castriota

Introduction

'Symptomatic severe atherosclerotic stenoses of the carotid bifurcation and/or the internal carotid artery, if medically treated, have a high probability of causing disabling strokes within a few years.'

Randomized studies in the United States (North American Symptomatic Carotid Endarterectomy, NASCET) and in Europe (European Carotid Surgery Trial, ECST)[1,2] have established that for symptomatic patients treated with carotid endarterectomy there is a considerable benefit if the stenosis is >70%. In the NASCET trial, the cumulative risk of stroke at 2 years was 26% in the medical group and only 9% in the surgical group, equivalent to an absolute risk reduction of 17%.[3] The absolute risk reduction of ipsilateral stroke with carotid endarterectomy was higher for older age groups (28.9 for >75 years of age; 15.1% for 65–74 years, and 9.7% for people <65 years of age).[4]

In asymptomatic male patients with carotid stenosis >60%,[5] surgical intervention may be of some benefit if their life-expectancy is more than 2 years, while in female patients with the same characteristics benefit has not been demonstrated.

All the patients selected for these trials had to meet strict inclusion requirements, such as: being fit for carotid endarterectomy; having had a transient ischaemic attack (TIA) or a non-disabling ischaemic stroke within 180 days prior to admission; having a severe stenosis of ipsilateral carotid artery visible on angiogram. Exclusion criteria included patients with: an age over 79 only for the first 3 years; organ failure; cardiac disorders (unstable angina or myocardial infarction within the last 6 months); uncontrolled hypertension; cancer; diabetes. On the basis of the best surgical results, the American Heart Association, has suggested that morbidity and mortality rates after carotid endarterectomy should be less than 5% for symptomatic and less than 3% for asymptomatic patients.

At the time of these studies, no endovascular alternative to the surgical therapy for carotid stenosis existed and therefore the question could only be whether to operate or not. Being the only procedure, surgery was able to evolve into a very refined and a highly sophisticated technique. The best results are reported from centres of excellence where carotid endarterectomy is performed in many cases every year and where low mortality and morbidity results can thus be achieved.[6,7,8]

Percutaneous transluminal angioplasty (PTA) of the carotid arteries was started in 1979 by Mathias, as reported by Jaeger,[9] but only in the early 1990s did it begin to be performed, though as yet in a very limited number of centres and with questionable results.[10,11] In the late 1990s, it gained a wider popularity because of the improved quality of the materials employed, increased experience, and the initial use of stents already accepted for peripheral arteries. The technique therefore became more popular and, because of the encouraging reports from many centres, it started to challenge surgery.

In the last two/three years of the 1990s, the materials improved considerably, special stents were purposely designed for carotid stenosis, and distal cerebral protection began to be used with a reduction of complications, thus making the procedure even more acceptable.

Undoubtedly, in the 1990s, these two invasive techniques, carotid endarterectomy and carotid artery stenting, for the treatment of carotid artery stenosis were not comparable for their different level of development and the results obtained with carotid endarterectomy could not be matched by early results obtained by carotid artery stenting. A comparison was, however, attempted by several randomized trials, with such unacceptable results for carotid artery stenting that two trials were discontinued before their completion: one because of an excessively high complication rate for endovascular therapies[12] and the other because of procedural and recruitment difficulties.[13]

These results, although seemingly unfavourable for carotid artery stenting, were an accurate evaluation of the technique at that moment, thus preventing an uncritical application of the procedure.

A recent trial, lasting from 1992 to 1997, is known as the Carotid and Vertebral Artery Transluminal Angioplasty Study (CAVATAS). Its 30-day results, published by *The Lancet* in June 2001,[14] far beyond all expectations, reported an equal and high incidence of disabling strokes and deaths for PTA/stenting and surgery; for this reason, this trial has not been interrupted.

In the CAVATAS trial, 'major outcome events within 30 days with disabling stroke or death were 6.4% for endovascular therapies vs 5.9% for surgery and 10% vs 9.9%, respectively, for any stroke lasting more than seven days; these data are not statistically significant. However, the incidence of restenosis at one year for endovascular therapy (14%) and for surgery (4%) is very important ($p<0.001$), as well as the cranial neuropathy reported in 8.7% of patients ($p<0.0001$) only after surgery. No substantial difference in the rate of ipsilateral strokes was however noted with the survival analysis up to three years after randomisation.'

The results of this trial were criticized by surgeons, many of whom had achieved results in their own centres extremely different from those reported here. It is not yet completely clear why surgery in this trial had a complication rate so much higher than those reported in other series, despite the fact that the same centres participated both in the CAVATAS and in the ECST with its very different results. However, a similar criticism was also made by interventionalists.

This difference is probably due to the fact that the sole inclusion criterion for patients to enrol in the CAVATAS was that they be suitable for both the endovascular and the surgical therapy. This recruitment policy led to a population of subjects at higher than average risk for treatment complications, because the process of patient selection was less restrictive than in other studies.[14,15]

In addition, the complication rates described in the CAVATAS for carotid artery

PTA and stenting are much higher than in other recent reports[16-20] where they were around 2–3%. This might reflect that many of the CAVATAS endovascular operators had to be trained rapidly in the procedure so that they were not at the peak of their 'learning curve', and they had less sophisticated techniques and materials than those available today, only a few years later.

The CAVATAS had the great merit of indicating that when **no patient selection is made stenting and surgery yield similar results.**

A more recent randomized trial Carotid Revascularization Endarterectomy versus Stent Trial (CREST)[15] is comparing endovascular therapy – incorporating the routine use of stents and distal cerebral protection – with surgery in symptomatic patients who are considered at 'low-risk' for endarterectomy.

To ensure state-of-the-art results, great emphasis has been placed on credentialing of both surgeons and stent operators. Notably, stent operators must have completed successfully up to 20 carotid stent cases to be considered for CREST and 50 cases for the new uncontrolled trial CARESS" (Carotid Revascularization with Endarterectomy or Stenting System).[15] The Food and Drug Administration (FDA) approved in March 2001 the Investigation Device Exemption (IDE) for CARESS. Several category B IDE trials have received FDA approval and are currently enrolling patients. These include: the SAPPHIRE controlled trial with AngioGuard protection (with approximately 300 patients who have been randomized to date); the CAVATAS II (in progress); the Acculink for Revascularization of Carotids in High-risk patients (ARCHeR) trial; and the Stenting of High-risk Extracranial Lesions Trial with Emboli Removal (SHELTER) trial. Category B IDE trials currently in the approval process include the Evaluation of the Medtronic AVE Self-Expanding Carotid Stent System with Distal Protection in the Treatment of Carotid Stenosis (MAVErIC) trial.

The problem is that the results of these randomized trials will not be available for 4–5 years, and during this period we will be unable to reach an evidence-based opinion as to the true value of carotid artery stenting.

In the meantime, a step forward was nonetheless made by proponents of endovascular therapy with the report by Roubin[18] a 5-year prospective analysis of carotid artery stenting in 528 patients with symptomatic and asymptomatic carotid artery stenoses. In this paper, the author reported a 30-day outcome of 2.6% major non-fatal strokes or deaths and 4.8% minor non-fatal strokes; he also indicated that cases with a high number of co-morbidities, such as coronary insufficiency, high blood pressure, bilateral carotid occlusion, and age >80, were also included. The importance of age is well documented by Table 3, where the number of strokes and deaths increases when the patients are over 80 years of age (p >0.01). The result of this study compares very well with surgical results.

Evidence

The problem now is whether we still consider carotid endarterectomy a gold standard therapy or whether we should consider it proper to suggest endovascular therapies as an alternative, without forgetting that the real goal of treatment is the prevention of a stroke.

Without any doubt, it is not ethical to suggest a therapeutic modality based only on one group's experience, anecdotal reports, or personal experience; we must, however, consider that today's experience with endovascular therapies is much better than what was reported in the past; we cannot go on forever citing the results of old trials which compare two techniques not at the same level of development.

The results from 1995 to 2001 are reported in the following tables, which show a continuous improvement of carotid artery stenting outcomes.

From the analysis of the data reported in Tables 1 and 2, there has been a substantial decrease in the 30-day mortality and morbidity rates, without considering minor neurological events lasting less than 7 days.

Data reported in those papers reflecting the experience in the late 1990s are without any doubt equal to surgical data, while they are absolutely better in those papers reflecting studies done in the years 1999–2000.

Table 1. Carotid artery stenting results (1990–1997)

Author	Patients	Success	30-day mortality and morbidity	Restenosis
NACPTAR Investigators[11]	147	83%	9% 3% deaths 6% strokes	22%
Diethrich *et al.*[10]	110		3.6% 1.8% deaths 1.8% major strokes 4.5% minimal strokes	
CAVATAS Study[14] (completed in 1997)	504		6.4% + 10% strokes lasting more than 7 days	14%

Table 2. Late carotid artery stenting results (1997–2001)

Author	Patients	Success	30-day mortality and morbidity	Restenosis
Mathur *et al.*[30] (Sep. 1994–Jan. 1997)	204	99%	1.03% deaths + major complications 7.41% minor complications	5% 14% stenosis + stent deformity
Dangas *et al.*[16] (Oct. 1995–Aug. 1998)	37	100%	2.6% death or any stroke	
Leger *et al.*[31] (Aug. 1996–Aug. 1998)	8	100%	0 major complications 1 TIA	12.5% 3 months 37.5% 6 months 62.5% 1 year 75.0% 2 years
Cremonesi *et al.*[20] (1997–Dec. 1999)	119	99.16%	0 death + major complications 3.36% minimal complications	5.4%
Roubin *et al.*[18] *Circulation* 2001 (Sep. 1994–Sep. 1999)	528		2.6% deaths and major complications 4.8% minor complications	
Mathias *et al.*[19] (Jan. 2000)	800	97%	2% major strokes + mortality	10%
D'Audiffret *et al.*[32] results in 3 stages (Sep. 1995–Feb. 2000)	79	1st-2nd stage: 82% 3rd stage: 100%	1st-2nd stage: 2.9% major strokes, reversed with urokinase; 1.5% minor strokes. 3rd stage: no complications	7.5%
Chakhtoura *et al.*[33] (Sep. 1996–May 2000)	46	100%	1 death no major stroke	8%
Jaeger *et al.*[9] (Dec. 2000)	20	100%	major complications 0 minimal complications = 3 (less than 1-cm infarctions, seen by diffusion MR only)	

In a very recent paper currently under review, Castriota *et al.*[21] (personal communication) reported their data on 275 cases: at 30 days there were no major strokes or deaths but only minor neurological events; their results showed improvement with cerebral protection. This group's number of cases has now risen to 335, among which there has been one major postoperative stroke with embolization of the ophthalmic artery and complete loss of the visual function of eye.

All in all, it is fair to say that these most recent reports suggest a trend towards a considerable decrease of major complications which is surely due to the remarkable increase in the experience and routine use of cerebral protection.

However, these results showing the almost complete disappearance of complications have been reported by single institutions and are therefore open to criticism because of the lack of supervision by an independent party; only if they can be duplicated by other institutions will they have more credibility.

Prospective innovations and conclusions

Why, then, am I in favour of carotid artery stenting and believe that it will become the gold standard? Because I strongly believe in two points: the *technical evolution* and a *better patient selection*.

Technical evolution

Both technique and technology are rapidly evolving and today's results, although not definitive, are very reassuring; this opinion derives also from my own experience.

The medical device industry is committing substantial resources to developing and improving devices for carotid artery stenting and supporting scientific studies to document efficacy.

Major innovations in the past several years which induce optimism for the future include:

Cerebral protection

Cerebral protection, first suggested by Theron 10 years ago, is now considered mandatory in every case of carotid stenting. There are two types of devices: balloon occlusion devices and with filters (which permit recovery of all the particles detached during balloon inflation and deflation) and the proximal protection. A third type of protection described by Parodi provides protection reversing flow in the carotid artery through occlusion of both the external and the common carotid arteries in conjunction with an arteriovenous communication with the femoral vein by an interposed filter;[22,23] this technique although more invasive is very efficient.

In a recent editorial, Diethrich[24] stated that 'cerebral protection is not 100% with any type of system,' but if it would reach only 88%, as shown by Ohki,[25] it would still represent a considerable improvement in patient safety.

Stents

New stents with lower profile, in conjunction with monorail delivery systems, have been developed specifically for carotid applications. New 'Carbonstents' which are

63

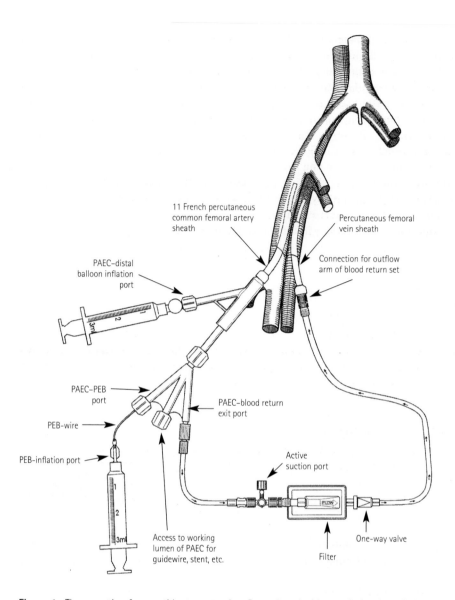

Figure 1. The operation for carotid artery stenting. Reproduced with permission from Ref. 34.

now available for coronary application, are made with a new cellular design and equipped with a carbon film permanent thromboresistant coating and are proving able to reduce the restenosis rate from 26 to 11%.[26]

Moreover, there is currently considerable excitement among interventionalists with drug-eluting stents showing success in the prevention of coronary restenosis. The rationale for drug-eluting stents is to maintain the lumen of the artery open and to deliver drugs where they are required, thus maximizing the drug effect and potentially decreasing systemic toxicity.

Although many agents are being investigated, the two most advanced in clinical studies are Sirolimus (Cordis) and Paclitaxel or Taxol (Cook, Boston Scientific, Guidant). Sirolimus (rapamycin) is a naturally occurring macrocyclic lactone which is a potent immunosuppressive agent originally developed for prevention of renal transplant rejection. Sirolimus induces cell cycle arrest in the late gastrointestinal phase, thus preventing proliferation of smooth muscles cells.[27] The results of one randomized trial called RAVEL[28] in coronary artery stenting have been reported with no restenosis at 6 months compared with 26% incidence in the placebo arm and no sign of edge effect.

Event-free survival at 6 months was close to 97% after coronary drug-eluting stenting and significantly superior (p<0.0001) to the 72% event-free survival of patients treated with bare stents.

If this type of drug-eluting stent can prevent restenosis after carotid stenting (which currently varies from 3 to 20%), then we can say that a considerable problem will be eliminated.

Patient selection

In the selection of candidates for carotid artery stenting we have to consider the plaque morphology and the predictors of stent complications. It is very well known that plaque morphology may be an indicator for risk of cerebral embolization during carotid artery stenting, according to ultrasound findings: a hypoechoic plaque indicates soft material which can easily fragment and produce microemboli, while as hyperechoic plaque indicates calcification, with less embolization risk.[29] This is only a theoretical possibility and not a proven fact.

In the presence of heavily calcified plaques with a horseshoe appearance on computed tomography, patients are probably better treated with surgery rather than with endovascular repair.[19]

The presence of thrombus and/or lengthy, severe, and multiple lesions should also be considered, since these factors undoubtedly increase the risk of complication for carotid artery stenting.[30]

The age of the patients should be also taken into the account: at ages >80, there is an increased risk of complications with both endovascular techniques and surgery, compared with the results obtained in younger patients.

In conclusion, if we analyse the most recent endovascular therapy results (2–3 years) and compare them with present surgical results, we discover that these are very competitive, if not even better. Although they cannot yet be said to have been proven by scientific evidence, they still represent an evolving technique whose promise cannot be dismissed during the waiting time (3–4 years) before results from new randomized trials will become available.

For these reasons, and also on the basis of my personal experience, I am definitely confident that carotid artery stenting will be the gold standard for the treatment of symptomatic carotid artery stenoses.

Finally, I would like to recall the effort that was required in the late 1970s in order to establish PTA of the iliac, renal, and coronary arteries, now considered the first-choice treatment for stenotic lesions of these arteries. It should also be remembered that carotid endarterectomy was done for several years without any evidence-based studies, and it was not until NASCET and ESCT that data were proven compared with the medical therapy.

Summary

- The CAVATAS study shows equal complications for carotid artery stenting and carotid endarterectomy.

- All the comparisons between carotid artery stenting and carotid endarterectomy are based on old studies.

- Endovascular stenting is improving and becoming better than surgery.

- Randomized controlled trials are needed.

- Indication for carotid artery stenting cannot be only for patients at high surgical risk.

- Validity of surgery or stenting for asymptomatic stenoses should be reconsidered only after the results of new trials.

References

1. North American Symptomatic Carotid Endarterectomy Trial Collaborators. Beneficial effect of carotid endarterectomy in symptomatic patients with high-grade carotid stenosis. *N Engl J Med* 1991; **325**: 445–53.

2. European Carotid Surgery Trialists' Collaborative Group. Randomised trial of endarterectomy for recently symptomatic carotid stenosis: final results of the MRC European Carotid Surgery Trial (ECST). *Lancet* 1998; **351**: 1379–1387.

3. Hobson II RW. Carotid angioplasty-stent: clinical experience and role for clinical trials. *J Vasc Surg* 2001; **33**: S117–S123.

4. Alamowitch S, Eliasziw M, Algra A, Meldrum H, Barnett HJM for the NASCET group. Risk, causes, and prevention of ischaemic stroke in elderly patients with symptomatic internal-carotid-artery stenosis. *Lancet* 2001; **357**:1154–1160.

5. ACAS (Executive Committee for the Asymptomatic Carotid Atherosclerosis Study) Endarterectomy for asymptomatic carotid artery stenosis. *JAMA* 1995; **273**: 1421–1428.

6. Zarins CK, Carotid endarterectomy: the gold standard. *J Endovasc Surg* 1996; **3**: 1411–1413.

7. Golledge J, Cuming R, Greenhalgh RM, Davies AH. Systematic comparison of the early outcome of angioplastry and endarterectomy for symptomatic carotid artery disease. *Stroke* 2000; **31**: 1439–1443.

8. Naylo AR, Hayes PD, Alroggen H *et al.* Reducing the risk of carotid surgery: a seven year audit of the role of monitoring and quality control assessment. *J Vasc Surg* 2000; **32**: 750–759.

9. Jaeger H, Mathias K, Drescher R, Hauth E *et al.* Clinical results of cerebral protection with a filter device during stent implantatoion of the carotid artery. *CVIR* 2001; **24**: 249–256.

10. Diethrich EB, Ndiye M, Reid DB. Stenting in the carotid artery: initial experience in 110 patients. *J Endovasc Surg* 1996; **3**: 42–62.

11. The NACPTAR Investigators: Feruson R, Schwarten D, Purd P *et al.* Restenosis following cerebral percutaneous angioplasty (Abstract) *Stroke* 1995; **26**: 186.

12. Naylor AR, Bolia A, Abbott RJ, *et al.* Randomized study of carotid angioplasty and stenting versus carotid endarterectomy: a stopped trial. *J Vasc Surg* 1998; **28**: 326–334.

13. Alberts MJ, McCann R, Smith TP *et al.* A randomized trial: carotid stenting versus endarterectomy in patients with symptomatic carotid stenosis, study designs. *J Neurovasc Dis* 1997; Nov. Dec. : 228–234.

14. CAVATAS investigators. Endovascular versus surgical treatment in patients with carotid stenosis in the carotid and vertebral artery transluminal angioplasty study (CAVATAS): a randomised trial. *Lancet* 2001; **357**: 1729–1737.

15. Roubin GS, Hobson II RW, White R *et al.* CREST and CARESS to evaluate carotid stenting: time to get to work! *J Endovasc Ther* 2001; **8**: 107–110.

16. Dangas G, Laird JR, Mehran R *et al.* Carotid artery stenting in patients with high-risk anatomy for carotid endarterectomy. *J Endovasc Ther* 2001; **8**: 39–43.

17. Shawl FA, Kandro W, Domanski MJ *et al.* Safety and efficacy of elective carotid artery stentino in high risk patients. *J Amer Coll Card* 2000; **35**: 1721–1728.

18. Roubin GS, New G, Iyer SS *et al.* Immediate and late clinical outcomes of carotid artery stenting in patients with symptomatic and asymptomatic carotid artery stenosis. A 5-year prospective analysis. *Circulation* 2001; **103**: 532–537.

19. Mathias K, Jager H, Hennigs S *et al.* Endoluminal treatment of internal carotid artery stenosis. *World J Surg* 2001; **25**: 328–336.

20. Cremonesi A, Castriota F, Manetti R *et al.* Endovascular treatment of carotid atherosclerotic disease: early and late outcome in a non-selected population. *Ital Heart J* 2000; **1**: 801–809.

21. Castriota F, Cremonesi A, Manotti R *et al.* Endovascular treatment of carotid atheroscle-rotic disease: the cerebral protection impact on early clinical outcome (personal communication). Submitted for publication.

22. Parodi JC. Initial evaluation of angioplasty and stenting using three different cerebral protection devices (abstract). *J Endovasc Ther* 2000; **7**(Suppl.): 1-30-31.

23. Parodi JC, Bates M. How to recover emboli and other particles from the middle cerebral artery: will this be valuable in carotid stenting and carotid endarterectomy? *Endo Cardio Vascular Multimedia Magazine* 2001; **5**: 167.

24. Diethrich EB. Characterizing the carotid revascularization candidate: will plaque morpho-logy be important? *J Endovas Ther* 2001; **8**: 44–45.

25. Ohki T, Marin ML, Lyon RT *et al. Ex vivo* human carotid artery bifurcation stenting: correlation of lesion characteristics with embolic potential. *J Vasc Surg* 1998; **27**: 463–471.

26. Bartorelli AL, Fabiocchi F, Loaldi A *et al.* Clinical and angiographic evaluation of the carbonstent: a new cellular design carbonfilm coated coronary stent. *Am J Cardiol* 1999; **84**: 109.

27. Sousa JE, Costa MA, Abizaid A *et al.* Lack of neointimal proliferation after implantation of Sirolimus-coated stents in human coronary arteries. *Circulation* 2001; **103**: 192–195.

28. Serruys PW, Morice MC, Sousa JE *et al.* The RAVEL study : a randomized study with the sirolimus coated Bx velocity balloon-expandable stent in the treatment of patients with de novo native coronary artery lesions. *Europ Heart J* 2001; **22**: 484.

29. Biasi GM, Ferrari ST, Nicolaodes AN *et al.* The ICAROS registry of carotid artery stenting. *J Endovasc Ther* 2001; **8**: 46–52.

30. Mathur A, Roubin GS, Iyer SS *et al.* Predictors of stroke complicating carotid artery stenting. *Circulation* 1998; **97**: 1239–1245.

31. Leger AR, Neale M, Harris JP. Poor durability of carotid angioplasty and stenting for treatment of recurrent artery stenosis after carotid endarterectomy: an institutional experience. *J Vasc Surg* 2001; **33**: 1008–1014.

32. d'Audiffret A, Desgranges P, Kobeiter H, Becquemin J-P. Technical aspects and current results of carotid stenting. *J Vasc Surg* 2001; **33**: 1001–1007.

33. Chakhtoura EY, Hobson RW, Goldstein J *et al.* In-stent restenosis after carotid angioplasty-stenting: incidence and management. *J Vasc Surg* 2001; **33**: 220–225.

33. Parodi JC, Bates MC. Angioplasty and stent with reversal of internal carotid flow as cerebral protection device. In *Vascular and Endovascular Surgical Techniques* 4th edn. Greenhalgh RM (ed). London: WB Saunders, 2001: 63–66.

Carotid stenting will become the gold standard

Against the motion
P Bergeron

Introduction

From its beginning, carotid angioplasty and stenting has been seen as a very competitive method in vascular surgery. Moreover, this feeling has been strengthened by the improvement of its technique, essentially due to the development of embolic cerebral protection.

On their side, vascular surgeons, not aware of this technique, try to protect themselves from it whereas most interventional radiologists and cardiologists use it to present carotid artery stenting as the best way to treat carotid stenosis.

As we lack comparative studies, no one can assert that carotid artery stenting will become the gold standard. To answer that question, we must wait for the results of randomized studies running in Europe and America. Let us describe the current situation of carotid artery stenting.

To become the gold standard, carotid artery stenting should meet several criteria and gain the support of both patients and practitioners:

1. Its non-invasive aspect and the short hospital stay is certain to appeal to patients.
2. Unlike the general public, endovascular therapists probably will not accept it so easily. Most surgeons will consider carotid artery stenting of interest only if they lose control of the carotid recruitment. Instead, they will keep on using a well proven technique they can control and will only accept learning the carotid artery stenting technique if it is simplified.
3. Carotid artery stenting will stand out if the superiority of its clinical results becomes obvious in precise indications. These results, based on short- and long-term scientific arguments, must be obtained by comparative studies, especially with medical treatment and conventional surgery.

To discuss the claim that carotid artery stenting will become a gold standard procedure, we must analyse the short-term results, according to types of patients, and long-term benefits.

Background

Determining groups of patients who benefit from carotid surgery and those where the surgical benefit remains questionable

Symptomatic patients

Over the last 10 years, in large randomized trials, carotid endarterectomy has been compared favourably with medical treatment for *symptomatic patients*.

For example, NASCET[1] randomized 659 symptomatic patients with moderate-to-severe carotid stenosis (70–99%); 328 were randomly placed in the surgical group and 331 in the medical group treated with aspirin. The study was interrupted after 18 months follow-up because of the superiority of carotid surgery.

In the surgical group, there were 5.8% perioperative stroke/deaths with 2.7% major stroke/deaths. The life-table analysis for any fatal or non-fatal stroke at 2 years was 9%.

In the medical group, the rate of stroke/death of any kind was 3.3% with 1.2% of major stroke/death. Life-table analysis at 2 years for any stroke/death was 26%.

Thus we can see that the absolute risk reduction after surgery is 17% at 2 years and the initial disadvantage of surgery was overcome in a few months. For symptomatic patients with moderate stenosis (50–69%), the 5-year ipsilateral stroke rate was respectively 15.7% and 22.2% for the surgical and medical arms.[2]

In the ECST,[3] symptomatic patients were randomized in the same groups as mentioned for NASCET. The surgical group consisted of 778 patients and led to 7.5% of perioperative morbidity/mortality. Life-table analysis at 3-year follow-up showed a risk of disabling stroke of 3.7% and 8.4% for the surgical and medical groups respectively.

Asymptomatic patients

On the other hand, the situation for *asymptomatic patients* seems to be very different.

The Asymptomatic Carotid Artherosclerosis Study (ACAS)[4] concerned 1662 patients with asymptomatic carotid stenosis >60%. The 30-day perioperative morbidity/mortality was 2.3% and life-table analysis at 5-year follow-up showed an ipsilateral stroke risk of 5.1% for the surgical group (including 1.2% of stroke morbidity due to arteriography) compared with 11% for the medical group. Thus, the absolute risk reduction is here 5.9%, i.e. 1.2% per year. Compared with symptomatic patients, the benefit of surgery seemed not to be so conclusive. Perhaps this was due to the reduced efficacy of surgery for men or women with a short life expectancy.

However, the natural risk of stroke for asymptomatic patients depends on the degree of stenosis.[5] For high grade stenosis >80%, the annual ipsilateral risk of stroke is 2% while it is only 1.4% for stenosis between 50 and 80%. The total annual risk of stroke/death is respectively 8.5% and 2.4% for lesions >80% and <80%. In other words, the only cases to be discussed are those with very tight asymptomatic stenosis.

Besides 1292 symptomatic subjects, the ACE trial (Aspirin and Carotid Endarterectomy)[6] also enrolled 1512 asymptomatic patients. In this group, the 30 days perioperative stroke/death was 4.6%. This rate of surgical complications for asymptomatic patients cannot compete with medical therapy.

Moreover, statistical data indicate that to prevent one stroke in 2 years, the number of asymptomatic patients needing CEA is 67 whereas the number of patients needed to treat for symptomatic patients is only 6 in NASCET. However, nobody should forget that these results strictly depend on the efficiency of surgical teams, whose rate of major perioperative stroke should not exceed 2–3%.

The National Stroke Association[7] and the American Heart Association[8] established guidelines concerning the stroke/death rate after carotid endarterectomy. For asymptomatic and symptomatic patients; the reference rates are respectively 3% and 6%; for patients presenting recurrent stenosis, it is increased to 10%.

Until now, there are relatively few consistent data on immediate and long-term results of carotid artery stenting. Only randomized, controlled trials, showing clinical equality or superiority of carotid artery stenting may place it as a new gold standard for carotid stenosis treatment. But today, no study can assess the superiority of carotid artery stenting compared with surgery or medical treatment. If we suppose, on the basis of preliminary results, that angioplasty brings similar results to surgery, then it should only be used for symptomatic or 'high-risk' patients, taking into account their co-morbidity (particularly cardiac co-morbidity).

A first conclusion is evident: carotid artery stenting will probably not be the gold standard for asymptomatic patients for a long time.

What about the other cohorts of patients? Carotid surgery has demonstrated its efficiency globally. However, particularly for surgical 'high-risk' patients its benefit still remains controversial. Such cases were seen, for example, in the NASCET with patients who presented contralateral carotid stenosis, in the ACAS in women with a perioperative rate of 3.6% and with patients in poor health. It is this subset of patients that carotid artery stenting could benefit.

The evaluation of complications is different whether it is carried out by neurologists or surgeons,[9] and this factor must be taken into account for carotid artery stenting evaluation. The selection of patients influences the selection of identified risky lesions which need surgery, as mentioned in ACST.[10]

Evidence

What could be the claims of carotid artery stenting?

1. Some preliminary feasibility studies have proved the tolerance of carotid angioplasty on selected patients. The CAST study[11] was carried out by vascular surgeons who selected 100 patients with short internal stenosis out of the carotid bifurcation. Unprotected angioplasty on these selected patients led to a 4% transient ischaemic attack rate, without stroke or neurological death.

2. Unprotected carotid artery stenting for symptomatic patients, based on individual series, shows a rate of neurological complications of approximately 10%. This was confirmed by the CAVATAS trial.[12] This study did not mention a single prevalence between the two methods, but demonstrated that angioplasty may reduce nerve injury and cardiac complications. In future, there is less chance that the CREST[13] study may prove the superiority of carotid artery stenting compared with surgery, despite the cerebral protection.

3. On the contrary, 'high-risk' patients, such as those with contralateral carotid occlusion or those presenting a deficiency of the Circle of Willis, are undoubtedly an evident target for angioplasty. According to McCrory et al.,[14] the presence of at least two risk factors is associated with a two-fold increase in the risk of adverse events.

Defining high-risk patients

Some groups of patients cannot join classical randomized studies and ideally should be entered into specific randomized studies concerning surgery vs carotid angioplasty. These patients have a high cardiological risk (NYHA Class III and IV; LVEF <30%; open heart surgery in the last 6 weeks; myocardial infarction in the last 4 weeks; unstable angina; synchronous severe carotid artery disease and carotid stenosis) as well as those presenting severe pulmonary disease, contralateral carotid occlusion, laryngal palsy, post X-ray exposure, previous carotid endarterectomy, common carotid artery lesions below the clavicle, high cervical internal carotid artery and severe tandem lesions. The SAPPHIRE trial (Stenting and Angioplasty with Protection in Patients at High Risk for Endarterectomy) is randomizing 600–900 'high surgical risk' patients relating to carotid endarterectomy or to carotid artery stenting. Other studies such as the CHRS (Carotid High Risk Study) sponsored by Boston Company work in the same field. These specific studies may show a superiority of carotid artery stenting, but for instant current data do not allow us to conclude precisely nor to defend carotid artery stenting as a gold standard for this subset of patients.

Can the short-term results of carotid artery stenting compete with surgery?

The first carotid stent implantation was due to Mathias[15] in 1989, who worked with a Wallstent. J. Theron talked about a carotid Strecker stent in 1990 (personal communication) and we reported in 1993[16] a Palmaz stent implanted in 1991.

The first series were small, and the patients were hardly selected, mainly presenting recurrent stenosis. At this time, elective stenting was used for dissection or residual stenosis after balloon angioplasty. It only became routine in the beginning of 1994 with our experiments and cerebral protection has only been applied since 1999. With Dietrich[17] in 1996 and Roubin[18] in 1997, the series has grown to include more than 100 patients. Tables 1 and 2 summarize the data for unprotected and protected carotid artery stenting.

Table 1. Immediate results of unprotected carotid artery stenting.

Author	Year	No. of patients	Method	TIA (%)	Minor stroke (%)	Major stroke (%)	Death (%)	Major stroke/death (%)
Mathias[23]	1983	3	PTA			1		1
Tsai[24]	1986	27	PTA	0	0	0	0	0
Kachel[25]	1991	35	PTA	1	0	0	0	0
Bergeron[26]	1996	28	PTA 17	17.8				
			Stent 11		3.6	0	3.6	3.6
Diethrich[27]	1996	110	Stent	4.5	4.5	1.8	1.8	2.7
Criado[28]	1997	1–3%	33 Stent	0	0	0	0	0
Yadav, Roubin[29]	1997	NR	107	6.5	1.8	0.9	2.8	
Wholey[30]	1997	108	Stent	4.6	1.9	1.9	1.9	4.6
Mathias (pers. comm.)	2001	1026	Stent	6.9	2.9	1.1	0.5	3.7

Table 2. Immediate results of protected carotid arterial stenting

Author	Year	No. of patients	Method	Minor stroke (%)	Major stroke (%)	Death (%)	Major stroke/death (%)
Kachel[31]	1996	74	Kachel balloon	2.8	1.4	0	1.4
Parodi, Bates[32]	2001	127	PAES	2 Contro-lateral	2 Reperfusion bleeds	2	2.4
Al–Mubarak, Roubin[33]	2001	80 8% cont. occlusion	Filter	1	0	0	1.25
Mathias (pers. comm.)	2001	284	Filter	1.3	0	0	1.3
Bergeron	2001	64	Filter and balloon occlusion	0	1.5	4.4	5.9
Henry/ Amor[34]	2001	148	Balloon Filter	1.2	0	0	1.2
CAFE study	2001	122	Balloon	2.4	1.6	0.8	4.8

It seems that the cerebral protection has reduced ipsilateral strokes. However, in one sense, due to contralateral strokes and reperfusion syndromes, the global neurological complications did not change in our experience. As these series are not controlled ones, the results should be carefully analysed. They cannot be compared with important surgical trials which bring scientific proofs on another level. Nevertheless, these series show us that carotid angioplasty can be competitive.

Limiting factors of carotid artery stenting

Anatomical features
Complex aortic arches are difficult to manage and they represent sources of embolism in both cerebral hemispheres, as reported by DW-magnetic resonance imaging, studies and transcranial Doppler records. Access to the common carotid artery is impossible in some tortuous arteries (Fig. 1).

Protection systems have their own limitations
1. Occlusion balloons interrupt blood supply during the procedure,
2. Flux reversion also interrupts the blood flow but avoids crossing the carotid stenosis,
3. Filters cross the lesion but allow blood flow supply during the procedure.

A comparative study is necessary, both in experimental and clinical fields. In an international registry, Wholey[19] has collected all the experiments of the biggest world centres. Amongst the 7034 patients and 7464 stents, only 736 (15%) were led by cerebral protection with a stroke/death rate of 5.38% including 0.94% of non-procedural death. This proved that protected carotid artery stenting is not exempt from neurological complications.

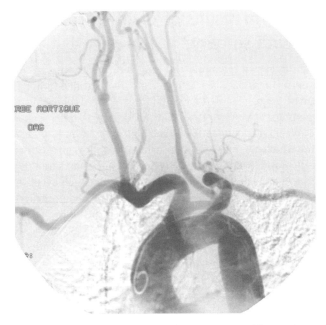

Figure 1. Some tortuous arteries make access to the common carotid artery impossible.

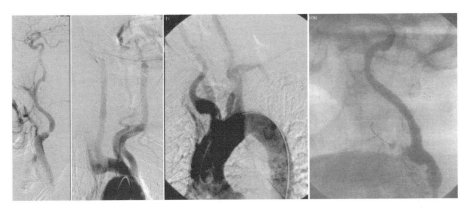

Figure 2. Conversion of protection. Example of a patient who needed two different protective devices. After the failure of the placement of a filter, a reverse flow system was used.

Stents are not perfect

This is particularly true for carotid bifurcation, covering the external carotid artery which is often immediately occluded or compressed. In addition, classical stents do not protect from restenosis which is a real issue with a rate of 8%. Coated stents will probably reduce this rate.

Conclusion

Carotid artery stenosis by itself is not applicable to all situations. Therefore, it should be accepted as an adjunctive method for carotid repair, and not as a method competitive with surgery.

Are the long-term results of carotid artery stenting competitive with surgery?

Very few publications report medium- and long-term results of carotid artery stenting. When they exist, these data are derived from uncontrolled individual series.

We have reviewed the results of 186 carotid artery stents, achieved since the beginning of our experiments in April 1991, date of our first stent implantation, up to September 2001. We have excluded from the results, based on Kaplan-Meïer evaluation, 13 cases for which we had less than 6 months follow-up, 12 deaths within 6 months following carotid artery stenting, five early conversions and two early occlusions. Thus, we have considered 154 carotid artery stents achieved on 119 patients with 180 stents. The average age was 70.5 years and the male/female ratio was 3/1. Amongst the patients, 49% were symptomatic. The mean follow-up was 42 months and ranged from 6 to 113 months. We analysed the long-term benefit of carotid artery stenting in terms of efficacy of stroke prevention, fate of the stented carotid artery, survival rate and causes of death.

Survival rate and causes of death

The life-table analysis of survival rate at 5 years was 50% (Fig. 3); 27 deaths occurred and are reported in Table 3.

Stroke prevention

The late (> 6 months) neurological events included four deaths (2.6%) among them three contralateral strokes at 8, 31 and 52 months and one intracerebral haemorrhage, one major ipsilateral stroke (0.65%) related to extensive in-stent restenosis at 12 months and four transient ischaemic attacks (2.6%). Among these, one was stent-related due to a traumatic crush of the cervical stent, two were contralateral and one was ipsilateral non-stent related. This last was due to an ulcerated plaque below the stent and surgery confirmed that the stent was perfectly recovered (Fig. 4). The ipsilateral stroke freedom was 95% (Fig. 5). In the literature, Roubin[20] reported that in 523 patients, similar results were obtained with 95% stroke freedom. Mathias (personal communication, Dortmund 2001) reported 91.2% of late stroke freedom.

What is the fate of stents in term of patency, deformation and restenosis rate?

Looking into 180 stents, we observed no late occlusion, ten stents with complications (5.5%) including five in-stent restenoses (2.7%) and five stents with deformation

Table 3. Causes of death during follow-up.

Causes of death	No. of deaths	%
Cancer	10	8.4
Heart disease	3	2.5
Lung disease	2	1.6
Visceral disease	5	4.2
Natural causes	3	2.5
Neurological causes	4	3.3
Total	27	17.5

Table 4. Percentage of in-stent restenosis.

Author	%	Type of stent
Henry	4	BE
Bergeron	2.2	BE
Wholey	2.2	BE
Roubin	6	BE+SE
Diethrich	8	BE+SE
Hobson	8	SE
Mathias	8	SE

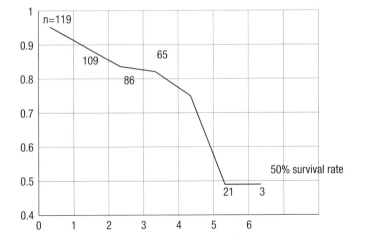

| | | | | LIFE TABLE ANALYSIS OF SURVIVAL RATE
Kaplan & Meïer method | | | | | |
Interval	Alive entering the interval	Presented the event	Alive excluded	Dead excluded	Lost	Exposed to risk	Probability of occuring event in the interval	Survival probability	95% confidence interval
1	119	4	0	0	6	116.00	0.97	0.97	0.03
2	109	6	1	0	16	100.50	0.94	0.91	0.06
3	86	5	0	0	16	78.00	0.94	0.85	0.07
4	65	1	1	0	15	57.00	0.98	0.83	0.08
5	48	3	0	0	24	36.00	0.92	0.77	0.10
6	21	5	1	0	12	14.50	0.66	0.50	0.20
7	3	0	0	0	2	2.00	1.00	0.50	0.20

Figure 3. Life table analysis of survival rate.

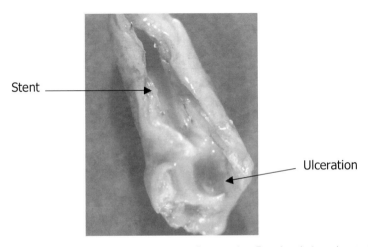

Figure 4. Internal carotid artery resection 2 years after stenting. Transient ischaemic attack was related to a huge ulceration. Note the perfect aspect of the stent.

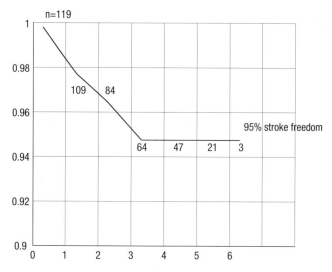

Figure 5. Ipsilateral stroke freedom.

Interval	Alive entering the interval	Presented the event	Alive excluded	Dead excluded	Lost	Exposed to risk	Probability of occuring event in the interval	Stroke freedom probability	95% confidence interval
1	119	0	0	4	6	114.00	1.00	1.00	0.00
2	109	2	1	6	16	97.50	0.98	0.98	0.03
3	84	1	0	5	14	74.50	0.99	0.97	0.04
4	64	1	1	1	14	56.00	0.98	0.95	0.05
5	47	0	0	2	24	34.00	1.00	0.95	0.05
6	21	0	1	5	12	12.00	1.00	0.95	0.05
7	3	0	0	0	2	2.00	1.00	0.95	0.05

(2.7%) with a narrowing lumen exceeding 50%. Five patients (2.7%) underwent a redilatation under intravenous ultrasound guidance, three times for compression (1.6%) and twice for in-stent restenoses (1.1%). Patency rate was 91% for primary stent patency and 98% assisted primary patency.

This allows us to say that for short Palmaz stents, crushing is not an issue, and that in-stent restenosis is relatively low. Others authors have reported an in-stent restenosis rate up to 8% (Table 4) depending on the use of expandable balloon (BE) or self-expandable (SE) stents.

These long-term results are encouraging ; the stent appears to be well stuck to carotid and the plaque seems healed. For more than 90% of cases, the stent has turned an evolving lesion into a stable one. This makes the removal of the plaque during surgery an acceptable challenge.

Whatever may happen in the future, the long-term data are too few today to permit a detailed examination of this technique. There are no specific arguments which can assert that carotid artery stenting will become the gold standard. Nevertheless, this technique seems obvious today for precise indications, particularly for high surgical risk patients.

What will be the sharing between carotid artery stenting and surgery?

The New York consensus[21] held in November 1999 under the initiative of Veith and Amor has gathered a panel of 17 leaders in the field of carotid angioplasty (seven interventional radiologists, three interventional cardiologists, six vascular surgeons and one neurosurgeon from five countries). The panel members agreed that angioplasty is justified to treat selected patients but did not support it as the standard of care. Angioplasty was defined as contraindicated in patients with difficult access or recent stroke.

Conclusion

In our opinion, both symptomatic and asymptomatic patients may be candidates for carotid stenting if the endovascular option appears of better benefit or leads to fewer complications. In our institution, carotid artery stenting and surgery are performed by vascular surgeons and the selection is based on the patient's risk factors. The decision for carotid artery stenting or surgery is taken by a team of vascular surgeon, anaesthetist, neurologist and cardiologist to determine the patient's fitness for one or the other treatment. This situation eliminates all competitive factors between practitioners.

Except when associated thrombus is suspected, we rarely consider the carotid plaque composition as a determining factor. The ICAROS registry (Imaging Carotid Angioplasty and Risk Of Stroke)[22] is correlating the plaque composition based on a computerized grey scale with the risk of brain embolization and restenosis at 1 year. This trial may identify lesions not suitable for CAS.

In conclusion, carotid artery stenting will not become the gold standard for a while. It will be considered for selected situations where surgery is prone to a high rate of complications and it can provide greater benefit.

Summary

1. *CAS will not be the gold standard for:*
- Asymptomatic patients.
- Low risk patients.
- Patients with a recent cerebrovascular accident or crescendo transient ischaemic accident.
- Extensive lesions including of the common carotid artery from the aortic arch to the carotid bifurcation.
- Lesions highly calcified.
- Lesions associated with carotid tortuosities.
- Lesions containing intraluminal thrombus.
- Lesions presenting difficult access with emboligenous risk during catheterization.
- Cases where stents and cerebral protection systems cannot be used, whatever the reason.

2. *CAS is dedicated to become the gold standard in particular situations where patients are unlike for surgery:*

- Anatomic cases leading to difficult or high risky surgery

  - All hostile necks
      radical neck surgery with tracheotomy,
      re interventions after carotid endarterectomy,
      cervical radiotherapy,
      radiation carotid stenosis,
      frozen necks,
      short and large necks with high carotid bifurcation,
      stenosis on carotid by-pass.

  - All highly situated lesions on internal carotid artery.

  - All lesions of common carotid artery and of the aortic arch.

- Clinical cases where surgery offer less good results

  - Contralateral carotid occlusions.

  - Dysfunction of Circle of Willis.

  - Tandem lesions with associated intracerebral or proximal stenosis.

  - Patients with severe coexisting carotid and coronary artery disease.

  - Patients with established previous neurological deficit.

  - Patients with cardiac heart failures or waiting for coronary angioplasty or by-pass.

- Patients with a short life expectancy due to malignancy or aging are relative indications.

References

1. North Amican Symptomatic Carotid Endarterectomy Trial Collaborators. Beneficial effect of carotid endarterectomy in symptomatic patients with high-grade carotid stenosis. *N Engl J Med* 1991; **325**: 445–453.
2. Barnett HJ, Taylor DW, Eliasziw M, *et al*. Benefit of carotid endarterectomy in patients with symptomatic moderate or severe stenosis. North American Symptomatic Carotid Endarterectomy Trial Collaborators. *N Engl J Med* 1998; **339**: 1415–1425.
3. European Carotid Surgery Trialists' Collaborative Group. Medical Research Council European Carotid Surgery Trial: Randomized trial of endarterectomy for recently symptomatic carotid stenosis: Final results of the MRC European Carotid Surgery Trial (ECST). *Lancet* 1998; **351**: 1379–1387.
4. The Executive Committee for the Asymptomatic Carotid Atherosclerosis (ACAS) Study. Endarterectomy for asymptomatic carotid artery stenosis. *JAMA* 1995; **273**: 1421–1428.
5. Mackey AE, Abrahamowicz M, Langlois Y *et al*. and the Asymptomatic Cervical Bruit Study Group. Outcome of asymptomatic patients with carotid disease. *Neurology* 1997; **48**: 896–903.
6. Taylor DW, Barnett HJM, Haynes RB *et al*. for the ASA and Carotid Endarterectomy (ACE) Trial Collaborators. Low-dose and high-dose acetylsalicylic acid for patients undergoing carotid endarterectomy: a randomized controlled trial. *Lancet* 1999; **353**: 2179–2184.
7. Gorelick PB, Sacco RL, Smith DB *et al*. Prevention of a first stroke: a review of guidelines and a multidisciplinary consensus statement from the National Stroke Association. *JAMA* 1999; **281**: 1112–1120.
8. Biller J, Feinberg WM, Castaldo JE *et al*. Guidelines for Carotid Endarterectomy: A statement for Healthcare Professionals from a Special Writing Group of the Stroke Council, American Heart Association. *Stroke* 1998; **29**: 554–562.

9.   Rothwell PM, Slattery J, Warlow CP. A systematic review of the risks of stroke and death due to endarterectomy for symptomatic carotid stenosis. *Stroke* 1996; **27**: 260–265.

10. Halliday AW, Thomas D, Mansfield A. The asymptomatic carotid surgery trial (ACST) rationale and design. *Eur J Vasc Surg* 1994; **8**: 703–710.

11. Bergeron P, Becquemin JP, Jausseran JM *et al.* Percutaneous stenting of the internal carotid artery: the European CAST I Study. Carotid Artery Stent Trial. *J Endovasc Surg* 1999; **6**: 155–159.

12. Brown MM. Vascular surgical society of Great Britain and Ireland : results of the carotid and vertebral artery transluminal angioplasty study. *Br J Surg* 1999; **86**: 710–711.

13. Hobson RW 2ⁿᵈ. Carotid angioplasty-stent: clinical experience and role for clinical trials. *J Vasc Surg* 2001; **33** (Suppl 2): S117-S123.

14. McCrory DC, Goldstein LB, Samsa GP *et al.* Predicting complications of carotid endarterectomy. *Stroke* 1993; **24**: 1285–1291.

15. Bockenheimer SAM, Mathias K. Percutaneous transluminal angioplasty in arteriosclerotic internal carotid artery stenosis. *Am J Neuroradiol* 1983; **4**: 791–792.

16. Bergeron P, Rudondy P, Poyen V *et al.* Abstract: Experience with carotid angioplasty and use of intervascular stents. *Endovascular Interventions. International Congress VI-Tomorrow's Technology Today.* Phoenix, Arizona, USA, 1993.

17. Dietrich EB, Ndiaye M, Reid DB. Stenting in the carotid artery: initial experience in 110 patients. *J Endovasc Surg* 1996; **3**: 42–62.

18. Yadav JS, Roubin GS, Iyer S *et al.* Elective Stenting of the extracranial carotid arteries. *Circulation* 1997; **95**: 376–381.

19. Wholey MH, Wholey M, Mathias K *et al.* Global experience in cervical artery stent placement. *Cathet Cardiovasc Interv* 2000; **50**: 160–167.

20. Roubin GS, New G, Iyer SS *et al.* Immediate and late clinical outcomes of carotid artery stenting in patients with symptomatic and asymptomatic carotid artery stenosis: a 5-year prospective analysis. *Circulation* 2001; **103**: 532–537.

21. Veith FJ, Amor M, Ohki T *et al.* Current status of carotid bifurcation angioplasty and stenting based on a consensus of opinion leaders. *J Vasc Surg* 2001; **33**(Suppl 2): S111–S116.

22. Biasi GM, Sampaolo A, Mingazzini P *et al.* Computer analysis of ultrasonic plaque echolucency in identifying high risk carotid bifurcation lesions. *Eur J Vasc Endovasc Surg* 1999; **17**: 476–479.

23. Bockenheimer SAM, Mathias K. Percutaneous transluminal angioplasty in arteriosclerotic internal carotid artery stenosis. *AJNR* 1983; **4**: 791–792.

24. Tsai FY, Matovich V, Hieschima G *et al.* Percutaneous transluminal angioplasty of the carotid artery. *AJNR* 1986; **7**: 349–358.

25. Kachel R, Basche S, Heerklotz I, Frossmann K, Endler S. Percutaneous transluminal angioplasty of supra-aortic arteries, especially the internal carotid artery. *Neuroradiology* 1991; **33**: 191–194.

26. Bergeron P, Chambran P, Bianca S, Benichou H, Massonat J. Traitement endovasculaire des artères à destinée cérébrales. *J Mal Vasc* 1996; **21**(Suppl A): 123–131.

27. Dietrich EB, Ndiaye M, Reid DB. Stenting in the carotid artery: initial experience in 110 patients. *J Endovasc Surg* 1996; **3**: 42–62.

28. Criado FJ. Wellons E. Clark NS. Evolving indications for and early results of carotid artery stenting. *Am J Surg* 1997; **174**: 111–114.

29. Yadav JS, Roubin GS, Iyer S *et al.* Elective stenting of the extracranial carotid arteries. *Circulation* 1997; **95**: 376–381.

30. Wholey MH, Wholey M, Jarmolowski CR *et al.* Endovascular stents for carotid occlusive disease. *J Endovasc Surg* 1997; **4**: 326–338.

31. Kachel R. Results of balloon angioplasty in the carotid arteries. *J Endovasc Surg* 1996; **3**: 22–30.

32. Parodi JC, Bates MC, Schonholz C *et al.* International multi-center Parodi anti-embolism study: preliminary results *Am J Cardiol* 2000; **86**(Supp 1, 8a): 33i.

33. Al-Mubarak N, Roubin GS, Vitek JJ, New G, Iyer SS. Procedural safety and short-term outcome of ambulatory carotid stenting. *Stroke* 2001; **32**: 2305–2309.

34. Henry M, Amor M, Klonaris C *et al.* Angioplasty and stenting of the extracranial carotid arteries. *Tex Heart Inst J* 2000; **27**: 150–158.

Carotid stenting will become the gold standard

Charing Cross Editorial Comments towards Consensus

Will it or will it not become the gold standard? By the time one sees the arguments of Fogarty, Gaines, and Rossi there can be no doubt in the eyes of the reader that this is a technique here to stay, but Greenhalgh, Bell and Bergeron throw doubt upon this concept. At the time of writing, perhaps the most telling issue is that approximately 8% only of Europe's carotid procedures are managed by angioplasty and stenting. In time, the more difficult cases will be presented for both procedures and then we shall know how well they do. It certainly will not be satisfactory to expect angioplasty and stenting to be used for the easy cases and then to say angioplasty and stenting is a superior technique. To do that would be to argue that in fact carotid endarterectomy is the safest technique and has to be used on the more difficult cases. The logic of that argument is that it should be used on the easy cases in order to provide the greatest certainty of a good result. The arguments of these chapters understandably take into account the developing nature of carotid angioplasty and stenting. Already there has been an enormous step forward for the use of cerebral protection. The trend towards success can be seen but at the time of writing it is simply too early to know how the latest angioplasty with stenting will compare with best carotid endarterectomy in the trials. For some years this argument will rage. The total numbers of carotid procedures will need to be tracked. We are extremely grateful to the European Vascular and Endovascular Monitor and the EVEM panel for data on the total numbers of procedures in Europe and this has helped put the matter into some perspective.

I will make one assumption. If a patient can get an equally good result without a scar on the neck, without an anaesthetic, and be out of hospital in record time, it necessarily follows that that procedure would be preferred. But will the procedure be as risk-free as careful carotid surgery? That is the question.

Roger M Greenhalgh
Editor

First rib excision is seldom required

For the motion
David Bergqvist

Introduction

Thoracic outlet syndrome is defined as symptoms caused by compression of nerves and/or vessels when passing through the thoracic outlet to the arm.[1] The dominating form is neurogenic (>95%), arterial and venous only 1–3 % each. The relative frequency of the two vascular types very much depends on how many patients with thoracic outlet syndrome there are in the investigated population. As neurogenic thoracic outlet syndrome may be diffuse in symptomatology the frequencies vary. This compression syndrome has had various names over the last 150 years or so: cervical rib syndrome, scalenus anticus syndrome, costoclavicular syndrome and thoracic outlet syndrome (used since 1956).[2] The names partly reflect various views on anatomical and pathophysiological factors of importance. The anatomy of the thoracic outlet shows a number of variations concerning muscles, bands and ligaments, skeletal structures and vessels. This has led to a number of operative options, when surgery has been considered the therapeutic solution to decompress the neurovascular bundle in the thoracic outlet. The most common method has been first rib resection, introduced in 1962,[3] but described by Murphy in 1910.[4] It may be performed via a supraclavicular approach or via a transaxillar approach, the latter being introduced by Roos.[5]

Arterial thoracic outlet syndrome

Compression of the subclavian artery by bony abnormalities or congenital bands or hypertrophic muscles, results in a localized stenosis of the artery. With time and repetitive trauma the arterial wall becomes thick and fibrotic, and a post-stenotic dilatation develops, which may actually develop into a fusiform aneurysmal structure. Turbulence and endothelial damage through the repetitive trauma lead to thrombus formation within the aneurysmal sack. The thrombotic process may give rise to distal microembolization, which when repeated may destroy the distal vasculature with tissue loss and aggrevation of ischaemia.[6]

In patients with microembolization or unilateral Raynaud's phenomenon arterial thoracic outlet syndrome must be suspected until otherwise proven. Some form of angiographic evaluation is necessary together with an anatomical analysis of the thoracic outlet. Arterial reconstruction is indicated to prevent further embolization together with first rib or cervical rib resection to open up the thoracic outlet. This is not the place to present further details which may be found in any textbook on vascular surgery. Thus, in patients with arterial thoracic outlet syndrome first rib resection is indicated in most of the cases, but the frequency is very low.

Venous thoracic outlet syndrome

Deep vein thrombosis in the upper extremitity comprises only a few percent of all deep vein thrombosis.[7-9] The so called Paget-von Schroetter's syndrome or 'effort thrombosis' may sometimes be caused by a narrow thoracic outlet passage. The cause relationship has, however, been difficult to establish. An anatomical defect (skeletal or muscular) is frequently found in patients with a primary deep vein thrombosis,[10,11] but we do not know how often deep vein thrombosis develops in patients with those anatomical defects.

Patients with subclavian-axillary vein thrombosis without occlusion or after successful thrombolysis should undergo provocative manoeuvres to analyse the presence of a thoracic outlet compression. This is not the place to discuss various treatment options of deep vein thrombosis, but usually the long-term results are fairly good, whatever option is chosen in the first place, also without first rib excision.[12]

If there is a thoracic outlet compression and the vein is not occluded with a good collateral situation, it is reasonable to surgically decompress the thoracic outlet. The earlier the treatment is instituted (today thrombolysis and first rib resection), the better the results.[13] Again the frequency of this operation is very low.

Neurogenic thoracic outlet syndrome

Whereas surgical decompression with first rib resection seems indicated in the majority of arterial outlet syndromes and in many of the venous there are some fundamental problems related to the neurogenic thoracic outlet syndrome and surgical treatment of it:

1 Criteria for the diagnosis of neurogenic thoracic outlet syndrome are not well defined and there are no reliable objective tests to establish the diagnosis.
2 Criteria for follow-up of neurogenic thoracic outlet syndrome are not well defined and follow-up times are often rather short.
3 Follow-up is rarely performed by an independent examiner.
4 The prevalence of neurogenic thoracic outlet syndrome is unclear.
5 Inclusion criteria into various clinical series differ, meaning variations in case-mix which will influence the outcome.
6 The natural history of untreated thoracic outlet syndrome is basically not known. The condition is rarely seen in elderly patients, indicating a rather favourable course.
7 There are no prospective randomized studies on the effect of surgical treatment.
8 First rib resection is not without complications (vascular injuries, pneumothorax, paraesthesia, paresis etc).

The symptoms are again related to compression of the neurovascular bundle by anatomical abnormalities. The diagnosis is essentially clinical and much of the diagnostic efforts are performed to exclude other conditions, which may also explain the symptoms. The rather diffuse symptoms together with difficulties in differential diagnosis, may explain the often long delay before treatment, almost 2–4 years in recent studies.[14–16]

Lepäntalo et al.[14] performed a long-term follow-up after first rib resection (average 6.1 years (range 2.5–13.5)). The examiners (one neurologist and one specialist in physical medicine and rehabilitation) were independent from the surgeons. One month postoperatively 77% were found to be improved whereas at long-term follow-up this frequency was only 37%. The authors stressed the importance of long-term follow-up and the use of independent examiners. The results were unfavourable compared with studies not having this design.

After a mean follow-up of 4.2 years Landry et al.[16] compared a surgically treated group (n=15) with 64 patients who had received non-operative treatment. Those undergoing surgery had seen more previous physicians and had been prescribed more medications; otherwise the groups were comparable. The current level of symptoms did not differ (severe or moderate symptoms present in 54 and 66% respectively and compared with baseline minimal and no improvement or worsening in 66 and 69% respectively). Total work time missed was statistically longer in the operated group (27.6 ± 6.0 months vs 14.9 ± 2.6 months; $p = 0.04$). The frequency of patients having returned to work did not differ, nor did current medication. The authors concluded that first rib resection did not improve functional outcome in patients with neurogenic thoracic outlet syndrome.

A history of trauma as a factor in the development of thoracic outlet syndrome seems to have significant negative impact to return to pre-illness activities.[17]

Franklin et al.[18] investigated outcome of surgery in injured workers 1 year postoperatively; 60% were still work-disabled, the strongest predictor being work disability preoperatively. Compared with non-operated patients, those having undergone surgery had 50% greater medical costs and were more than three times more likely to be work-disabled.

Lindgren et al.[19] found that the duration of preoperative sick leave was significantly associated with duration of postoperative sick leave after thoracic outlet syndrome operation, that is patients with longer preoperative sick leave had longer postoperative sick leave.

Although several series have claimed beneficial effects of surgery for neurogenic thoracic outlet syndrome[20] most of them have several of the methodological defects mentioned initially in this section. This together with the much less optimistic results of the studies discussed above motivate the view that first rib resection in patients with neurogenic thoracic outlet syndrome is only rarely indicated.

Conclusion

First rib resection for neurogenic thoracic outlet syndrome should not be performed outside randomized studies, which are urgently needed to solve the controversy whether conservative treatment or surgery is the best therapeutic option. Such a study should have a long-term follow-up (at least 2 years) with at least two independent outcome examiners. It must be in the interest of patients as well as their doctors to have this problem solved in a scientifically based way.

Summary

- First rib excision is required in arterial thoracic outlet syndrome.

- First rib excision may be required in venous thoracic outlet syndrome.

- Arterial and venous thoracic outlet syndromes are rare.

- Randomized trials are needed to evaluate the effect of first rib excison in neurogenic thoracic outlet syndrome.

References

1. Roos DB. Historical perspectives and anatomic considerations. *Semin Thorac Cardiovasc Surg* 1996; 8: 183–189.
2. Peet RM, Hendriksen JD, Andersen TP, Martin GM. Thoracic outlet syndrome: Evaluation of a therapeutic exercise program. *Proc Mayo Clin* 1956; 31: 281–287.
3. Clagett OT. Research and prosearch. Presidential address. *J Thorac Cardiovasc Surg* 1962; 44: 153–166.
4. Murphy T. Brachial neuritis caused by pressure of first rib. *Austral Med J* 1910; 15: 582–585.
5. Roos DB. Transaxillary approach for first rib resection to retrieve thoracic outlet syndrome. *Annl Surg* 1966; 163: 354–358.
6. Gelabert HA, Machleder HI. Diagnosis and management of arterial compression at the thoracic outlet. *Annl Vasc Surg* 1997; 11: 359–366.
7. Adams JT, McEroy RK, De Weese JA. Primary deep venous thrombosis of upper extremity. *Arch Surg* 1965; 91: 29–42.
8. Coon W, Willis PW. Thrombosis of axillary and subclavian veins. *Arch Surg* 1967; 94: 657–663.
9. Nordstrom M, Lindblad B, Bergqvist D, Kjellstrom T. A prospective study of the incidence of deep-vein thrombosis within a defined urban population. *J Int Med* 1992; 232: 155–160.
10. De Weese JA, Adams JT, Gaiser DL. Subclavian venous thrombectomy. *Circulation* 1970; 42: 158–163.
11. Thompson RW, Schneider PA, Nelken NA, Skioldebrand CG, Stoney RJ. Circumferential venolysis and paraclavicular thoracic outlet decompression for 'effort thrombosis' of the subclavian vein. *J Vasc Surg* 1992; 16: 723–732.
12. Lindblad B, Tengborn L, Bergqvist D. Deep vein thrombosis of the axillary-subclavian veins: Epidemiologic data, effects of different types of treatment and late sequelae. *Eur J Vasc Surg* 1988; 2: 161–165.
13. Urschel HC, Jr., Razzuk MA. Paget-Schroetter Syndrome: What is the best management? *Annl Thorac Surg* 2000; 69: 1663–1669.
14. Lepantalo M, Lindgren KA, Leino E *et al.* Long term outcome after resection of the first rib for thoracic outlet syndrome. *Brit J Surg* 1989; 76: 1255–1256.
15. Jamieson WG, Chinnick B. Thoracic outlet syndrome: Fact or fancy? A review of 409 consecutive patients who underwent operation. *Can J Surg* 1996; 39: 321–326.
16. Landry GJ, Moneta GL, Taylor LM Jr, Edwards JM, Porter JM. Long-term functional outcome of neurogenic thoracic outlet syndrome in surgically and conservatively treated patients. *J Vasc Surg* 2001; 33: 312–319.
17. Green RM, McNamara J, Ouriel K. Long-term follow-up after thoracic outlet decompression: An analysis of factors determining outcome. *J Vasc Surg* 1991; 14: 739–746.
18. Franklin GM, Fulton-Kehoe D, Bradley C, Smith-Weller T. Outcome of surgery for thoracic outlet syndrome in Washington state workers' compensation. *Neurology* 2000; 54: 1252–1257.
19. Lindgren SH, Ribbe EB, Norgren LE. Two year follow-up of patients operated on for thoracic outlet syndrome. Effects on sick-leave incidense. *Eur J Vasc Surg* 1989; 3: 411–415.
20. Sanders RJ. Results of the surgical treatment for thoracic outlet syndrome. *Semin Thorac Cardiovasc Surg* 1996; 8: 221–228.

First rib excision is seldom required

Against the motion

Jörg-Dieter Gruss, C Geissler, D Hanschke,
H Prescher

Introduction

This report is based on 2013 patients with a compression of the superior thorax aperture who we observed between 1973 and 2000. In all, 968 operations to decompress the neurovascular bundle were carried out in 744 patients. The figures document that a surgical decompression was only required in rather more than one-third of our patients whereas decompression could be achieved more or less correctly with physical measures in almost two-thirds.

Cervical ribs occur in about 6% of the overall population compared with 13% of our thoracic outlet syndrome patients who had cervical ribs. In the thoracic outlet syndrome patients treated surgically, this proportion rises to 18%, whereas it amounts to 90% of patients with aneurysm of the subclavian artery treated surgically.

All compression syndromes at the superior thorax aperture used to be diagnosed and treated under various names such as costoclavicular syndrome, scalene muscle syndrome, smaller pectoral muscle syndrome, hyperabduction syndrome, Paget-von-Schroetter syndrome etc. Today, these are all subsumed under the collective term thoracic outlet syndrome. Paradoxically, thoracic outlet syndrome also includes the thoracic inlet syndrome as a special form. Many further conditions might be added to the syndromes listed above such as cervical rib syndrome or scalenus minimus syndrome etc. The question as to whether these are or were indeed discrete clinical entities will remain open. All syndromes subsumed under the term thoracic outlet syndrome have in common the feature that they can be treated and cured by complete removal of the first rib. The objective of treatment is always complete decompression of the neurovascular bundle. It is self-evident that cervical ribs and congenital as well as acquired fibromuscular ligament anomalies are also eliminated during surgery. It follows from this definition that the head of the humerus syndrome cannot be classified under thoracic outlet syndrome, since in this clinical picture the axillary artery fixed to the head of the humerus with two major branches is compressed by the head of the humerus in overhead work or sport.[1]

Even today, it has not yet been possible to present definitive data on the incidence of thoracic outlet syndrome, since this disease is still largely unknown at least in German-speaking countries, so that patients with thoracic outlet syndrome symptoms are misdiagnosed and wrongly treated in many places. A survey of around 1500 patients treated a few years ago showed that an average of 6.5 physicians needed 4.3

years to make the diagnosis.[2] Many of the patients have therefore received orthopaedic, chiropractor, rheumatological or hand surgery pretreatment. Many patients have scars following surgical treatment of carpal tunnel syndrome, an ulnar groove syndrome, radial or ulnar epicondylitis etc. Our own patients may not be regarded as representative: many patients consult us from the whole of the Federal Republic of Germany, so that the figure we gave on the incidence of thoracic outlet syndrome would doubtless be too high.

Aetiology

According to our present-day knowledge, four factors appear to play a role in the aetiology of thoracic outlet syndrome: postural anomaly (phenotype), congenital osseous and fibromuscular anomalies, physiological lowering of the shoulder girdle and traumata.

On first presentation, thoracic outlet syndrome patients are between 20 and 50 years old with a peak age of 30 years. We have observed an onset of the disease before the 10th year of life in two cases, and after the 50th year of life in six cases.

The physiognomic type of female thoracic outlet syndrome patients is asthenic or leptosomic. The female phenotype is characterized by a slouching posture with drooping shoulders and the corners of the mouth pointing downwards. The pelvis is tilted to ventral, in consequence of which lumbar lordosis, thoracic kyphosis and cervical lordosis are largely abolished. The tips of the shoulder blades point outwards, so that the clavicles rotate downwards via the connection of the acromioclavicular joint. The pale careworn face with its disgruntled expression often reflects the prior unsuccessful attempts at therapy which not uncommonly have already caused these patients to consult psychiatrists, non-medical practitioners or faith healers. In contrast, one is at first disinclined to believe that the male patient, with his athletic phenotype and very well-developed musculature who is apparently bursting with health and vitality, has these symptoms. Our patients are often active competitive sportsmen (tennis, sailing, hang-gliding, surfing), bodybuilders, hand-to-hand combat trainers with the police or the federal army or engaged in heavy work, mostly in former East German industrial enterprises.

The most frequent congenital anomaly is complete or incomplete cervical ribs. Synostoses between the cervical rib and the first rib or the first rib and the second rib are very much rarer. The most frequent fibromuscular anomaly involves the smallest scalene muscle, which originates from the cervical spine and passes between the subclavian artery and the plexus and inserts at the upper border of the first rib. The remaining fibrous anomalies were classified by Roos in nine types which will not be further discussed here. Merely the T3 ligament will be mentioned as the most frequent ligament that can pass from the dorsal to the ventral rib circumference, traversing the superior thorax aperture.

Postural anomalies or phenotype as well as the congenital osseous and fibrous anomalies become pathogenetically relevant when the physiological lowering of the shoulder girdle occurs in our third decade of life. The already existing bottleneck now becomes too narrow, so that the structures passing through the ventral and dorsal scalene space are compressed to different extents and cause corresponding symptoms.

Traumata act in the same way; they are reported by about two-thirds of our patients when the history is recorded meticulously.[3-7] Not only the typical whiplash trauma of the cervical spine, but any blow, jolt, strain or contusion trauma in the region of the cervical spine, the neck and the superior thorax aperture (falling sideways from a horse or from a surfboard at a high speed, a boxing blow to the temple, burial alive, rear collision accident) is an adequate trauma. All traumata which lead to ruptures in the musculature (subclavian muscle, anterior scalene muscle, middle scalene muscle) must be considered. The fine muscle ruptures lead to local haematomas which heal with cicatricial fibrous atrophy.[2,7-12] The cicatricial shrinkage of the musculature leads to a corresponding contraction of the affected muscles and consecutive narrowing of the scalene space. In discussing a traumatic cause or for expertise purposes, separate exploratory excisions should be taken from the subclavian muscle, the anterior and middle scalene muscle during surgery, and these should be worked up histologically. In this way, we have also forensically demonstrated triggering by trauma or indicative deterioration of a pre-existing thoracic outlet syndrome. Traumata can lead to acquired fibrous trabeculae in the region of the superior thorax aperture which cannot be classified in the ten types according to Roos. The overshoot callus formation after clavicular fracture or clavicular fracture which has healed in a malposition should be mentioned as aetiological factors.

Symptomatology and clinical features

Two-thirds of our patients are female, and one-third is male. As a rule, the symptoms begin between the 20th and 30th year of life. Symptoms are diverse, since they are caused by compression of the plexus, artery and vein to varying degrees. Whereas the symptoms may be exceedingly multifarious overall, they are always relatively constant in individual patients. According to Roos,[12] Urschel,[13] and Session,[14] neurological symptoms are found in 97–98% of patients when they are examined meticulously. We distinguish between the rare high plexus compression which affects the roots C5, C6 and C7, and lower plexus compression which affects the roots C8 and Th1. The symptoms of upper plexus compression can be triggered or intensified by rotation and/or tilting the head to the opposite site. The symptoms of lower plexus compression can be triggered or intensified by abduction of the arm and by pulling the arm. These patients suffer pain in the region of the dorsal side of the shoulder and the axilla with radiation to the inside of the arm, the elbow joint and finally fingers four and five. These patients often complain of tingling paraesthesias at night and that the arm goes to sleep. The simultaneous presence of irritation of sympathetic fibres lead to increased sweat secretion and a cold feeling. In both types of compression, the symptoms occur more intensely at night and at rest. Especially severe nocturnal symptoms are complained of after strenuous bodily exertion or sport of above-average intensity on the previous day. In both types of compression, weakness and a feeling of heaviness in the affected arm, loss of dexterity and loss of the ability to coordinate finger movement occur later. Characteristically, patients report dropping objects unexpectedly or that they are unable to hold them for a long time. Increasing impairment of fine motor activity leads to difficulties in writing, in using a computer or in playing a musical instrument (violin, piano). Atrophy of the small muscles of the hand becomes visible at a relatively late stage. If compression of the subclavian artery predominates, then rapid fatigability, claudication-like pain in overhead work, pallor and coldness of the hand are most prominent. Thrombotic deposits of the locally damaged subclavian artery arise as a result of small local intimal lesions.[2,4-6,15,16] Mural thrombi can also arise in a post-stenotically dilated subclavian artery and in a post-stenotic aneurysm of the subclavian artery and become the cause of peripheral emboli. Our own investigations have shown that about 75%

of patients with a thoracic outlet syndrome show peripheral embolic occlusions of the digital arteries. Such emboli can cause punctiform necrosis in the skin and also lead to the loss of individual fingers or even the entire forearm.

In mainly venous compression, the patients complain of heaviness and a feeling of tension in the entire affected arm. They often wake up in the morning with an arm that is swollen and blue. The feeling of heaviness can be quite painful in overhead work, and the veins on the hand, forearm, upper arm, shoulder are prominent.

In the majority of cases, there are neurological, arterial and venous symptoms of varying degrees of severity side by side that can hardly be distinguished from each other.

Vascular complications

Thoracic outlet syndrome is not uncommonly diagnosed only on occurrence of an arterial or venous complication.

The episodic multiple small infarcts (microembolizations) were already referred to in the previous section. Large emboli from a post-stenotically dilated subclavian artery or a subclavian aneurysm can cause the occlusion of main arteries such as the ulnar, radial and brachial artery. These emboli are remarkable and dangerous, since as a rule they encounter an arterial vascular system which has already been subject to prior damage, i.e. it is already largely blocked peripherally. The minimal or entirely absent reflux from the periphery in embolectomy is typical. It is important to consider intraoperative lytic treatment in good time. Without intraoperative lysis, recurrence of the thrombotic occlusion almost always occurs. In addition, these microemboli are often followed by true recurrences when a thoracic outlet syndrome or a subclavian aneurysm was not considered in preoperative diagnostics, so that angiography was not performed. The constant flow of thrombotic material from the afferent vessels in the operation automatically entails suspicion of a subclavian aneurysm.[2]

Acute thrombosis of a subclavian aneurysm continues to be a serious arterial complication. This practically always leads to complete ischaemia of the affected arm. The complete occlusion of the subclavian artery results in major difficulties in diagnosis, since angiography does not point to the aetiology. Sometimes, the corresponding symptoms on the contralateral side or a positive AER (abduction, elevation, rotation) test on the opposite site may provide important indications. First of all, treatment must comprise deobliteration of the periphery. For this purpose, an access route from the angle of the elbow is to be recommended. Besides the obliteration of the inflow and outflow tract, this also allows specific catheter lysis of the radial and ulnar artery. Transaxillary exarticulation of the first rib or a cervical rib is carried out as the next step. The same access route allows elimination of the subclavian aneurysm and interposition of a venous transplant.

Acute thrombosis of the subclavian vein is very much more frequent than acute thrombosis of the subclavian artery. The affected arm is a vivid blue with increased circumference and is firmer; the veins of the skin are prominent. The patient has often engaged in prior strenuous overhead work or strenuous sport such as cross-country skiing, volley ball or surfing. After phlebographic or duplex sonographic corroboration of the diagnosis, restoration of the venous vascular bed is the first step in the treatment schedule. Formerly, this was often achieved by thrombectomy via the bicipital sulcus or by systemic fibrinolysis. Recently, locoregional lysis has become established because of the very much lower rate of complications. At all events, com-

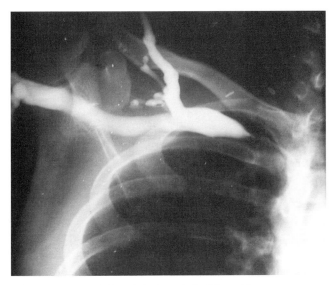

Figure 1. Filiform compression of the subclavian vein in AER position.

pression must be documented by phlebography or digital subtraction angioplasty as cause of the thrombosis after restoring the venous circulation. If the underlying compression has been demonstrated, transaxillary exarticulation of the first rib is carried out during the next 24 hours.[6,17]

An insufficiently or inadequately treated subclavian vein thrombosis leads to a post-thrombotic syndrome of the upper limb that is relevant in terms of clinical angiology in 12% of cases.

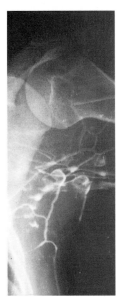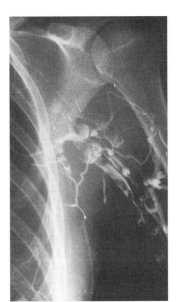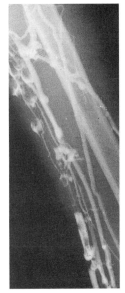

Figure 2. Acute subclavian vein thrombosis.

(a)

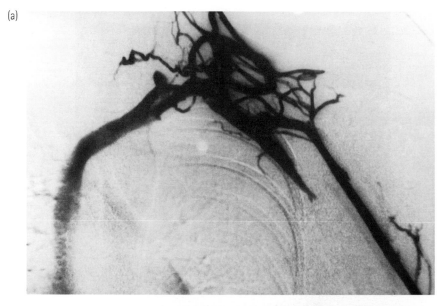

(b)

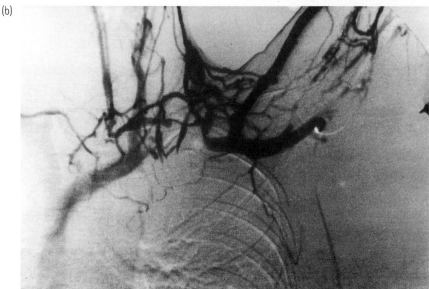

Figure 3a,b. Post-thrombotic syndrome of the upper extremity with documented compression of the original vein and the collaterals.

Neurological complications

Corresponding to the post-stenotic dilation of the subclavian artery or the subclavian aneurysm and corresponding to the post-thrombotic damage of the subclavian vein, definitive damage may also occur in the region of the plexus in consequence of pressure, contusion and kinking. The transition from an only functional compression-induced disorder to definitive structural damage can be diagnosed only with exceeding difficulty or not at all. The reduction of the proximal nerve impulse conduction velocity of the ulnar nerve and the median nerve in the segment

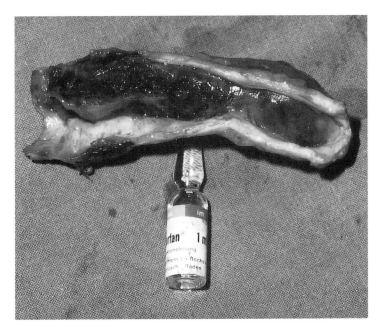

Figure 4. Thrombi in the subclavian artery.

plexus/axilla provides a pointer. Compression and strain of the lower parts of the plexus lead to microhaemorrhages from the blood vessels supplying the nerve into the tissue of the perineural sheath. The microhaematomas heal leaving connective-tissue scars with cicatricial contraction; sometimes there is ingrowth of connective tissue trabeculae and septae between the fibrils. Decompressing the neurovascular bundle too late by removal of the outwardly compressing substrates (ribs, fibromuscular trabeculae, scar plates recognizable from the outside) cannot induce reversal of this process, so that persistent neurological symptoms result.[13,18-21]

Diagnostics

Careful recording of the patient history is of crucial importance. In view of the multitudinous results of previous investigations and X-rays the patients bring with them, this is sometimes a very time-consuming task, but is often very worthwhile. The examination starts with the patient standing up, since only then does a postural anomaly become apparent. Skin colour, skin temperature and secretion of sweat are compared as well as increase in circumference and consistency, increased venous marking, trophic disorders and muscular atrophies are registered. The crude strength in shaking hands and in splaying of the fingers is recorded. In palpation, the plexus is often painful to pressure in the axilla and above the supraclavicle. The shoulder joint and cervical spine are investigated with regard to their mobility. The contracture of the upper part of the trapezoid is characteristic: palpation is reported to be painful. A cervical rib can often be palpated supraclavicularly as a retractile resistance. A simple test has proved to be effective in distinguishing thoracic outlet syndrome from disk injury or a disk prolapse: the patient is asked to rotate his/her head to the opposite side and to tilt it to dorsal. Thoracic outlet syndrome can be very probably ruled out if pressure of both hands on the head of the seated patient causes radicular pain and paraesthesias. A vertebragenic cause of the symptoms can then be assumed.

The angiological investigation comprises the pulse status, vascular auscultation and measurement of the Doppler occlusion pressures on both sides. Absence of the pulse in elevation and abduction of the arm can be evaluated as part of the diagnostic mosaic only in corresponding clinical features. Asymptomatic loss of the pulse, which according to the literature is present in 30–60% of young adults is not tantamount to diagnosis of thoracic outlet syndrome.[2,3,5,6,9,12] Attenuation or loss of the pulse can be documented using acral oscillography or Doppler sonography. The AER test is of crucial importance for clinical diagnostics. Both arms are abducted by 90 degrees and rotated outwards. In this position, the patient clenches his/her fist every 2 seconds for 3 minutes. This must be carried out slowly and powerfully. Pain and tingling paraesthesias in the fingers often occur before 3 minutes have elapsed. Fatigue and a feeling of heaviness follow. In arterial compression, there is long-lasting painful paling of the fingers in addition. A mainly venous compression leads to engorged distention of the veins of the hand and arm. The AER test is negative in carpal tunnel syndrome, in ulnar groove syndrome and in degenerative lesions of the cervical spine.

X-Rays of the cervical spine are taken routinely in four planes with a special X-ray of the superior thorax aperture. Digital subtraction angiography follows to image the subclavian artery and vein in the normal and horizontal position as well as in elevation and abduction of the arm. If the compression does not become apparent during this investigation despite corresponding clinical features with positive AER test, the digital subtraction angiography must be repeated in the sitting position. It reveals deposits in the subclavian artery, post-stenotic dilations, subclavian aneurysms and post-thrombotic wall lesions of the subclavian vein with corresponding collateralization. In patients with clinical relevant post-thrombotic syndrome, not only the

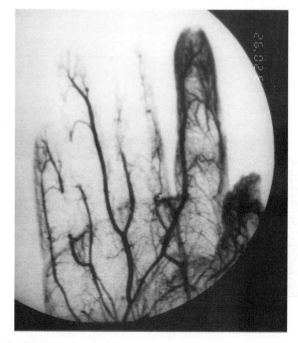

Figure 5. Embolic digital artery occlusions.

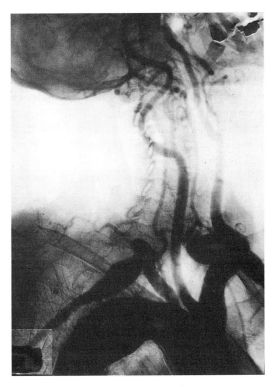

Figure 6.   Subclavian artery aneurysm.

recanalized subclavian vein, but all collateral vascular vessels are often shut off in elevation and abduction of the affected arm. Direct brachialis angiography with imaging of the digital arteries is carried out in addition if morphological changes in the region of the subclavian artery can be demonstrated on digital subtraction angiography and clinical signs of peripheral ischaemia are present.

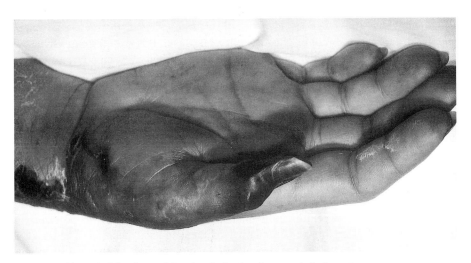

Figure 7.   Necrosis following peripheral embolization from a subclavian artery aneurysm.

All patients with clinically detectable thoracic outlet syndrome undergo neurological investigation comprising electromyographic measurement of the proximal conduction velocities in the ulnar and median nerve. At all events, reduction of the proximal ulnar and/or median nerve conduction velocities in the plexus/axilla segment proves the presence of underlying compression, whereas the absence of a reduced conduction velocity does not rule out thoracic outlet syndrome. Especially when these are combined with already demonstrable atrophy of the small muscles of the hand, highly reduced nerve impulse conduction velocities indicate structural plexus damage and must therefore be rated as prognostically unfavourable.[2,13]

Therapy

Rather more than one-third of patients with diagnosed thoracic outlet syndrome have to undergo surgical treatment. In mild-to-moderately severe cases, it is justified to attempt conservative physical therapy first. Conservative therapy will not be dealt with in this chapter. Nevertheless, as many as two-thirds of the patient group described above can be rendered largely free of symptoms by conservative measures. Surgery is indicated when morphological lesions of the subclavian artery are present or when clinically manifest peripheral embolization has already occurred. A reduced proximal ulnar and/or median nerve conduction velocity is an absolute indication for surgery. However, we also operate on patients with neurological compression syndromes and normal conduction velocities when they have very severe pain at night and heavy analgesic intake. Moreover, surgery is indicated in filiform compression of the subclavian vein and in clinically relevant post-thrombotic syndrome with demonstrated compression of the collateral vessels in elevation and abduction.

Surgical treatment is also indicated when conservative therapy has been unsuccessful or has led to deterioration. This is the case especially often after chiropractic measures such as reductions or treatment with the Glisson sling.

The objective of surgical treatment is complete decompression of the neurovascular bundle. A further goal must be to avoid recurrences and thus second operations. At the same time, the surgical access route should enable treatment of the vascular complications, i.e. elimination of subclavian aneurysm and venous thrombectomy as well as simultaneous performance of thoracic sympathectomy. The transaxillary access route has proved to be ideal for this purpose.[10,15,23] Only the parascapular approach[7] provides a similarly good overview: however, this requires extensive severance of the dorsal shoulder girdle musculature, is often very bloody and can be accompanied by appreciable postoperative pain. Neither the supraclavicular nor the infraclavicular anterior access route fulfil the above conditions.

The patients are positioned on their side for the operation. The affected arm is sterile-packed and held by an assistant standing on a raised platform at the head end of the patient. This enables the arm to be moved to ventral and dorsal and slight traction to be applied if this should be required in order to get a better overview. Continuous traction on the arm and suspending the arm under traction on a frame should both be avoided. During the operation, the arm is kept predominantly in an approximately 110 degrees abduction position. It is completely relaxed for several minutes between the individual stages of the operation (this procedure is repeated again and again) and put down in the adducted position. The surgeon stands at the patient's back. The arcuate cutaneous incision at the margin of the lower axillary hair passes from the posterior margin of the greater pectoral muscle to the anterior margin of the latissimus dorsi muscle. The smiling incision of the skin and subcutaneous tissue is continued vertically up to the thorax wall. Afterwards, the axillary glandular body is pushed back *en bloc* to cranial. Damage to the intercostal brachial nerve is avoided if possible. The scalene spaces are clearly exposed. The following structures are severed one after the other from upper border of the first rib: 1. the tendon of the subclavian muscle, 2. the anterior scalene muscle, 3. the middle scalene muscle. Details of the surgical procedure are given in Breitner's surgical manual.[23] The intercostal musculature is severed from the lower border of the first rib so that the rib is clearly exposed between the manubrium of the sternum and the spine. The pleural cupula is cautiously pushed back with the fingers or with a dissection swab from the back of the first rib and Sibson's fascia. An Overhold clamp or a renal pedicle clamp are passed under the rib. By rotating the clamp, Sibson's fascia is perforated and is then further incised to ventral and dorsal with a curved scissors.

Ligament anomalies can now be discerned and accordingly resected with the curved scissors. The first rib is now completely exposed, so that it can be severed and removed ventrally and dorsally with the corresponding rib scissors according to Roos. The difficult part of the surgical operation is the next step, which consists in complete exarticulation of the dorsal rib stump. The dorsal stump is initially dissected up to both its articulations with the vertebral body using a nerve spatula to protect the plexus. A right angled Luer or a special pistol-shaped rongeur have proved effective for exarticulation. In the exarticulation of the dorsal stump, no traction may be applied to the arm, so that the plexus is completely relaxed. In some cases, it is easier to exarticulate the medial rib process between the individual fascicles of the plexus than to proceed strictly from dorsal. The ventral rib stump is shortened with a Luer up to the cartilage of the manubrium of the sternum. Care must be taken to excise scar callus tissue which envelopes the subclavian vein. In the presence of a cervical rib, this is dissected like the first rib up to the spine. The connection of the cervical rib with the first rib should be maintained under all circumstances. After severing the first rib ventrally and dorsally, the cervical rib can be manipulated better by pulling on the first rib. The cervical rib is first of all severed as far dorsally as possible and removed *en bloc* with the first rib. Afterwards, both rib stumps are exarticulated as described above. It is just as important to leave a wide area of surgery which is absolutely free of blood as it is to correctly exarticulate of the dorsal rib stumps. In about one-third of the cases, the pleura is opened accidentally. A Bülau drainage is set up in these cases for 24 hours. A redon drainage for 24 or 48 hours is sufficient in the remaining cases.

After the operation, care must be taken preferentially to use the unaffected arm for 8 weeks. Massages, exercise and physiotherapy are to be avoided under all circumstances. The first follow-up examination is 6 weeks after discharge from the hospital and the patients may resume their work or sporting activity only when they are completely free of symptoms. If symptoms persist, avoiding use of the affected arm and inability to work must be prolonged. In very severe cases, this can last for up to 6 months. In patients with a reduced proximal nerve impulse conduction velocity, it has proved to be worthwhile to repeat the measurement at intervals of 4 weeks after the operation. As a rule, an improvement of the clinical status and a decline of the symptoms accompanies amelioration of the nerve impulse conduction velocities. Patients in whom an acute subclavian vein thrombosis was the indication for surgery receive anticoagulant treatment with a dicumarol preparation for 6 months after the operation and are provided with a compression sleeve of compression class III at the same time.

Persistent and recurrent compression syndromes

The specific and often difficult problems of these special cases of disease will only be dealt with here in passing.[12,19,20,23,26] Persistent compression syndromes are characterized in that the first operation was not suitable for complete decompression of the neurovascular bundle. These include operations such as partial resection of a cervical rib, resection of a cervical rib, partial resection of a first rib and combination of partial resection of both a cervical rib and a first rib, partial resection of the clavicle, hollowing out the first rib, fenestration of the lateral thorax wall, severance of the smaller pectoral tendon or severance of the anterior scalene muscle etc. The most important causes for a persistent compression syndrome are long dorsal rib stumps, a long ventral rib stump and a re-attachment of the anterior scalene muscle to the first rib and on the pleural cupula with subsequent atrophy.[12,19] True recurrences are relatively rare compared with persistent compression syndromes, but are observed time and again and also in our own patients after correct adequate prior operation. The causes of a true recurrence are a matter of speculation. There are the following possibilities: an area of surgery which was not sufficiently dried of blood at the first operation, development of a postoperative haematoma in the region of surgery, physiotherapy started too early or insufficient postoperative avoidance of using the affected arm as was recommended. The surgical procedure in persistent compression syndromes depends on the first operation. If the first operation is carried out from a dorsal subclavicular or infraclavicular approach, the second operation is carried out from a transaxillary access route. At all events, the objective of the operation is complete decompression of the neurovascular bundle with exarticulation of the dorsal rib stumps and if appropriate also of the ventral rib stumps (rare), elimination of the entire scar tissue which has arisen postoperatively including elimination of residual fibromuscular ligaments.

In recurrent compression syndrome, we always choose a supraclavicular access route, since the recurrence always involves the plexus, more rarely the artery and very rarely the vein. Use of a nerve stimulator to identify the phrenic nerve and to identify the individual parts of the plexus is indispensable. Employing a magnifying glass is recommended. The anaesthetist must not administer muscle relaxants in use of the nerve stimulator. The operation consists of dissecting the plexus out of a whitish hard callus more or less sharply and freeing it of the whole of the compressing scar tissue. The anterior scalene muscle is carefully dissected away from the pleural cupula and resected as high as high possible. A pleural opening with subsequent insertion of a Bülau drainage sometimes cannot be avoided. Decompression of the subclavian vein is the most difficult in technical terms, especially because lesions of the vein lead to profuse haemorrhages which can only be stopped with great difficulty. It is practically impossible to stop the haemorrhage by applying vascular clamps. Use of the cell saver is imperative and may save the patient's life.

Additive methods of treatment with the attempt to prevent a second or third recurrence in the form of cortisone irrigation of the plexus or in the form of sheathing the individual fascicles with polytetrafluoroethylene films have produced disappointing results up to now. Operation of a persistent or recurrent thoracic outlet syndrome is an undertaking of 3–5 hours duration.

Results of treatment

Finally, the results of surgical treatment will be reviewed briefly. After the first operation, 85% become completely free of symptoms, 12% are unequivocally improved and 3% have remained the same or become worse. Compared with this, the results of treatment in the persistent and recurrent compression syndromes are very much poorer and disappointing. Only 48% became completely free of symptoms whereas 31% were at least substantially improved, but 21% remained unchanged or became worse in this group. Against this background, it is interesting to observe that in the period during which we have been involved with thoracic outlet syndrome, the number of second and multiple operations has significantly increased. We only had 0.8% second operations between 1973 and 1985, whereas this figure has risen to 18% between 1986 and 2000. The reported results of treatment are a strong argument in favour of adequate first operation.[2,16]

Table 1. Outcome of 972 thoracic outlet syndrome-operations (1975–2000).

Symptom-free	Improved	Unchanged or deteriorated
79%	16%	5%

Conclusion

Today, the term thoracic outlet syndrome subsumes all compression syndromes at the superior thorax aperture. This report is based on 2013 thoracic outlet syndrome patients of whom 744 received surgical treatment. The number of operations to decompress the neurovascular plexus is 968. Two-thirds of the thoracic outlet syndrome patients show adequate trauma in their history. With appropriate symptoms and a positive AER test, further instrumental diagnostics must be undertaken. This comprises X-rays of the cervical spine in four planes, a special X-ray of the superior thorax aperture, digital subtraction angiography to image the subclavian artery and vein in the normal position and in elevation and abduction in the seated patient. In signs of ischaemia of the hand, direct brachialis angiography must be performed in addition. A neurological investigation with measurement of the proximal ulnar and median nerve impulse conduction velocities is indispensable. Grave vascular complications are embolizing subclavian arterial aneurysm and acute thrombosis of the subclavian vein. The first-line therapy is transaxillary exarticulation of the first rib and if appropriate of a cervical rib. After 882 transaxillary rib exarticulations (first operations), 85% of cases were entirely free of symptoms, 12% showed substantial improvement and 3% have remained the same or become worse. In persistent recurrent compression syndromes, the results are very much poorer: only 48% became completely free of symptoms, 31% substantially improved but 21% remained unchanged or have deteriorated.

Summary

Our indications for first rib exarticulation:

- High degree (filiform) stenosis of the subclavian vein in AER-position.

- The subclavian vein thrombosis with reopening and documented underlying compression.

- Thrombi or irregularities in the subclavian artery.

- Subclavian artery aneurysm.

- Reduced ulnar nerve conduction time.

- Reduced median nerve conduction time.

- Severe pain in the neck, the shoulder and the arm causing abuse of analgesics (inspite of normal nerve conduction velocities).

- The disabling PTS of the upper extremity with proven compression of the recanalized vein and the collaterals.

- The first rib and/or the cervical rib should be eliminated completely.

- Aneurysms repair and/or thoracic sympathectomy can be done simultaneously.

References

1. Durham JR, Yao JST, Pearce H, Nuber GM, McCarthy WJ. Arterial injuries in the thoracic outlet syndrome. *J Vasc Surg* 1995; 21: 57–61.
2. Gruss JD, Geissler C. Über das Thoracic-outlet-Syndrom. *Gefäßchirurgie*. 1997; 2: 57–64.
3. Dongen van RJAM. Klinische Diagnostik und operative Erfahrung mit dem transaxillären Zugang beim TOS. In *Läsionen des Plexus Brachialis*. Hase U, Reulen HJ (eds). Berlin, New York: Gruyter, 1984: 177–193.
4. Dunant JH. Trauma als ätiologischer Faktor beim Schultergürtelsyndrom. *VASA* 1980; 9: 74–75.
5. Gruss JD, Hiemer W, Bartels D. Klinik, Diagnostik und Therapie des Thoracic outlet Syndroms. *VASA* 1987; 16: 337–344.
6. Gruss JD. Thrombectomie veineuse axillo-sous-claviere. In *Les Syndromes de la Traversé Thoraco-Brachiale*. Kieffer E (ed.) Paris: AERCV, 1989: 195–198.
7. Martinez NS. Traumatic thoracic outlet syndrome. *Contemp Surg* 1982; 21: 1–3.
8. Machleder HJ. Complications and recurrences. In *Vascular Disorders of the Upper Extremity*. Machleder HJ (ed). New York: Futura Publishing Company, 1989: 205–224.
9. Roos DB. Rédidives postopératoires des syndromes de la traversée thoraco-brachiale. In *Les Syndromes de la Traversée Thoraco-Brachiale*. Kieffer E (ed). Paris: AERCV, 1989: 317–328.
10. Roos DB. New concepts in the etiology, diagnosis and surgical treatment of thoracic outlet syndrome. In *Pain in Shoulder and Arm*. Greep JM, Lemmens HAJ, Roos DB, Urschel HC (eds). Dordrecht: Nijhoff, 1979: 201–217.
11. Roos DB. Thoracic outlet syndromes: Update 1987. *Am J Surg* 1987; 154: 568–573.
12. Roos DB. Overview of thoracic outlet syndromes. In *Vascular Disorders of the Upper Extremity* 2nd edn. Machleder H (ed). New York: Futura Publishing Company, 1989: 155–177.
13. Urschel HC, Razzuk MA, Albers JE. Reoperation for recurrent thoracic outlet syndrome. *Ann Thorac Surg* 1976; 21: 19–25.
14. Session RT. Recurrent thoracic outlet syndrome: causes and treatment. *South Med* 1982; 75: 1453–1462.

15. Dongen van RJAM. Behandlung des neurovaskulären Kompressionssyndroms des Schultergürtels – Transaxilläre Resektion der ersten Rippe und einer Helsrippe. In *Neurovaskuläre Kompressionssyndrome*. Hepp W (eds). Oxford, London: Blackwell, 1996: 37–45.

16. Gruss JD, Vargas-Montano H, Bartels D, Simmenroth H, Haider A. Results achieved in the surgical treatment of the thoracic outlet syndrome. *Int Angiol* 1984; 2: 179–184.

17. Gruss JD, Bartels D, Karadedos C *et al*. Unser Behandlungskonzept bei akuten Verschluß der Vena subclavia. *Phlebol Proktol* 1981; 10: 25–29.

18. Barwegen MGMH, van Dongen RJAM. Neurovaskuläre Kompressionssyndrome an der oberen Thoraxapertur und ihre vaskulären Komplikationen. In *Gefäb-chirurgie*. Herberer G, van Dongen RJAM (eds). Berlin, Heidelberg, New York: Springer, 1996: 571–584.

19. Machleder HI, Moll F, Nuwer M, Jordan SJ. Somatosensory evoked potentials in the assessment of thoracic outlet compression syndrome. *J Vasc Surg* 1987; 6: 177–184.

20. Mellière D, Kassab M, Salion E, Becquemin JP, Etienne G. Complications graves de la chirurgie des syndromes de la traversée thoraco-brachiale. In *Les Syndromes de la Traversée Thoraco-Brachiale*. E. Kieffer (ed). Paris: AERCV, 1989: 309–316.

21. Roos DB. Thoracic outlet syndromes. In *Vascular Disorders of the Upper Extremity*. Machleder HJ (ed). New York: Futura Publishing Company, 1983: 91–106.

22. Urschel HC, Razzuk MA. The failed operation for thoracic outlet syndrome: the difficulty of diagnosis and management. *Ann Thorac Surg* 1986; 42: 523–528.

23. Gruss JD. Zweiteingriffe bei Kompressionssyndromen an der oberen Thoraxapertur. In *Neurovaskuläre Kompressionssyndrome*. Hepp W (ed). Oxford, London: Blackwell, 1996: 55–64.

24. Gruss JD, Geissler C, Hiemer W. Zweiteingriffe bei Thoracic outlet Syndrom. *Angio* 1990; 12: 49–55.

25. Lindgren SHS, Ribbe EB, Norgren LEH. Two years follow up of patients operated on for thoracic outlet syndrome. Effects on sick-leave incidence. *J Vasc Surg* 1989; 3: 411–415.

26. Sanders RJ, Monsour JW, Gerber WF *et al*. Scalenotomy versus first-rib resection for treatment of the thoracic outlet syndrome. *Surgery* 1979; 85: 109–121.

First rib excision is seldom required

Charing Cross Editorial Comments towards Consensus

Here an erudite Scandinavian is pitted against a first rib excision enthusiast with teutonic zeal.

There can be little doubt that first rib excision produces patient satisfaction in those patients carefully selected for the procedure. It is also noteworthy that the operation is performed in large quantities in certain parts of the world, and very infrequently in other areas. The overall indications for first rib excision are probably quite small. David Bergqvist indicates that it should be performed under certain circumstances but overall his argument is that this amounts to a small number of the whole population. I believe that the message from Jörg-Dieter Gruss is not dissimilar. Where an arterial venous or venous obstruction can be demonstrated first rib excision has value. Also where there is a pressure upon a nerve root again, symptomatic relief follows a careful removal of the pressure on the nerve. There remains a variety of enthusiasm for first rib excision and these authors rehearse the arguments well.

Roger M Greenhalgh
Editor

Subclavian artery stenosis is best managed by PTA and stent

For the motion
Jim A Reekers

Introduction

Percutaneous treatment of stenotic or occlusive disease of the subclavian and innominate arteries has been reported in the literature starting in the early 1980s.[1] No series were reported but only case reports about treatment of the subclavian steal syndrome. In these early days treatment of the innominate artery was done even less frequently. In the first reports about larger series of patients the indications for treatment also included arm ischaemia next to vertebrobasilar insufficiency. In the most recent reports coronary steal and anticipated coronary artery bypass grafting using the internal mammary artery are also indications for treatment. Because aorteritis (Takayasu's arteritis) which also leads to supra-aortic lesions, is very rare, and the treatment more complex, these lesions are not included in this presentation. It has to be taken into consideration that the early and late reports probably cannot be compared, as stenting was not done in these early series. Both from the perspective of the aetiology of the majority of these lesions and the possible cerebral complications, encountered in these early series, stenting is done in our practice in most cases.

As the aetiology is atherosclerosis, lesions at the origin of the subclavian or innominate artery should be considered to be lesions of the wall of the aortic arch, similar to ostial lesions of the renal arteries, and primary stenting is therefore mandatory to obtain a durable result. Lesions not at the origin are true atherosclerotic lesions of the vessel itself, and stenting is not mandatory. In those cases were there is still normal antegrade vertebral flow and no retrograde flow (steal), cerebral embolic complications have been reported both in the early and late reports. Cerebral protection is therefore recommended by some authors.[2]

Detection of a stenosis is always after a clinical suspicion of either arm ischaemia or vertebrobasilar insufficiency. A duplex ultrasound can in most cases be helpful to establish the diagnosis of the lesion. Other modalities like magnetic resonance angiography (MRA) can be used, however, angiography is still the gold standard to make the final diagnosis and treatment plan.

Technique

There are several techniques, which can be used to treat these lesions, and preference is dictated by local anatomy and lesion morphology.

Lesions, which carry a risk for cerebral embolization, like those in the innominate artery, should probably best be treated with primary stenting, in line with the current policy on angioplasty of carotid lesions. As these lesions are often heavily calcified and/or rigid, predilatation is recommended to assure safe stent placement. For lesions at the origin of the artery precise stent placement is a must, and therefore balloon expandable stents are used. A control angiography to guide precise placement is always necessary and therefore a second diagnostic catheter has to be installed. Although an approach coming from the brachial artery is most often more easy, one has to take into account the size of the brachial artery, which is sometimes hypoplastic. To recanalize occlusions the brachial approach is in our opinion always by far the most successful. To treat stenotic subclavian lesions, which still have an antegrade vertebral flow, primary stenting is in our view the safest procedure. For lesions with a retrograde vertebral flow – steal – simple percutaneous transluminal angioplasty (PTA) can be performed. So the decision about how to treat a subclavian or innominate artery lesions is guided by the localization of the lesion, flow, the morphology and the symptomatology.

Figures 1 and 2 show the technique of primary stenting of a lesion at the origin of the innominate artery. (A second agiographic catheter should be in position for control angiography during stent placement.)

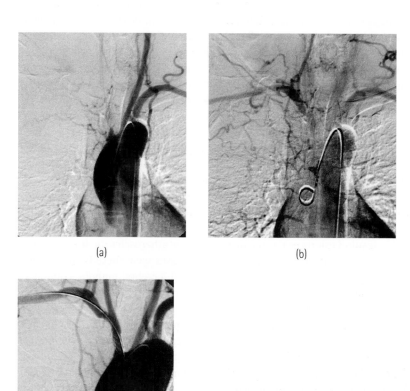

(a)

(b)

(c)

Figure 1. A 46-year-old patient with a combination of vertebrobasilar insufficiency and right arm ischaemia. (a) Early arterial phase shows occlusion of the innominate artery. (b) Late arterial phase shows retrograde filling of the right vertebral and subclavian artery. (c) After 8mm balloon-expandible stent (Corinthian, Cordis, J&J) through the right brachial artery. At follow-up there was total relief of symptoms previously complained of.

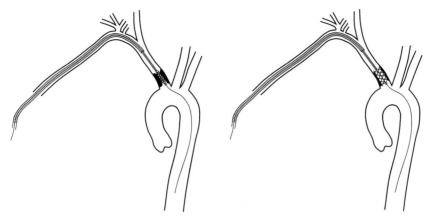

Figure 2. The sheath is withdrawn and then the stent deployed. Reproduced with permission from Ref. 10.

Evidence

There are no systemic reviews and there are no Cochrane data available. Disregarding the early and late case-reports, the few published available series were analysed. A division was made between series with and without stents, for this could be of influence on the results. Finally only five studies were suited for multistudy analysis.[3–7] These data are presented in Table 1.

There is one study with 46 innominate occlusions and stenting on indication.[8] The results from this study are too different from the other studies and will therefore not be analysed further here.

There is one study, which compared the long-term results with and without stenting.[9]

Of the total of 156 patients, in this multistudy analysis, only 5% were treated for an innominate lesion. There were 9% occlusions and 91% stenosis. The strongest indication for treatment was arm ischaemia. For stenosis there was an initial success rate of 91%, but for occlusions it was only 41%. During follow-up the reported relief of symptoms was 77%. Serious complications can be expected in 4.5% (neurological) and minor complications in 7%.

We compared these results with another study published (113 patients) where both stand-alone angioplasty and stenting was used; there were strong similarities.[8] The second study also showed an initial result for subclavian stenosis of 91% and a low success for occlusions (53%). Major complications were 2.6%, primary patency rates without stent 69% and with stent 87% (not significant).

In conclusion, the evidence for percutaneous treatment of subclavian and innominate artery lesions is not overwhelming; however, from the available data it seems justified to advise angioplasty as a first choice option for symptomatic subclavian artery stenotic lesions. The success rate is high (>90%) and the follow-up results are acceptable, being >70%. For occlusions, the expected success rate is much lower and the general patient condition should play a major role in final discussions between surgery and angioplasty. There is no evidence that stenting will improve the long-term outcome in these lesions. In agreement with the data on renal artery ostial

Table 1

Year	No. of patients	Subclavian lesions	Innominate lesions	Occlusion	Stenosis	Ischaemia	Steal	Combination	Success stenosis	Occlusion	Relief	Mean follow-up	Serious complications	Minor complications
1990(3)	27	33	2	3	34	15	8	5	27(28)		25(27)	24 M	2	1
1991(4)	7	9	2	3	4		3		4(6)	0(3)	4(6)	10 M	1	2
1992(5)	52	52	0	9	43	52	39	39	40(43)	5(9)	28(39)	29 M	?	?
1994(7)	33	36			36			31(33)	?		?		0	5
1999(8)	37	38	4		33	26	14		32(37)		20(28)	100M	4	3

lesions, a stent might be useful in lesions at the level of the aortic arch. For all other lesions stents should only be used if there is a suboptimal initial result after angioplasty.

There is a great need for a well controlled randomized trial. Because angioplasty of subclavian and innominate arteries is not performed very frequently the first step should be an international registry.

Summary

- Multistudy analysis shows that subclavian artery angioplasties are not performed very frequently.

- For subclavian artery stenosis, angioplasty is the first treatment choice.

- For occlusions a high percentage of initial failure has to be expected.

- There is no evidence for stents in subclavian or innominate artery lesions.

- Stents can be used after suboptimal initial angioplasty result.

References

1. Bachman DM, Kim RM. Transluminal dilatation for subclavian steal syndrome. *AJR* 1980; **135**: 995–996.
2. Staikov IN, Do DD, Remonda L *et al*. The site of atheromatosis in the subclavian and vertebral arteries and its implication for angioplasty. *Neuroradiolology* 1999; **41**: 537–542.
3. Insall RL, Lambert D, Chamberlain J *et al*. Percutaneous transluminal angioplasty of the innominate, subclavian and axillary arteries. *Eur J Vasc Surg* 1990; **4**: 591–595.
4. Sharma S, Kaul U, Rajani M. Indentifying high-risk patients for percutaneous transluminal angioplasty of subclavian and innominate arteries. *Acta Radiol* 1991; **32**: 381–385.
5. Hebrang A, Maskovic J, Tomac B. Percutaneous transluminal angioplasty of the subclavian arteries: long-term results in 52 patients. *AJR* 1992; **156**: 1091–1094.
6. Bogey WM, Demasi RJ, Tripp MD *et al*. Percutaneous transluminal angioplasty for subclavian artery stenosis. *Am Surg* 1994; **60**: 103–106.
7. Korner M, Baumgartner I, Do DD, Mahler F, Schroth G. PTA of the subclavian and innominate arteries:long-term results. *Vasa* 1999; **28**: 117–122.
8. Mathias KD, Luth I, Haarmann P. Percutaneous transluminal angioplasty of proximal subclavian artery occlusions. *Cardiovasc Intervent Radiol* 1993; **16**: 214–218.
9. Henry M, Amor M, Henry I *et al*. Percutaneous transluminal angioplasty of the subclavian arteries. J Endovasc Surg 1999; **6**: 33–41.
10. Cleveland TJ. Subclavian and auxillary artery angioplasty and stenting. In *Vascular and Endovascular Surgical Techniques* 4th edn. Greenhalgh RM (eds). London: WB Saunders, 2001: 295–304.

Subclavian artery stenosis is best managed by PTA and stent

Against the motion

Georg Kretschmer, T Sautner, C Domenig,
T Hölzenbein, R Ahmadi, M Schillinger,
P Peloschek, J Lammer, E Minar, P Polterauer

Introduction

Since the first report[1] various papers have appeared in the literature dealing with the successful treatment of occlusive changes at the carotid bifurcation, but only a few discuss the management of occlusive lesions in other sites within the brachiocephalic arterial vasculature. Various reasons are given for this. Lesions in the brachiocephalic region are less common, as only 14% of cerebrovascular angiograms show significant changes of the proximal subclavian and vertebral arteries.[2] The natural course of isolated proximal lesions involving the arch vessels is usually benign, lesions are frequently asymptomatic, and an ischaemic stroke is hardly ever observed.[3,4] The early transthoracic approaches to repair these proximal blocks were associated with substantial operative burden and mortality. Therefore it was impossible to offer a convincing argument for prophylactic surgical intervention and aggressive operative management was consequently discouraged.

Crawford et al. (1962) described local thrombendarterectomy,[5] Parrot (1964) introduced carotid-subclavian transposition[6] and Diethrich et al. (1967) advocated carotid-subclavian bypass.[7] Thereby a variety of extrathoracic techniques became available, all avoiding the thoracic cavity, propagating the extra-anatomic approach to the proximal subclavian vessels.[8-12] According to pooled data[13] and own experience[14] these procedures yield similar results, but carotid-subclavian transposition seems to offer superior patency rates than extra-anatomic bypass.[11,13,14]

These procedures gained wide acceptance over the following nearly two decades until 1980, when Mathias et al.[15,16] and others, mostly based in Europe,[17-20] as well as Bachman and Kim,[21] introduced transluminal angioplasty as an endovascular method to treat lesions of the brachiocephalic trunk and the proximal subclavian vessels, an alternative, which has gained widespread acceptance since. Both kinds of treatment, endoluminal interventions and open surgery are employed concurrently.

Because active operative or endoluminal intervention is rarely considered to be indicated, a prospective trial comparing these two options is lacking.

The purpose of this contribution is to evaluate the treatment results of proximal subclavian lesions with subclavian-carotid transposition – obviously the surgical method of choice – compared with transluminal angioplasty with and without stent placement (PTA) as achieved in our institution.

Since this is an analysis of the clinical series but not a prospective trial we have endeavoured to demonstrate an equal balance of risk factors[22] and an equal probability of postoperative survival to emphasize particularly the statistical comparability of both groups of patients.

Technique

Open surgery: subclavian–carotid transposition

The operation is carried out through a supraclavicular approach, which allows sufficient exposure of the subclavian as well as the common carotid arteries. The incision is 5–10 cm in length traversing 2.0 cm above the clavicle, starting medially between the two heads of the sternocleidomastoid muscle and extends into the supraclavicular fossa. The platysma and the clavicular portion of the muscle are dissected. The scalenic fat pad is mobilized and retracted cephalad. The phrenic nerve is carefully identified upon the anterior scalenic muscle and moved out of the way. The subclavian artery is identified and mobilized; some of its branches are encircled; some are divided to ease exposure. Usually it is unnecessary to divide the internal mammary artery, the preservation of which might be of importance in patients with potential coronary artery diease. The vertebral artery is the first proximal branch of the subclavian artery and without any branches, which is important for identification. A part of the subclavian artery proximal to the origin of the vertebral artery has to be dissected free. Care has to be taken not to injure the recurrent laryngeal nerve. The patient is anticoagulated by administering heparin sodium usually 100U per kg bodyweight. After clamping and transection the proximal part of the subclavian artery (the stump) has to be secured appropriately.

The common carotid artery is exposed, thereby retracting the internal jugular vein, being aware of the vagus nerve. An inlaying shunt is hardly ever necessary.

The anstomosis is constructed with 6 x 0 running monofilament suture in side-to-end technique. Loop magnification may be helpful. After completion of the anastomosis the anticoagulation should not be reversed. Suction drainage is used and the wound closed in layers. The mean anaesthesia time is 180 minutes (from induction to end of anaethesia), carotid cross-clamping time 15–25 minutes. In general we follow the recommendations as published by Edwards and Mulherin.[23] Figure 1 demonstrates the postoperative control using the DSA-technique. Usually patients receive an antithrombotic treatment indefinitively or until contraindications develop.

Percutaneous transluminal angioplasty (PTA) with or without stent placement

The procedure may be performed through a femoral and brachial access route. In case of femoral access a 6 French introducer sheath is inserted, for stents a 7 F sheath is necessary. A pigtail angiography is performed to document the lesion and the direction of flow in the vertebral artery. In the case of a right subclavian artery stenosis being present an RAO 30 degrees projection is used, for a left subclavian artery stenosis an LAO 30 degrees projection is preferred. Prior to the recanalization 5000 IU of heparin are administered through the sheath. The obliteration is passed with a

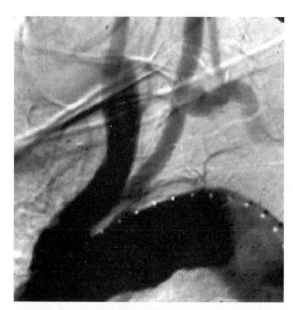

Figure 1.   Control-angiography in DSA-technique following subclavian-carotid transposition. A calibrated catheter is lying in the aortic arch; the proximal stump of the subclavian artery opposite to the catheter is oversewn. Note the common trunk of brachiocephalic and left common carotid artery. The anastomosis is widely patent; the vertebral artery is in cerebropetal perfusion. A .brachiocephalic trunk' on the left side has been constructed.

sidewinder Simmons 2 or a headhunter catheter and a straight or 45 degrees angeled guidewire and is dilated with a 7-9 mm balloon for 30–60 seconds. The result is sufficient if the residual narrowing is less than 30%, the trans-stenotic mean pressure gradient is less than 10 mmHg and an antegrade flow into the vertebral artery is seen. In case of a significant residual stenosis, stent placement is indicated. Both balloon-expandable and self-expandable stents can be used. It is important not to cover the ostium of the vertebral artery. For accurate stent placement between the aortic arch (right common carotid artery on the right side) and the vertebral artery roadmapping should be used. For recanalization of total subclavian artery occlusions a brachial access is recommended. This enables a better manoeuvreability of guidewires and catheters. After PTA, medical treatment with low-dose acetyl salicylic acid (100 mg/day) is recommended. After stent placement a combination of low molecular weight heparin for 2 days and clopidogrel for 6 weeks (Plavix 75 mg/day) is prescribed.

Evidence

The presented evidence is based upon a comparative re-evaluation of our own clinical series and published data[14,22,28] as well as various publications dealing with the topic summarized in the **Discussion** (p. 112) and listed in the **References** (p. 115).

Patients and methods

From 1 January 1975 to 31 December 1998 all consecutive patients were included in the series who were treated at the Divisions of Angiology, Interventional Radiology and Angiography as well as Vascular Surgery in a European 2200-bed tertiary-care university hospital for atherosclerotic arterial disease of the proximal subclavian artery; i.e. from orifice of the aortic arch or brachiocephalic trunk to the origin of ipsilateral vertebral artery.

The results of subclavian artery PTA with and without stenting as achieved in the Department of Angiology have been published previously in part[22] as well as the results of subclavian–carotid transposition and carotid–subclavian bypass in the Department of Vascular Surgery.[14]

All patients with angiographically proven subclavian artery stenosis or occlusion were eligible for evaluation. Patency following either method of treatment was defined as the presence of an anastomosis perfused in an orthograd direction – or the absence of a haemodynamically relevant subclavian artery stenosis at the time of follow-up (as indicated by a < 50% diameter reduction in the treated arterial segment).

Standard laboratory methods were employed to check for the typical risk factors in obliterative arterial disease (e.g. hypertension: > 160/90 mmHg, diabetes mellitus, dyslipidaemia).

Eligible patients were identified from the respective department's databases, surgical reports, operational notes and notes and reports at discharge. Patients charts were reviewed systematically, data were collected, clinical signs and symtoms including cardiovascular risk factors were registered. Patient complaints on exercise of the upper limb were noted, like arm claudication, arm paraesthesia and weakness of the extremity and were distinguished from symptoms of cerebral hypoperfusion like syncope, vertigo and transient visual impairment due to subclavian steal phenomenon. Oscillography, bilateral blood pressure measurements, ultrasonography as well as results of surgery and interventional procedures were documented.

Reversal of blood flow in the vertebral artery as proven by duplex scanning and/or angiography was considered as presence of subclavian steal phenomenon. Results of interventions and operations as well as periprocedural complications were collected.

Follow-up

Immediately following any procedure the reduction in pressure gradient between both upper extremities was determined. The morphological result was usually assessed by duplex scanning, angiography or magnetic resonance angiography prior to discharge in order to judge the procedure from a technical point of view. Scheduled on an outpatient basis follow-up included clinical examination, pulse palpation and blood pressure measurement in both upper extremities at 3-monthly intervals during the first postoperative year, twice a year thereafter or whenever it was felt to be indicated, but at least once a year. Restenosis was suspected whenever a blood pressure difference of 20 mmHg or more was noted and the patients were scheduled for respective control examinations.

Statistical methods

For univariate analysis of continuous variables the Mann-Whitney U test was used. The probability of function as well as survival was estimated employing the Kaplan–Meier method;[24] possible differences were checked using the non-parametric tests according to Mantel[25] and Breslow.[26]

For the graphic representation of the Kaplan–Meier plots the recommendations of the Ad Hoc Committee regarding reporting standards were used.[27] An univariate Cox proportional hazard model was applied to assess the effect of treatment at the time of follow-up. The results of the model are expressed as the Hazard ratio (HR) and the 95% confidence interval (95% CI).

An additional Cox proportional regression model was employed to detect possible factors influencing survival. The distribution of risk factors in the comparative groups was assessed using a Chi-square test. All tests were employed bitailed; p-values < 0.05 were considered statistically significant. The intention to treat principle was used. Calculations were performed with Statview version 5.0 for Macintosh.

The most recent information regarding the survival was conveyed through the Austrian Central Bureau of Statistics (Österreichisches Statistisches Zentralamt) Vienna, Austria and transferred to the main frame computer at the Medical Faculty in Vienna at least once a year by electromagnetic tape. In order to obtain this information data collection was terminated 1998. See in addition the Appendix (p. 114) for current legislation in Austria, regarding reporting of residency and cause of death, as well as obtaining permission for postmortem examination.

Results

For comparable evaluation 211 patients were available; 84 patients underwent subclavian-carotid transposition, 127 patients received primary PTA; of these 36 additional stent placements were necessary. The median age of the patients was 60 years; 108 patients were female. The distribution of various risk factors within both groups is summarized in Table 1, solely hypertension showing an uneven pattern of distribution. In the Cox-model diabetes mellitus (p = 0.007) and coronary artery disease (p = 0.041) adversely influenced survival, but these factors were found evenly distributed.

The probability of survival between the two comparative groups is shown in Fig. 2.

It was impossible to show a statistical significant difference between groups (p = 0.379 Mantel; p = 0.409 Breslow). So the assumption was made that comparable groups of patients were evaluated.

Surgery

A total of 84 patients received a primary subclavian-carotid transposition. The procedure was successful in all patients. One patient died within 30 days of surgery (1.2%). Severe complications were observed in three patients (3.6%), minor complications occured in 19 patients (22.6%).

Transient peripheral neurological deficits accounted for the maiority of complications. These lesions resolved during admission due to conservative management (Table 2).

Table 1.   Distribution of various risk factors in the surgical vs endovascular group

Variables	PTA with (without stent)	Surgery	p value
	n = 127	n = 84	
Median age (IQR)	59.7 (16.2)	59.7 (16.3)	0.9
Male gender (%)	54 (43%)	44 (52%)	0.1
Left-sided lesion (%)	98 (77%)	69 (82%)	0.4
Smoking habits (yes)	76 (60%)	57 (60%)	0.3
Diabetes mellitus (yes)	33 (26%)	15 (18%)	0.2
Arterial hypertension (yes)	66 (52%)	16 (19%)	0.001
Peripheral occlusive arterial disease (yes)	60 (47%)	38 (45%)	0.8
Coronary arterial disease (yes)	44 (35%)	30 (36%)	0.9
Subclavian steal phenomenon (yes)	95 (75%)	60 (71%)	0.8
Peripheral symptoms	74 (58%)	37 (44%)	0.1

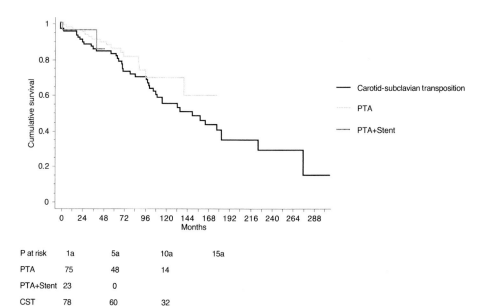

Figure 2. Probability of patient survival, Kaplan–Meier estimates; comparison between groups (the symbols refer to subclavian-carotid transposition, PTA with and PTA without stent placement). The numbers indicate patients at risk entering a certain time interval. P: patients.

Table 2. Summary of complications

	Number of events	
	Minor	Severe
SCT	plexus[a]; n = 2 phrenic[a]; n = 6 recurrens[a]; n = 5 Horner[a]; n = 1 lymphatic[b]; n = 2 chylus[b]; n = 2 haematoma; n =1	Carotid thrombosis; n = 2[c] brachial embolism; n = 1
%	22	4
PTA	PSA; n = 1 stent loss; n = 2	TIA; n = 1 brachial thrombosis; n = 2 haematoma; n = 1
PTA (Stent)	PSA; n = 1 stent loss; n = 1	brachial embolism; n = 1 stent loss; n = 1
%	5	5
Complications Total (%)	27	9

Minor complication: conservative treatment.
TIA: transient ischaemic attack.
Severe complication: operative management necessary.
PSA: pseudoaneurysm.
[a] Transient peripheral neurological deficit.
[b] Fistula.
[c] One died in hospital.

The median follow-up was 73 months; eight patients were lost to follow-up (9.5%). The primary success following subclavian-carotid transposition was 100%; 42 patients died during follow-up from their underlying arterial disease.

All the anastomoses remained patent with one exception, reocclusion occurring after 144 months of follow-up.

Endovascular treatment

The intention was to treat 127 patients with PTA, but the procedure was only feasible in 116 (92.8%) with or without stent placement. In 36 patients stenting was considered necessary (28% of PTA patients). The mortality within 30 days was 0.

Minor complications (4.5%) occured in six patients (pseudoaneurysms, haematoma, hypotensive episodes during the procedure). Major complications occurred in six patients (4.5%), as transient ischaemic attacks, emboli into the superior mesenteric artery and left renal artery dislodged during catheter placement; stent loss and displacement into the iliac artery followed by successful surgical retrieval from the right groin; pseudoaneurysm at the puncture site needing surgical correction (see Table 2).

The median follow-up was 46 months for PTA alone and 23 months for stent plus PTA, overall 37 months. Six patients (5%) were lost to follow-up. Restenosis occured in 22 patients (19%). Cumulative patency at 1, 3, 5 and 7 years was 85%, 80%, 70% and 62% and 93%, 80%, 0%, 0% for PTA plus stent respectively. During follow-up 20 patients died due to unrelated causes.

Comparison of treatment

Open surgery showed a significantly better primary technical success rate than either technique of endoluminal repair (p = 0.001). Overall complications occurred significantly more often in the surgical group (26%), vs 10% in the PTA – and in the PTA with stent group, the difference being significant to the p = 0.001 level. Severe complications following both options of treatment were similar (p = 0.68).

Surgery demonstrated a statistically significant better primary patency than any form of PTA, as shown in Fig. 3 (p = 0.0001 Mantel; p = 0.0001 Breslow).

Following subclavian-carotid transposition the relative risk of restenosis or reocclusion at the time of follow-up was 0.026 (98% CI 0.004–0.189).

Discussion

The proximal part of the subclavian artery between its orifice in the aortic arch or the brachiocephalic trunk and the origin of the vertebral artery is located in a transition area responsible for the perfusion of the central nervous system and the upper extremity. Obliterative lesions sited here may cause impaired blood supply in both vascular districts. The reason for flow disturbances in the upper extremity, such as arm claudication or tissue loss due to embolic showers originating from proximal stenosis are well understood.[28,29] The pathophysiology of flow reversal in the vertebral artery either remaining completely asymptomatic for many years staying a silent phenomenon or causing cerebral and/or arm symptoms – thereby mutating into the well known syndrome – is less obvious.

Arterial reconstructions for upper extremity ischaemia constitute 1–4% of all arterial interventions. Obliterative lesions of the proximal part of the subclavian artery

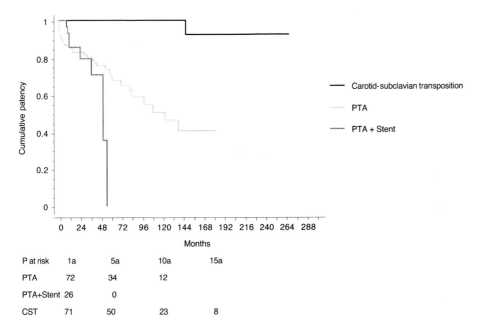

Figure 3. Probability of primary function, Kaplan–Meier estimates; comparison between groups (the symbols refer to subclavian-carotid transposition, PTA with and PTA without stent placement). The numbers indicate reconstructions at risk entering a certain time interval. Note that following subclavian-carotid transposition one reocclusion occurred after 144 months of observation. P: patients.

are the most commonly seen blocks involving the supraaortic branches. Due to this low number no randomized trials are available comparing various therapeutic options, either surgical or interventional or conservative. Therefore comparative analyses directed to formulate therapeutic recommendations might be acceptable, but should be interpreted with caution. It may be possible to give a Grade C recommendation only.[30]

If the ipsilateral common carotid artery is undiseased, the currently accepted surgical method is the extrathoracic extra-anatomic carotid subclavian bypass[31,32] using short either autologous or alloplastic grafts. Nevertheless at this site in contrast with other locations vein grafts yield more inferior results than alloplastic conduits.[33] Carotid-subclavian bypass grafts demonstrate good results with acceptable mortality and morbidity, but as always following implantation of vascular substitutes a certain annual attrition rate has to be accepted.

Following Parrot's initial report of subclavian-carotid transposition, interest was encouraged by the series of Sandmann and others.[34–36] The procedure avoids the implantation of any vascular substitutes, creates a 'left' brachiocephalic trunk and seems to be a near ideal operation. Several retrospective analyses demonstrated low mortality and superior patency.[31,34,35] Both procedures have in common the necessity of carotid cross-clamping for a short period of time with the rare danger of producing a central neurological deficit.[32]

At present, PTA of the great vessels, subclavian arteries in particular, is performed with increasing frequency. Articles report less invasiveness, high but not 100% early success rate, moderate long-term patency with or without stenting and superior comfort for the patient by avoiding an open operation.

As demonstrated in Fig. 2 the probability of long-term survival following both methods of treatment is without statistically significant difference. Since the distribution of risk factors between groups is similar, it seems reasonable to assume that equal groups of patients were compared.

Neither the operative burden during open surgery nor the fact that PTA is less invasive have influenced postoperative survival significantly.

Previously we have demonstrated[14] that patients following operative extrathoracic treatment of subclavian lesions (n = 51) have a significantly longer life-expectancy than patients operated upon for internal carotid stenosis in the clinical state I or II (n = 273) (p = 0.002 Breslow; p = 0.0002 Mantel).

Various authors including ourselves have reported gratifying results demonstrating long-term patency for 10 and even more years[12-14,34,35] following subclavian-carotid transposition. Therefore this has to be considered the most durable treatment procedure for subclavian artery repair,[11-14,31,32,34,36,37] in cases where active intervention is indicated.

Summary

- Subclavian–carotid transposition is a near ideal operation for focal proximal subclavian lesions.

- One single anastomosis between two neighbouring arteries is required.

- The primary success rate is 100%.

- The probability of function approaches 100% over 10 years of follow-up.

- The probability of function following transposition is significantly better than following PTA. The probability of survival following both methods of treatment is similar; the life expectancy of patients with subclavian lesions is significantly longer than those who have had internal carotid artery surgery.

- Therefore the most durable method of therapy should be employed, if active intervention is indicated.

Appendix

In Austria under the Act on Reporting Residency, residents are obliged to report their place of residence (and all changes thereof) to the local authorities or the police. In addition, if a person dies in hospital, then the director of the clinic or the physician, who performed the coroner's inquest, has to report to the local authorities the cause of death to enable the local authorities to pass on that information to the Austrian Central Statistical Office. This leads to an estimated postmortem examination frequency of 70-75%, thereby rendering accurate information about patient survival and causes of death possible.

Acknowledgement

We wish to thank the Austrian Central Bureau of Statistics, Vienna, Austria, for making available to us the survival data of the patients.

References

1. Eastcott HHG, Pickering GW, Robb C. Reconstruction of internal carotid artery in a patient with intermittent attacks of hemiplegia. *Lancet* 1954; ii: 994–996.
2. Edwards WH, Mulherin JL. The surgical approach to significant stenosis of vertebral and subclavian arteries. *Surgery* 1980; **87**: 20–27.
3. Hennerici M, Klemm C, Rautenberg W. The subclavian steal phenomenon: a common vascular disorder with rare neurologic deficits. *Neurology* 1988; **38**: 669–673.
4. Hennerici M, Rautenberg W, Mohr S. Stroke risk from symptomless extracranial arterial disease. *Lancet* 1982; ii: 1180–1183.
5. Crawford ES, De Bakey ME, Jordan GL jr *et al.* Segmental thombo-obliterative disease of the great vessels arising from the aortic arch. *J Thorac Cardiovasc Surg* 1962; **43**: 38–43.
6. Parrot JD. The subclavian steal syndrome. *Arch Surg* 1964; **88**: 661–665.
7. Diethrich EB, Garett HE, Ameriso J *et al.* Occlusive disease of the common carotid and subclavian arteries treated by carotid subclavian bypass. Analysis of 125 cases. *Am J Surg* 1967; **114**: 800–808.
8. Hafner CD. Subclavian steal syndrome. *Arch Surg* 1976; **111**: 1074–1080.
9. Crawford ES, De Bakey ME, Morris GC, Powell GC. Surgical treatment of the innominate, common carotid, and subclavian arteries: a 10 year experience. *Surgery* 1969; **65**: 17–31.
10. Crawford ES, Stowe CL, Powers RW jr. Occlusion of the innominate, common carotid and subclavian arteries: long term results of surgical treatment. *Surgery* 1983; **94**: 781–791.
11. Mannick JA. Extrathoracic operations for lesions of the vessels arising from the aortic arch. In *Indications in Vascular Surgery*. Greenhalgh RM (ed). London: WB Saunders 1988: 63–69.
12. Mehigan JT, Buch WS, Pipkin RD, Fogarty TJ. Subclavian–carotid transposition for subclavian steal syndrome. *Am J Surg* 1978; **136**: 15–20.
13. Criado FJ. Extrathoracic management of aortic arch syndrome. Proffered review. *Br J Surg* 1982; **69** (Suppl): 45–51.
14. Kretschmer G, Teleky B, Marosi L *et al.* Obliterations of the proximal subclavian artery: to bypass or to anastomose? *J Cardiovasc Surg* 1991; **32**: 334–339.
15. Mathias K, Steiger J, Thron A *et al.* Perkutane Katheterangioplastie der Arteria subclavia. *Dtsch Med Wochenschr* 1980; **105**: 16–18.
16. Mathias KD, Luth I, Haarman P. Percutaneous transluminal angioplasty of the proximal subclavian artery occlusions. *Cardiovasc Intervent Rad* 1993; **16**: 214–218.
17. Kachel R, Basche ST, Heerklotz I *et al.* Percutaneous transluminal angioplasty (PTA) of supraaortic arteries, especially the internal carotid arteries. *AJNR* 1991; **33**: 191–196.
18. Jaschke W, Menges HW, Ockert D *et al.* PTA of the subclavian and innominate artery: short and long term results. *Ann Radiol* 1989; **32**: 29–34.
19. Henry M, Amor M, Henry I *et al.* Percutaneous transluminal angioplasty for subclavian arteries. *J Endovasc Surg* 1996; **6**: 33–41.
20. Korner M, Baumgartner I, Do DD, Mahler F, Schroth G. PTA of the subclavian and innominate arteries: long term results. *J Vasc Dis* 1999; **28**: 117–122.
21. Bachman DM, Kim RM. Transluminal dilatation for subclavian steal syndrome. *AJR* 1980; **135**: 995–996.
22. Schillinger M, Haumer M, Schillinger S, Ahmadi R, Minar E. Risk stratification for subclavian artery PTA: increased rate of restenosis after stent implantation? *J Endovasc Ther* 2001; **8**: 550–557.
23. Edwards WH, Mulherin JL. Direct vertebral revascularisation for proximal subclavian artery atherosclerosis causing cerebral steal syndrome. In *Current Therapy in Vascular Surgery*. Ernst CB, Stanley JC (eds). Oxford: Blackwell Scientific, 1987: 60–62.
24. Kaplan EL, Meier P. Nonparametric estimation for incomplete observations. *J Am Statist Assoc* 1958; **53**: 457–481.
25. Mantel N. Evaluation of survival data and two new order statistics arising in its consideration. *Cancer Chemother Reports* 1965; **50**: 163–165.
26. Breslow N. A generalised Kruskal–Wallis test for comparing K – samples for incomplete patterns of censorship. *Biometrika* 1970; **57**: 579–582.
27. Ad Hoc Committee on Reporting Standards; Society for Vascular Surgery/North American Chapter International Society for Cardiovascular Surgery. Suggested Standards for Reports dealing with lower Extremity Ischemia. *J Vasc Surg* 1988; **4**: 80–94.
28. Kretschmer G, Polterauer P, Waneck R, Wagner O, Marosi L. Ischämiesyndrom der oberen Extremität aus nicht kardialer Ursache. *Chirurg* 1982; **53**: 441–445.
29. Diethrich EB, Koopot R, Kinard SA, Futural JE. Treatment of microemboli of the upper extremity. *Surg Gyn Obstet* 1979; **184**: 584–587.

30. Clagett PG for the Ad Hoc Committtee on Clinical Research in Vascular Surgery. *J Vasc Surg* 1992; 15: 867–873.
31. Deriu GP, Milite D, Verlato F *et al.* Surgical treatment of atherosclerotic lesions of subclavian artery: carotid-subclavian bypass versus subclavian-carotid transposition. *J Cardiovasc Surg* 1998; 39: 729–734.
32. Cherry KJ Jr. Arteriosclerotic occlusive disease of brachiocephalic arteries. In *Vascular Surgery* 4th edn. RB Rutherford (ed). London: WB Saunders, 1995: 935–952.
33. Ziomek S, Quinones-Baldrich WJ, Busuttil RW *et al.* The superiority of synthetic arterial grafts over autologous veins in carotid-subclavian bypass. *J Vasc Surg* 1986; 3: 140–145.
34. Sandmann W, Kniemeyer HW, Jaeschock R, Hennerici M, Aulich A. The role of subclavian carotid transposition in surgery for supra-aortic occlusive disease. *J Vasc Surg* 1987; 5: 53–58.
35. Weimann S, Willeit H, Flora G. Direct subclavian-carotid anstomosis for the subclavian steal syndrome. *Eur J Vasc Surg* 1987; 1: 305–310.
36. Schardey HM, Meyer G, Rau HG *et al.* Subclavian carotid transposition: an analysis of a clinical series and a review of the literature. *Eur J Vasc Endovasc Surg* 1996; 12: 431–436.
37. Edwards WH, Tapper SS, Edwards SF *et al.* Subclavian revascularisation. A quarter century experience. *Ann Surg* 1994; 219: 673–677.

Subclavian artery stenosis is best managed by PTA and stent

Charing Cross Editorial Comments towards Consensus

There are pitfalls to avoid in the management of subclavian stenosis. First, if the stenosis occurs behind the clavicle it is thought not to be caused predominantly by atherosclerosis. Subclavian disease at the origin of the subclavian artery is classical evidence of an inflammatory type of arterial disease. The left subclavian off the arch is affected more than the right. The stenoses which occur behind the clavicle can sometimes be a part of an arteritis and the possibility of repeated trauma of the artery against the clavicle is thought to be an aetiological factor.

Experience indicates that angioplasty is frequently followed by a restenosis and stents have been used in this situation. Unfortunately stents have cracked and the restenosis process has also been demonstrated to grow through stents when placed in this situation. In general surgeons prefer an endovascular approach for these stenoses but use of a stent behind the clavicle has its problems. There are those who would go straight for direct excision or bypass as outlined in the preceding chapter.

Roger M Greenhalgh
Editor

Thoracic aneurysms and type B dissections should be treated by stent-graft

For the motion

Hüseyin Ince, Tim C Rehders, Christoph A Nienaber

Introduction

Aneurysms and dissections of the aorta represent a potential life-threatening situation. Surgical resection and interposition of vascular prostheses (Gortex or Dacron) have long been considered the only treatment option. Although great strides have been achieved during the past decades in the management of patients with thoracic aortic aneurysms and dissections by improving surgical techniques, postoperative morbidity and mortality still remain high. The afflicted population is usually of older age and present a variety of co-morbidities with significant impact on post-surgical outcome. Postoperative complications, such as paraplegia and renal insufficiency, contribute to prolonged hospital stay and higher medical costs.

Conversely, interventional stent-graft placement may be a promising non-surgical strategy for the treatment of thoracic aortic aneurysms and dissections. Endovascular stent-graft prostheses are based on the concept of a metal grid covered with vessel graft material. The initiation of the natural healing process by exclusion of an aneurysm or sealing of the proximal entry (in aortic dissection) induces both remodelling of the aortic wall and consolidation of the false lumen. Although the initial results of stent-graft treatment of thoracic aortic aneurysms and dissections are promising, the concept of non-surgical reconstruction must be subjected to a randomized long-term study.

Implantation technique

Stent-graft placement was performed in the cardiac catheterization laboratory with patients under general anaesthesia and receiving ventilation. Patients were prepared to undergo surgery in case the procedure failed. The procedure was begun by injecting 5000 units of heparin and introducing a 6-French pigtail catheter (Cordis, Hamburg, Germany) into the left subclavian artery for precise guidance near the subclavian artery and for intraprocedural aortography. In all patients, the femoral or distal iliac artery was surgically exposed, and a 0.89-mm (0.035-inch) guidewire was inserted. When the position of the wire in the true lumen of the aorta had been confirmed by fluoroscopy and ultrasonography, the sheath with the stent, a pusher, and a deflated large-bore latex balloon (the Talent prosthesis) was introduced. The compressed stent was advanced to the site of the interluminal communication, under guidance by simultaneous transoesophageal colour Doppler imaging.

Before the stent-graft was unloaded, systolic blood pressure was titrated to 50 mmHg with sodium nitroprusside; as soon as the position was found, the stent-graft was launched and struts expanded by balloon molding (by inflation of the balloon at 2–3 atm); when the stent-struts were fully extended and there was no flow into the false lumen, the infusion of sodium nitroprusside was discontinued. Care was taken to completely seal the entry with Dacron and to protect the left subclavian artery with the bare-spring end of the stent-graft. Both the sheath and the guidewire were then removed, and the incision was closed. No additional heparin or antiplatelet medication was administered after completion of the procedure.

Evidence

Thoracic aneurysms

In three of the largest studies totalling 264 patients with thoracic aneurysms who had not undergone surgery at the time of diagnosis, rupture of the aneurysm was the most common cause of death with rates ranging from 42 to 70%.[1-4] In all three series, the rate of rupture of dissecting aneurysms exceeded the rate for non-dissecting aneurysms with a 5-year survival rate from 13 to 39%.[5-7,8-16]

In patients undergoing surgery for descending thoracic aneurysm, the operative mortality for all cases (emergency or elective) averaged 11%.[5-7,8-16] Independent risk factors for early mortality and morbidity included emergency operation, congestive heart failure, advanced age (older than 70 years) and atherosclerotic aetiology. The acturial survival estimates were 70–79% at 5 years, 40–49% at 10 years and 25% at 20 years depending on whether or not the aneurysm resection was performed electively. Causes of late death included cardiovascular and cerebrovascular events in 41–59% of cases and rupture of another aortic aneurysm in an additional 20–25% of cases.

A number of important technical advances have reduced the surgical risk. These include the development of Dacron grafts impregnated with collagen or gelatin, which makes them impervious to blood; improved cardiopulmonary bypass circuits that reduce injury to blood elements; and better intraoperative protection of the myocardium.

However, even with improved surgical techniques, major operative complications include paraplegia (estimated incidence of 4%) and renal insufficiency (estimated incidence of 5%) due to hypoperfusion of both the anterior spinal cord tracts and renal arteries (kidneys) as well as acute left ventricular decompensation due to proximal hypertension.[5-7,8-16]

An alternative method to the treatment of descending thoracic aortic aneurysm is endovascular stent-grafting.[17-19] Fann *et al.* reported over 81 patients with descending thoracic aortic aneurysms treated with endovascular stent-grafting.[19] Approximately half of these patients were considered by cardiovascular surgeons suitable candidates for conventional repair.[18] There were seven procedure-related deaths (early mortality rate of 9%). The rates of paraplegia and stroke were 4 and 5%, respectively. No patient required conversion to open surgical approach. In 4%, thrombosis of the aneurysm was incomplete after stent-graft deployment. The acturial survival estimates were 87% at 1 year, 81% at 2 years and 81% at nearly 4 years.

In a recent study Ehrlich *et al.* compared endovascular stent-grafting with open surgical repair in a small group of 10 patients and reported a 30-day mortality in the conventional group with 31% vs 10% in the stent group.[20] The duration of the intervention was 320 minutes in the conventional group and 150 minutes in the stent group. Spinal cord injury occurred in 12% in the surgical group, whereas none of the stented patients developed any neurological sequelae. Mean hospital stay was 23 days with 13 days of intensive care, compared with 10 days with stents. Lachat *et al.* demonstrated similar results in nine patients treated with endovascular stent-grafting.[1] There was no operative or early mortality, and all aneurysms were successfully excluded with the endovascular technique.

Recent results in several series ranging from 40 to 260 patients per study with thoracic aneurysms presented in March 2001 were as follows. Operative mortalities were between 0 and 4%, technically successful device deployments occurred in 98–100% of cases, and immediate aneurysm thrombosis was achieved in 90–100%.[15–19] Paraplegia was a complication in 0–1.6%, and stroke occurred in a range of 0–2.8%. Conversion to open surgical repair occurred in 0–4% of cases, and late endoleaks were noted in 2–3%.[8–12]

Type B dissections

In a recent publication both safety and efficacy of elective transluminal endovascular stent-graft insertion in 12 consecutive patients with descending (type B) aortic dissection were compared with results of surgery in 12 matched controls.[21] In all 24 patients, aortic dissection was diagnosed by magnetic resonance angiography. In each group, the dissection involved the aortic arch in three patients and the descending thoracic aorta in all 12 patients. With the patient under general anaesthesia, either surgical resection was undertaken or a custom-designed endovascular stent-graft was placed by unilateral arteriotomy. Our findings suggest that non-surgical reconstruction may constitute a viable therapeutic option for patients with descending dissection of the thoracic aorta and one or more indications for surgical repair, such as an aortic diameter greater than 5.5 cm, a patent false lumen with potential for expansion, or recurrent pain.[22–25,29] In contrast to thoracic surgery for type B dissection, transfemoral stent-grafting was not associated with early or longer-term mortality or with serious morbidity. Our preliminary analysis even suggests that substantial cost savings could result from the reduced need for intensive care and the shorter hospital stay.

Whereas emergency surgical repair is lifesaving in ascending (type A) aortic dissection,[28–30] both emergency surgery and deferred surgery for descending (type B) dissection are associated with 6–67% mortality rate and offer no substantial advantage over medical therapy.[26,28,31,32] Also, paraplegia (or paresis) occurs in 7–36% of patients who undergo surgery, depending on the extent of aortic resection and the duration of cross-clamping.[14,26,28,33] Even with intraoperative atriodistal bypass, reattachment of all the critical intercostal arteries, and induction of mild hypothermia, early surgical mortality is 7.1% in patients with chronic type B dissection and 8.7% in those with acute type B dissection.[34–37] Similarly, surgery-related paraplegia or paresis occurs in 2.9% of patients with chronic type B dissection and in 19% of those with acute cases; again advanced age, excessive cross-clamping time, and inappropriate reattachment of the great anterior radiculomedullary artery are predictors of adverse outcome.[37–42]

Although spinal cord dysfunction was expected to develop in approximately 8% of our patients with stent-grafts,[40] no neurological complications were encountered, in contrast to the outcome in patients treated surgically. Preservation of the integrity of the aorta, rather than resection of the dissected segment, may be important to protect the spinal arteries. The use of short stent-grafts, from 80 to 150 mm in length, and deployment far from vertebrae T8 to L2, further minimize the risk of paraplegia, compared with the risk of surgical grafts, which were 220±74 mm in length (p<0.001). Most important, the stent-graft procedure took only 1.6±0.4 hours, compared with 8.0±2.0 hours for surgery (p<0.001); it circumvented the need for circulatory arrest and cross-clamping of the aorta, and the associated ischaemia and potential reperfusion injury.[14,32,37,41,43]

In the light of our initial promising results, we have expanded the use of non-surgical stent-graft placement for a series of 120 patients with type B dissection with suitable anatomical characteristics (an accessible proximal entry, at least one femoral artery without dissection, and no substantial tortuosity). Moreover, four patients with aortic intramural haematoma (IMH) and para-aortic leakage of blood, and 15 patients with a penetrating aortic ulcer have received an endovascular stent-graft (Table 1).

Table 1. Our results of stent-graft placement in type B dissection, IMH and penetrating atherosclerotic aortic ulcer

Entity	Success	30-day mortality	1-year mortality
Type B dissection (n = 120)	98%	2 (1.7%)	2 (1.7%)
IMH (n = 4)	100%	0	0
Penetrating aortic ulcer (n = 15)	100%	0	0

Tables 2 and 3 summarize the results of medical, surgical and endoluminal treatment of type B dissections as reported from recent literature.[21,44–47] In the light of disappointing prognostic figures with surgery, the endoluminal procedures seem promising even in a meta-analytic approach.

Table 2. Type B dissection: survival of non-operated vs operated patients[45]

Survival	Non-operated	Operated
1 year	73–92%	47%
3 years	63%	40%
5 years	58–89%	28%
10 years	25–76%	

Table 3. Type B dissection: surgical results vs endovascular results[21,44,46,47]

Events	Emergency surgery	Elective surgery	Endovascular stent-grafts
Mortality %	10–45	14–6	16
Paraplegia %	20	10	0
Respiratory insufficiency %	6–31	15–40	5
Stroke %	7	2	–

Conclusions

Although conceptually promising, the management of thoracic aneurysms and type B dissections by stent-graft placement requires the support of long-term follow-up data. On the other hand, over several years of follow-up after stent-graft placement for the treatment of abdominal aneurysms, late adverse effects were infrequent justifying the use of stent-grafts in patients too sick or multimorbid for classic surgery.[17,18]

Moreover, the custom design of each stent-graft currently limits the concept to patients undergoing elective procedures or requires a large stock and selection of stent-grafts to treat acutely ill patients. Finally, sophisticated imaging techniques, such as magnetic resonance angiography, intraprocedural transoesophageal echocardiography, and digital angiography, appear to be necessary to ensure optimal results. Stent-graft placement may be a promising non-surgical strategy for the treatment of thoracic aneurysms and type B dissections (Fig 1a, 1b).

The initiation of the natural healing process (false lumen thrombosis) by sealing of the proximal entry induces both consolidation of the false lumen and remodelling of the aortic wall. In a variety of cases of type B dissection and even in presence of distal malperfusion syndrome, interventional stent-graft placement may be offered to selected patients in lieu of surgical repair. With further refinement of the technique, more patients with severe coexisting conditions and high surgical risk may be considered for the procedure. Although the initial results of stent-graft treatment are promising, the concept of non-surgical reconstruction should be subjected to randomized long-term evaluation.

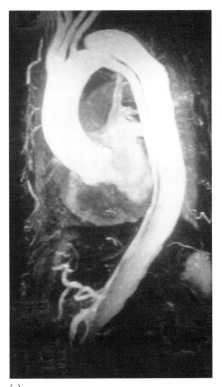 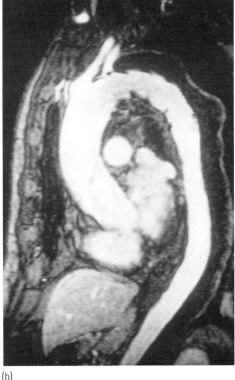

(a)   (b)

Figure 1.   Magnetic resonance angiography of type B dissection showing the communication between true and false lumen (a). Magnetic resonance angiography of type B dissection after stent-graft placement with complete reconstruction and remodelling of the aorta (b).

Summary

- Endovascular stent-grafts have potential to initiate a healing process of type B thoracic aortic dissection by sealing proximal entry sites to the false lumen.

- In selected cases of thoracic aneurysms and dissections, and even in presence of distal malperfusion, stent-grafts may be offered instead of surgical repair or medical treatment alone.

- The concept of non-surgical reconstruction of the aorta should be subjected to randomized evaluation.

References

1. Lachat M, Pfammatter T, Turina M. Transfemoral endografting of thoracic aortic aneurysm under local anesthesia: a simple, safe and fast track procedure. *Vasa* 1999; **28**: 204–206.
2. Pressler V, McNamara JJ. Thoracic aortic aneurysm: natural history and treatment. *J Thorac Cardiovasc Surg* 1980; **79**: 489–498.
3. Bickerstaff LK, Pairolero PC, Hollier LH *et al.* Thoracic aortic aneurysms: a population-based study. *Surgery* 1982 **92**: 1103–1108.
4. Perko MJ, Norgaard M, Herzog TM, Olsen PS, Schroeder TV, Pettersson G. Unoperated aortic aneurysms: a survey of 170 patients. *Ann Thorac Surg* 1995; **59**: 1204–1209.
5. Moreno-Cabral CE, Miller DC, Mitchell RS *et al.* Degenerative and atherosclerotic aneurysms of the thoracic aorta. *J Thorac Cardiovasc Surg* 1984; **88**: 1020–1032.
6. Pressler V, McNamara JJ. Aneurysm of the thoracic aorta. *J Thorac Cardiovasc Surg* 1985; **89**: 50–54.
7. DeBakey ME, McCollum CH, Graham JM. Surgical Treatment of aneurysms of the descending thoracic aorta. *J Cardiovasc Surg* 1978; **19**: 571–576.
8. Dake MD. The advent of thoracic aortic endografting. The First International Summit on Thoracic Aorta Endografting. Tokyo, Japan, 2001.
9. Ehrlich MP. Thoracic aorta endografting: the Austrian experience. The First International Summit on Thoracic Aorta Endografting. Tokyo, Japan, 2001.
10. Fattori R. Endovascular treatment of the thoracic aorta. The First International Summit on Thoracic Aorta Endografting. Tokyo, Japan, 2001.
11. Ischimaru S. Thoracic aorta grafting: the reliable treatment option. The First International Summit on Thoracic Aorta Endografting. Tokyo, Japan, 2001.
12. Livesay JJ, Cooley DA, Ventemiligia RA *et al.* Surgical experience in descending thoracic aneurysmectomy with and without adjuncts to avoid ischaemia. *Ann Thoracic Surg* 1985; **39**: 37–46.
13. Hamerlijnk RP, Rutsaert RR, DeGeest R, de la Riviere AB, Defauw JJ, Vermeulen FE. Surgical correction of descending thoracic aortic aneurysms under simple aortic cross-clamping. *J Vasc Surg* 1989; **9**: 568–573.
14. Borst HG, Jurmann M, Buhner B, Laas J. Risk of replacement of descending aorta with a standardized left bypass technique. *J Thorac Cardiovasc Surg* 1994; **107**: 126–133.
15. von Segesser LK, Killer I, Jenni R, Lutz U, Turina MI. Improved distal circulatory support for repair of descending thoracic aortic aneurysms. *Ann Thorac Surg* 1993; **56**: 1373–1380.
16. Najafi H. Update: Descending aortic aneurysmectomy without adjuncts to avoid ischemia. *Ann Thorac Surg* 1993; **55**: 1042–1045.
17. Dake MD, Miller DC, Semba CP, Mitchell RS, Walker PJ, Liddell RP. Transluminal placement of endovascular stent-grafts for the treatment of descending thoracic aortic aneurysms. *N Engl J Med* 1994; **331**: 1729–1734.
18. Mitchell RS, Dake MD, Semba CP *et al.* Endovascular stent-graft repair of thoracic aortic aneurysms. *J Thorac Cardiovasc Surg* 1996; **111**: 1054–1062.
19. Fann JI, Mitchell RS, Dake MD, Miller DC. Results of endovascular stent-grafting in patients with descending thoracic aneurysm. In *Progress in Vascular Surgery*. Yao JST, Pearce WH (eds). Stamford, CT: Appelton and Lange, 1997: 241–254.
20. Ehrlich M, Grabenwöger M, Grimm M *et al.* Endovascular stent graft repair for aneurysms on the descending thoracic aorta. *Ann Thorac Surg* 1998; **66**: 19–24.

21. Nienaber CA, Fattori R, Lund G. *et al.* Nonsurgical reconstruction of thoracic aortic dissection by stent-graft placement. *N Engl J Med* 1999; **340**: 1539–1545.

22. Dinis da Gama A. The surgical management of aortic dissection: from uniformity to diversity, a continuous challenge. *J Cardiovasc Surg (Torino)* 1991; **32**: 141–153.

23. Svensson LG. Natural history of aneurysms of the descending and thoracoabdominal aorta. *J Cardiovasc Surg* 1997; **12**(Suppl): 279–284.

24. Kato M, Bai HZ, Sato K *et al.* Determining surgical indications for acute type B dissection based on enlargement of aortic diameter during the chronic phase. *Circulation* 1995; **92**: Suppl II: II-107-II-112.

25. Glower DD, Fann JI, Speier RH *et al.* Comparison of medical and surgical therapy for uncomplicated descending aortic dissection. *Circulation* 1990; **82**: Suppl IV:IV-39-IV-46.

26. Miller DC. The continuing dilemma concerning medical versus surgical management of patients with acute type B dissections. *Semin Thorac Cardiovasc Surg* 1993; **5**: 33–46.

27. Masuda Y, Yamada Z, Morooka N, Watanabe S, Inagaki Y. Prognosis of patients with medically treated aortic dissections. *Circulation* 1991; **84**: Suppl III:III-7-III-13.

28. Svensson LG, Crawford ES, Hess KR, Coselli JS, Safi HJ. Dissection of the aorta and dissecting aortic aneurysms: improving early and long-term surgical results. *Circulation* 1990; **82**: Suppl IV:IV-24-IV-38.

29. Dinsmore RE, Willerson JT, Buckley MJ. Dissecting aneurysm of the aorta: aortographic features affecting prognosis. *Radiology* 1972; **105**: 567–572.

30. Rizzoli G, Mazzucco A, Fracasso A, Giambuzzi M, Rubino M, Gallucci V. Early and late survival of repaired type A aortic dissection. *Eur J Cardiothorac Surg* 1990; **4**: 575–583.

31. Fuster V, Halperin JL. Aortic dissection: a medical perspective. *J Card Surg* 1994; **9**: 713–728.

32. Svensson LG, Crawford ES. Aortic dissection and aortic aneurysm surgery: clinical observations, experimental investigations, and statistical analyses. *Curr Probl Surg* 1992; **29**: 913–1057.

33. Svensson LG, Crawford ES, Hess KR, Coselli JS, Safi HJ. Variables predictive of outcome in 832 patients undergoing repairs of the descending thoracic aorta. *Chest* 1993; **104**: 1248–1253.

34. Hagan P, Nienaber CA, Das S *et al.* Acute aortic dissection: presentation, management and outcomes in 1996 – results from the International Registry for Aortic Dissection (IRAD). *JAMA* 2000; **238**: 897–903.

35. Kouchoukos NT, Daily BB, Rokkas CK, Murphy FS, Bauer S, Abboud N. Hypothermic bypass and circulatory arrest for operations on the descending thoracic and thoracoabdominal aorta. *Ann Thorac Surg* 1995; **60**: 67–77.

36. Kouchoukos NT, Dougenis D. Surgery of the thoracic aorta. *N Engl J Med* 1997; **336**: 1876–1888.

37. Coselli JS, LeMaire SA, de Figueiredo LP, Kirby RP. Paraplegia after thoracoabdominal aortic aneurysm repair: is dissection a risk factor? *Ann Thorac Surg* 1997; **63**: 28–36.

38. Schepens MAAM, Defauw JJAM, Hamerlijnck RPHM, Vermeulen FE. Use of left heart bypass in the surgical repair of thoracoabdominal aortic aneurysms. *Ann Vasc Surg* 1995; **9**: 327–338.

39. Panneton JM, Hollier LH. Dissecting descending thoracic and thoracoabdominal aortic aneurysms. *Ann Vasc Surg* 1995; **9**: 596–605.

40. Acher CW, Wynn MM, Hoch JR, Popic P, Archibald J, Turnipseed WD. Combined use of cerebral spinal fluid drainage and naloxone reduces the risk of paraplegia in thoracoabdominal aneurysm repair. *J Vasc Surg* 1994; **19**: 236–248.

41. Svensson LG, Hess KR, Coselli JS, Safi HJ. Influence of segmental arteries, extent, and atriofemoral bypass on postoperative paraplegia after thoracoabdominal aortic operations. *J Vasc Surg* 1994; **20**: 255–262.

42. Svensson LG, Crawford ES, Hess KR, Coselli JS, Safi HJ. Experience with 1509 patients undergoing thoracoabdominal aortic operations. *J Vasc Surg* 1993; **17**: 357–370.

43. Schor JS, Yerlioglu ME, Galla JD, Lansman SL, Ergin MA, Griepp RB. Selective management of acute type B aortic dissection: long-term follow-up. *Ann Thorac Surg* 1996; **61**: 1339–1341.

44. Dake MD, Kato N, Mitchell RS, Sermba CP *et al.* Endovascular stent-graft placement for the treatment of acute aortic dissection. *N Engl J Med* 1999; **340**: 1524–1531.

45. Miller DC. The continuing dilemma concerning medical versus surgical management of patients with acute type B dissections. *Semin Thorac Cardiovasc Surg* 1993; **5**: 33–46.

46. Kato M, Hirano T, Kaneko M *et al.* Outcomes of stent-graft treatment of false lumen in aortic dissection. *Circulation* 1998; II305–II312.

47. Miller DC, Mitchell RS, Dake MD. Midterm results of first generation endovascular stent-grafts for descending thoracic aortic aneurysms. In *Proceedings of the Sixth Aortic Surgery Symposium, New York, April 30 May 1.* 1998: 34–35 [Abstract].

Thoracic aneurysms and type B dissections should be treated by stent-graft

Against the motion

Hans O Myhre, Jan Lundbom,
Alexander Wahba, Petter Aadahl,
Staal Hatlinghus, Jenny Aasland

Introduction

Open surgery for aneurysms and dissections of the descending thoracic aorta has been used for several decades.[1,2] In patients with type B dissection, surgery has mainly been a supplement to medical antihypertensive treatment.[3-5] The technique as well as the graft material have proved their sufficiency, and the results have improved over the years. Open surgery must therefore be regarded as the 'gold standard' against which new techniques should be evaluated. Recently stent-grafting has been applied to some extent for aneurysms and dissections of the descending thoracic aorta.[6,7] However, this must be regarded as an experimental procedure since the follow-up period is rather short and we have seen several problems with this method. Based on reviews of the literature and our own experience we wanted to evaluate the status of traditional surgical treatment of descending thoracic aortic aneurysms and type B dissections, which is the basis for comparison with more recent therapeutic options.

Open repair of descending thoracic aneurysms

Open repair is performed through a left thoracotomy. In most of our cases we have used direct cross-clamping of the aorta as our standard method. This method is simple, but expedient surgery is necessary to keep the aortic clamp time as short as possible.[8-10] Shunting or cardiopulmonary bypass is by many regarded as an advantage provided one is expecting a cross-clamp time longer than 30 minutes.[11,12]

Distal perfusion may improve circulation to the spinal cord and the visceral organs during this critical period.[11] Two methods are available to achieve this: atriofemoral bypass and partial cardiopulmonary bypass. The advantage of atriofemoral bypass lies in its simplicity. Heparin-coated equipment is used, minimizing the need for additional heparin. Distal body perfusion is achieved by a centrifugal pump. The set up of partial cardiopulmonary bypass in the groin is somewhat more complex (Fig.1). The full heart lung machine including heat exchanger, oxygenator, arterial line filter and cardiotomy suction is employed. The advantage of this approach lies in its versatility. The use of cardiotomy suction gives the surgeon additional safety in the case of bleeding. The system may be converted to full cardiopulmonary bypass with deep hypothermia if required, by inserting a cannula in the ascending aorta. Temperature control of the patient is easier obtained with this technique.

Today open surgery for descending aortic aneurysms has become a highly specialized mode of treatment for a relatively small group of patients with a serious disease. Frequently they suffer from significant co-morbidity. Several adjuncts to the operation have been developed. These include cerebrospinal fluid drainage, monitoring of evoked potentials, extracorporal circulation and pharmacological treatment, adding to the complexity of the surgical procedure. Nevertheless, reported results in large series are excellent.[13,14] The 30-day mortality varies from 5 to 12% in different series, but as expected the mortality is higher in patients who have pain due to expansion, or rupture. A mortality from 25–50% has been reported following emergency surgery.[13-15] There is reason to believe that continued research will improve the results of open surgery in dedicated units.

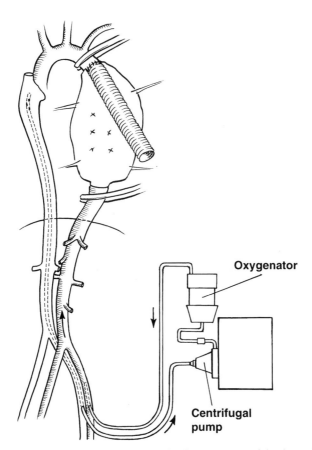

Oxygenator

Centrifugal pump

Figure 1. Schematic illustration indicating open repair of an aneurysm of the descending thoracic aorta. The proximal anastomosis has been completed. Partial cardiopulmonary bypass is installed via the femoral vessels. The system includes pump, oxygenator, heat exchanger, reservoir, bubble trap and cardiotomy suction.

We have treated 48 patients for descending thoracic aneurysm, 35 with open surgery and 13 with stent-grafting. In the first group 28 patients were operated on as emergency cases including nine with rupture and shock whereas seven were operated electively. Five patients died within 30 days; four with rupture and one with chest pain, giving a total 30-day mortality of 14%. There was no mortality in the elective group. Three patients (8.6%), all in the emergency group developed paraplegia post-operatively. The median operating time was 173 minutes (100–375) and the median aortic clamp time 45 minutes (15–110). No reoperations became necessary.

Following open surgery, management of the aneurysmal disease is completed when the patient is leaving the hospital since there is no need for sophisticated control investigations. The long-term results in large series are satisfactory[2] and the quality of life after operation is acceptable.[16] Following endovascular surgery on the other hand, the patients need to be followed at regular intervals with CT-scans and in selected cases arteriography, to investigate for leaks, dislocation or disintegration of the implant. This represents a burden to the patients and it adds to the costs of the treatment.

Neurological deficits

A paraplegia rate following elective open surgery from 0 to 8% has been reported.[2,8,13–15,17,18] It has been claimed that the incidence of paraparesis and paraplegia following endovascular treatment appears to be lower than the open technique. However, this could be the result of case selection. Reports of paraplegia following stent-grafting of descending thoracic aneurysms have recently emerged with reported incidences between 0 and 9 %.[19–22] Due to the pathogenesis of paraplegia following treatment of descending aortic aneurysms, this complication will necessarily occur in an undetermined percentage of patients. Failure to re-establish blood flow to critical segmental arteries of the spinal cord during repair has been identified as one of several causes of paraplegia following open surgery.[2] There is no indication that this can be avoided during endovascular treatment. In contrast, identification and revascularization of critical segmental arteries is impossible when using the endovascular approach, whereas significant progress has been made with regard to this problem in open procedures. The monitoring of motor evoked potentials during open surgery, however cumbersome and difficult it may be, has a potential to improve the results in these cases.[23,24] Further, in experimental investigations intraoperative Doppler ultrasound has been useful in identifying critical segmental arteries.[25] This method could have a potential during open surgery. At the present time one cannot draw firm conclusions as to whether open or endovascular surgery is preferable with regard to the problem of paraplegia and paraparesis.

Summary

- Open surgery has been used for several decades.
- The technique is standardized.
- The grafts are durable.
- The long-term results are known and are in general excellent.
- All patients can be operated by the same method.
- No special follow-up investigations are necessary.
- Open surgery is the gold standard.

Stent-grafting of thoracic aneurysms

It has been suggested that the operative trauma of endovascular aneurysm repair is less than following open surgery.[6,7,19,26] Recent investigations indicate that at least the systemic reaction following the implantation of an endoprosthesis could be quite dramatic.[27] The anatomy of the aneurysm must fulfill certain criteria before endovascular surgery can be performed. In general one would need an upper neck of more than 15 mm and the neck should not be too wide or angulated. There should be no thrombosis at the upper or distal points of fixation. Thus, stent-grafting can only be applied in some of the patients. In unstable patients with ruptured aneurysms,[27] a thorough radiological investigation to select a proper endoprosthesis may be contraindicated due to the time interval needed. Furthermore, there can be problems with access to the arterial system since one is using rather long and wide introducer systems. Tortuosity, stenosis or heavy calcification of the iliac arteries or the aorta may represent a contraindication against endovascular surgery (Figs 2a,b). In elderly patients the descending thoracic aorta usually has a more pronounced curvature than in younger people. Therefore it may be connected with problems to get around the aortic curvature with some introducer systems. Dislocation of atherosclerotic material and even perforation of the aorta has been reported. Also some of the endoprosthesis are rather stiff with the implication that it could be difficult to follow the curvature of the proximal part of the descending thoracic aorta.

The endoprosthesis consist of a metallic and a fabric part. The metallic part may break and in some cases tear holes in the fabric part with a type III leak as the result (Figs 3a,b). This is a serious complication, which immediately should lead to secondary intervention. The complication shown in Fig. 3 is to our knowledge the first reported case with disintegration of the fabric part of the Excluder® stentgraft (WL Gore & Ass. Flagstaff, AZ, USA) . The metal part at the landing zones can also lead to rupture of the aorta with fatal consequences.[29] In summary, endovascular surgery of the thoracic aorta is in general connected with the same problems as seen in other anatomical areas.[30] Graft malpositioning may be caused by imprecise deployment. This is a serious complication which could lead to upper extremity or visceral ichaemia.[22,31] The fixation may slip and lead to dislocation of the implant, especially at the proximal part, leading to type I leaks. In one of our cases the endoprosthesis had a tendency to kink and enter the aneurysmal sack (Fig. 4). Also type II leaks are seen in the thoracic aorta. An endoleak rate between 5.5 and 15% has been reported and also an incidence of stroke and transient ischaemic attack between 0 and 7% has been observed following stent-grafting.[22,31,32]

The supposed simplicity of the endovascular approach could lead to a spreading of such procedures to units lacking sufficient experience with care of patients with descending thoracic aortic aneurysms. The tendency of spreading stent-grafting of the thoracic aorta to more centres including non-teaching hospitals has been confirmed by the European Vascular and Endovascular Monitoring Panel, and initiative by Vascular News. During the last 12 months 4150 open operations were performed in 15 European countries for thoracic aneurysmal disease and dissection. During the last decade there have been between 30 000 and 35 000 procedures. In contrast 1280 endovascular procedures were reported the last year. It could give rise to concern that some of the 150 centres doing endovascular stent graft procedures had very small experience. An increase in endovascular procedures could be followed by reduction in the case volume for existing surgical programmes for descending thoracic surgery. The treatment of complications and patients unsuitable for endovascular repair could be even more diffused than today. This will render it more difficult to keep up a high standard within the unit as a whole. Training of new members of the surgical team in particular could be increasingly difficult.

An uncritical utilization of the endovascular approach may in the long run lead to inferior results for the group of patients with descending aortic aneurysms as a whole although an hitherto undefined subgroup of patients may benefit from stentgrafting. Endovascular treatment should therefore be restricted to units dealing with a reasonable case volume offering the full advantage of all treatment options.

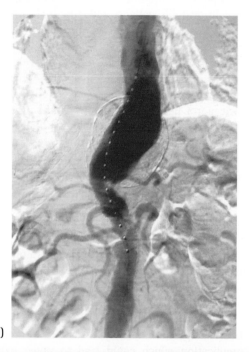

(a)

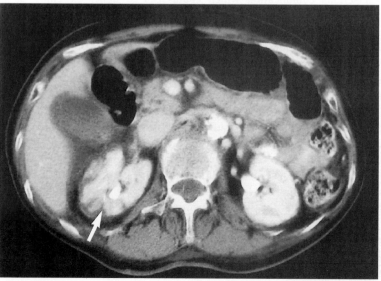

(b)

Figure 2. Aortography of a 74-year old patient, where endovascular treatment of a descending thoracic aortic aneurysm was planned. There was heavy calcification and stenosis of the abdominal aorta (a). During stent-grafting embolization to the kidneys (b) occurred (→).

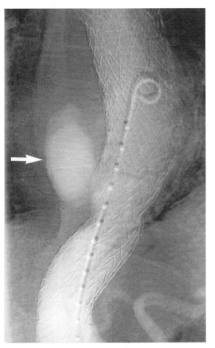
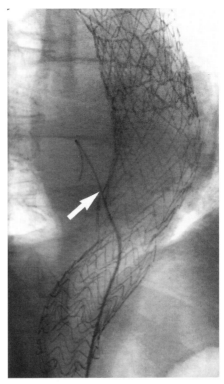

(a)   (b)

Figure 3. Arteriogram 12 months after the implantation of an Excluder® endoprosthesis for the treatment of an aneurysm of the descending thoracic aorta. Disintegration of the fabric part of the endoprosthesis had taken part and the contrast was filling the aneurysmal sac (→) (a). The guidewire was passing the hole (→) into the aneurysmal sac to verify the perforation (b). Endovascular repair was performed successfully.

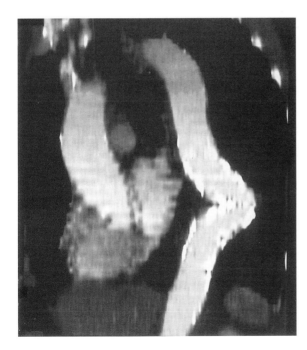

Figure 4. A 70-year-old woman was operated by endovascular technique for a saccular aneurysm of the descending thoracic aorta. A CT-scan 2½ year after treatment showed that the graft had kinked and entered the aneurysmal sac.

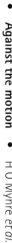

Thoracic aneurysms and type B dissections should be treated by stent-graft • **Against the motion** • *H O Myhre et al.*

We have treated 13 patients with stent-grafting for descending thoracic aneurysms. Eleven were treated electively whereas one had chest pain. There were no patients with rupture in this group. One patient had an open operation for infrarenal abdominal aortic aneurysm, with insertion of a bifurcation graft during the same procedure. One patient with pulmonary disease died from septicaemia 2 days following an uncomplicated implantation and another patient died 9 months after treatment due to perforated doudenal ulcer. This patient also had temporary paresis in the lower extremities following the stent-graft implantation, but the symptoms recovered following removal of cerebrospinal fluid. Finally, one patient with severe atherosclerosis of the aorta had embolization and infarctions in the kidneys and the spleen (Fig. 2b). The median operating time was 185 minutes (120–295). The case-mix of our two series indicate that it is difficult to make a meaningful retrospective comparison between the two treatment modalities since there were more emergency operations in the group of patients operated by open technique.

Summary

- Stent-grafting cannot be performed in all patients due to anatomical limitations.

- Access the with introducer system may be prohibited by tortuosity of the iliac arteries, stenosis, calcification etc.

- This treatment modality could be difficult to apply in some patients with ruptured aneurysms.

- The observation time of stent-grafting is short and the long-term results are unknown.

- There is a risk of endoleak, graft malpositioning or dislocation, disintegration etc.

- The patients must be followed at regular intervals with CT-scans and arteriography in selected cases.

- The follow-up examinations as well as the stent-grafts are expensive.

Type B dissections
Combined medical and surgical treatment

Because aortic dissection can be caused by hypertension, Marfan's disease and other conditions, most series contain a mixture of different diseases. Furthermore, dissections can be acute or chronic. The presented series are often heterogeneous and interpretation of the results can be difficult. Type B dissection of the aorta is a life-threatening condition. However, the risk of fatal complications during the acute phase is lower than for type A dissections. Patients with type A dissections should therefore undergo surgery as soon as possible.[5] In contrast, type B dissections tend to become chronic. Most authorities advocate medical treatment for acute uncomplicated type B dissections because of the high mortality and morbidity with surgery in the acute phase. Medical treatment aims at reducing blood pressure and heart rate in addition to treatment of congestive heart failure. Operations during the acute phase are used for treating complications of the dissections such as rupture, persisting pain, organ or lower limb ischaemia or aneurysm formation.[5,33,34] This may be achieved by resection and graft replacement of the diseased segment of the aorta, closing the original intimal tear, or fenestration of the intima to allow perfusion of occluded visceral arteries.[35]

Continued medical treatment and rigorous control with serial CT-scans are the mainstay of treatment for chronic type B dissections. It has recently been shown that long-term β-blocker therapy improves outcome in these patients.[36] A substantial number of patients with chronic dissection eventually require treatment for progressive dilatation of the diseased aortic segments.[37] Several risk factors for rupture or continued expansion have been identified; uncontrolled hypertension, high age, chronic obstructive pulmonary disease and patency of the false lumen.[35] Special reference has been made to the increased risk of patients with an aortic diameter of more than 40 mm and a patent false lumen. A more aggressive approach with early surgical intervention has been advocated in these patients.[37,38] The technique for surgical treatment of type B dissections follows similar lines as those of descending thoracic aortic aneurysms. It is mainly directed towards the relief of aneurysmal expansion and threatening or manifest rupture of the dissected segment.[5,39] From these statements it follows that treatment of acute and chronic type B dissections represents a difficult balance between medical and surgical treatment options. To achieve optimal results it is mandatory that treatment and follow-up should be assigned to a dedicated unit and primary treatment should be taken care of by the same centre where the follow-up is performed.

The early mortality following combined medical and surgical treatment of acute type B dissections varies from 0% to as high as 33%.[38-42] However, the results have improved significantly in recent series. Already in 1975 Reul et al.[43] achieved a decrease in early mortality from 21 to 6.5%. About the same results can be shown for combined medical and surgical treatment of chronic type B dissection. Whereas DeBakey et al. in 1965[1] reported a 19% mortality, Crawford in his series had improved to 7.4% in 1988.[33] The 5-year survival rate for patients operated for type B dissections has been relatively good, averaging 80%. After 10 years the mean survival is still around 65%. Although somewhat controversial this indicates a relatively good prognosis for those who are surviving an emergency operation. Also after chronic dissections survival after 5 years has varied between 60 and 95% decreasing to approximately 55% after 10 years.[5,40-42] The increased mortality depends on high age, hypertension and cardiovascular co-morbidity. The combination of medical and surgical treatment has become more sophisticated during recent years rendering better results. However, in spite of aortic dissection being a disease with high mortality and many controversial issues no randomized series have so far been performed.

Stent-grafting

Stent-grafting is a new strategy for treatment of type B dissections.[44] Although emerging results are encouraging, stent-grafting for type B dissection must be regarded as experimental and should be reserved for special situations and a restricted number of units. This follows from our general comment that the treatment is demanding and allocation of some treatment options to specialists who are otherwise not involved in the treatment of these patients may produce adverse results. Several concerns must be raised with regard to stent-grafting of type B dissections: Disintegration with breaks of the metal part has been observed in several types of the endoprosthesis and could in the long run lead to disastrous complications. The introducer system could cause serious damage in a fragile arterial system. In patients with Marfan's disease, where the endoprosthesis is deployed into an aorta of poor wall quality, one can speculate whether further dilatation will lead to dislocation of the endograft. In one series four of nine patients treated with stent-grafting for type B dissections developed saccular aneurysms in the proximal descending aorta requiring further treatment.[45] Thus the ultimate goal of the treatment; prevention of progressive aortic dilatation was not achieved in nearly half of the patients despite primary control of the intimal tear . There is concern that the stiff uncovered ends of the stent-grafts may tear the intimal flaps and thus weaken the aortic wall. Thus perforation of the intimal flap with a guidewire leading to abandoning of the procedure has been reported.[46]

Our own experience is based on 268 patients admitted for aortic dissection during the period 1987–2001. Only six of these have been treated by stent-grafting for type B dissection[47] and three of them were treated electively. One patient had chest pain whereas two had ruptured. There was no mortality in this group, but one patient who underwent a combined procedure developed paraplegia postoperatively. Further, two patients required secondary procedures due to type I leaks (Fig.5).

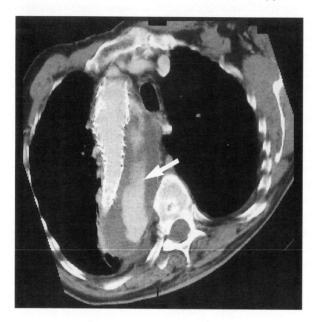

Figure 5. CT-scan 3 months after endovascular treatment of a type B dissection. There is contrast leak into the false lumen (→) at the proximal landing point indicating a type I leak.

Summary

- Type B dissections should be treated by medical antihypertensive regimen.

- Long-term β-blocker therapy is indicated.

- The patients must be followed by serial CT-scans.

- Open surgery is preferred for aneurysmal expansion, persisting pain, organ or lower limb ischaemia.

- The reservations regarding stent-grafting are the same as for descending thoracic aneurysms.

- Compared with aneurysmal disease the aortic wall has even poorer quality with potential complications and problems.

Conclusions

Open surgery for descending thoracic aneurysms is the gold standard and the preferred method today. This method can be used for most categories of patients. The standardization of the technique facilitates teamwork. Endovascular repair is a new technique without any randomized series and the long-term results are unknown. Serious complications with the method have been reported. The patients must be followed to investigate for endoleaks, retrograde filling of the aneurysmal sack and dislocation or disintegration of the endoprosthesis. This adds to the cost of the procedure. Stent-grafting for descending thoracic aortic aneurysms must at the present time be regarded as experimental.

For the time being, patients with acute type B dissections should receive rigorous medical treatment in a dedicated unit. After the early acute phase, long-term β-blocker therapy is recommended. The patients must be followed closely with serial CT-scans. Once an indication for surgery arises, open procedures are preferred. Randomized controlled series comparing the different treatment options are needed.

References

1. DeBakey ME, Henly WS, Cooley DA *et al.* Surgical management of dissecting aneurysms of the aorta. *J Thorac Cardiovasc Surg* 1965; **49**: 130–148.
2. Svensson LG, Crawford ES, Hess KR, Coselli JS, Safi HJ. Variables predictive of outcome in 832 patients undergoing repairs of the descending thoracic aorta. *Chest* 1993; **104**: 1248–1253.
3. Fann JI, Smith JA, Miller C *et al.* Surgical management of aortic dissection during a 30-year period. *Circulation*, 1995; (Suppl II), II 113–II 121.
4. Hagan PG, Nienaber CA, Isselbacher EM *et al.* The International Registry of Acute Aortic Dissection (IRAD). New insights into an old disease. *JAMA* 2000; **283**: 897–903.
5. Borst HG, Heinemann MK, Stone CD. *Surgical Treatment of Aortic Dissection.* New York: Churchill Livingstone, 1996.
6. Dake MD, Miller DC, Mitchell RC *et al.* The "first generation" of endovascular stent-grafts for patients with aneurysms of the descending thoracic aorta. *J Thorac Cardiovasc Surg.* 1998; **116**: 689–704.
7. Greenberg R, Resch T, Nyman U *et al.* Endovascular repair of descending thoracic aortic aneurysms: An early experience with intermediate-term follow-up. *J Vasc Surg* 2000; **31**: 147–156.
8. Cooley DA, Golino A, Frazier OH. Single-clamp technique for aneurysms of the descending thoracic aorta: report of 132 consecutive cases. *Eur J Cardio-Thoracic Surg* 2000; **18**: 162–167.
9. Biglioli P, Spirito R, Porqueddu M *et al.* Simple clamping technique in descending thoracic aortic aneurysm repair. *Ann Thorac Surg* 1999; **67**: 1038–1044.
10. Mauney MC, Tribble CG, Cope JT *et al.* Is clamp and sew still viable for thoracic aortic resection? *Ann Surg* 1996; **223**: 534–543.
11. Safi HJ, Miller CC, Yawn DH *et al.* Impact of distal aortic and visceral perfusion on liver function during thoracoabdominal and descending thoracic aortic repair. *J Vasc Surg* 1998; **127**: 145–153.
12. Kouchoukos NT, Masettei P, Rokkas CK *et al.* Safety and efficacy of hypothermic cardiopulmonary bypass and circulatory arrest for operations on the descending thoracic and thoracoabdominal aorta. *Ann Thorac Surg* 2001; **72**: 699–708.
13. Coselli JS, Plestis KA, La Francesca S, Cohen S. Results of contemporary surgical treatment of descending thoracic aortic aneurysms: Experience in 198 patients. *Ann Vasc Surg* 1996; **10**: 131–137.
14. Safi HJ, Subramaniam MH, Miller CC *et al.* Progess in the management of Type I thoracoabdominal and descending thoracic aortic aneurysms. *Ann Vasc Surg* 1999; **13**: 457–462.
15. Verdant A, Cossette R, Pagè A, Baillot R, Dontigny L, Pagè P. Aneurysms of the descending thoracic aorta: Three hundred sixty-six consecutive cases resected without paraplegia. *J Vasc Surg* 1995; **21**: 385–391.
16. Olsson C, Thelin S. Quality of life in survivors of thoracic aortic surgery. *Ann Thorac Surg* 1999; **67**: 1262–1267.

17. Estrera AL, Rubenstein FS, Miller CC *et al.* Descending thoracic aortic aneurysm: surgical approach and treatment using the adjuncts cerebrospinal fluid drainage and distal aortic perfusion. *Ann Thorac Surg* 2001; **72**: 481–486.

18. von Segesser LK, Tkebuchava T, Niederhäuser U *et al.* Aortobronchial and aortoesophageal fistulae as risk factors in surgery of descending thoracic aortic aneurysms. *Eur J Cardio-Thoracic Surg* 1997; **12**: 195–201.

19. Dake MD. Endovascular stent-graft management of thoracic aortic diseases. *Eur J Radiol* 2001; **39**: 42–49.

20. Reichart M, Balm R, Meilof JF *et al.* Ischemic transverse myelopathy after endovascular repair of a thoracic aortic aneurysm. *J Endovasc Ther* 2001; **8**: 321–327.

21. Tiesenhausen K, Amann W, Koch G *et al.* Cerebrospinal fluid drainage to reverse paraplegia after endovascular thoracic aortic aneurysm repair. *J Endovasc Ther* 2000; **7**: 132–135.

22. Mitchell RS, Miller DC, Dake MD. Stentgraft repair of thoracic aortic aneurysms. *Semin Vasc Surg* 1997; **10**: 257–271.

23. Sueda T, Morita S, Okada K *et al.* Selective intercostal arterial perfusion during thoracoabdominal aortic aneurysm surgery. *Ann Thorac Surg* 2000; **70**: 44–47.

24. de Haan P, Kalkman CJ, de Mol BA *et al.* Efficacy of transcranial motor-evoked myogenic potentials to detect spinal cord ischemia during operations for thoracoabdominal aneurysms. *J Thorac Cardiovasc Surg* 1997; **113**: 87–100.

25. Shibata K, Takamoto S, Kotsuka Y *et al.* Doppler ultrasonographic identification of the critical segmental artery for spinal cord protection. *Eur J Cardio-Thorac Surg* 2001; **20**: 527–532.

26. Ehrlich M, Grabenwoeger M, Cartes-Zumelzu F *et al.* Endovascular stent graft repair for aneurysms on the descending thoracic aorta. *Ann Thorac Surg* 1998; **66**: 19–25.

27. Moriage N, Esato K, Zenpo N, Fujioka K, Takenaka H. Is endovascular treatment of abdominal aortic aneurysms less invasive regarding the biological responses? *Surg Today* 2000; **30**: 142–146.

28. Semba CP, Kato N, Kee ST *et al.* Acute rupture of the descending thoracic aorta: repair with use of endovascular stent-grafts. *J Vasc Intervent Radiol* 1997; **8**: 337–342.

29. Malina M, Brunkwall J, Ivancev K *et al.* Late aortic arch perforation by graft-anchoring stent: complication of endovascular thoracic aneurysm exclusion. *J Endovasc Surg* 1998; **5**: 274–277.

30. Resch T, Koul B, Dias NV, Lindblad B, Ivancev K. Changes in aneurysm morphology and stent-graft configuration after endovascular repair of aneurysms of the descending thoracic aorta. *J Thorac Cardiovasc Surg* 2001; **122**: 47–52.

31. Mitchell RS, Dake MD, Semba CP *et al.* Endovascular stentgraft repair of thoracic aortic aneurysms. *J Thorac Cardiovasc Surg* 1996; **11**: 1054–1067.

32. Temudom T, D'Ayala M, Marin HL *et al.* Endovascular grafts in the treatment of thoracic aortic aneurysms and pseudoaneurysms. *Ann Vasc Surg* 2000; **14**: 230–238.

33. Crawford ES, Svensson LG, Coselli JS, Safi HJ, Hess KR. Aortic dissection and dissecting aortic aneurysm. *Ann Surg* 1988; **208**: 254–273.

34. Gandjbakhch I, Jault F, Vaissier E *et al.* Surgical treatment of chronic aortic dissections. *Eur J Cardio-Thorac Surg* 1990; **4**: 466–471.

35. Panneton JM, The SH, Cherry KJ *et al.* Aortic fenestration for acute or chronic aortic dissection: An uncommon but effective procedure. *J Vasc Surg* 2000; **32**: 711–721.

36. Genoni M, Paul M, Inni R *et al.* Chronic β-blocker therapy improves outcome and reduces treatment costs in chronic type B aortic dissection. *Eur J Cardio-Thorac Surg* 2001; **10**: 606–610.

37. Marui A, Mochizuki T, Mitsui N *et al.* Toward the best treatment for uncomplicated patients with type B acute aortic dissection. *Circulation* 1999; **100** (Suppl.II), II 275–II 280.

38. Juvonen T, Ergin MA, Galla JD *et al.* Risk factors for rupture of chronic type B dissections. *J Thorac Cardiovasc Surg* 1999; **117**: 776–786.

39. Safi HJ, Miller CC, Reardon MJ *et al.* Operation for acute and chronic aortic dissection: recent outcome with regard to neurologic deficit and early death. *Ann Thorac Surg* 1998; **66**: 402–411.

40. Schor JS, Yerlioglu ME, Galla JD, Lansman SL, Ergin MA, Griepp RB. Selective management of acute type B aortic dissection: long-term follow-up. *Ann Thorac Surg* 1996; **61**: 1339–1341.

41. Masuda Y, Yamada Z, Morooka N, Watanabe S, Inagaki Y. Prognosis of patients with medically treated aortic dissections. *Circulation* 1991; **84** (5 Suppl): III 7–13.

42. Doroghazi RM, Slater EE, DeSanctis RW *et al.* Long-term survival of patients with treated aortic dissection. *J Am Coll Cardiol* 1984; **3**: 1026–1034,

43. Reul GJ, Cooley DA, Hallman GL, Reddy SB, Kyger ER 3ʳᵈ, Wukasch DC. Dissecting aneurysm of the descending aorta. Improved surgical results in 91 patients. *Arch Surg* 1975; **110**: 632–640.

44. Nienaber CA, Fattori R, Lund G *et al.* Non surgical reconstruction of thoracic aortic dissection by stent graft placement. *N Engl J Med* 1999; **340**: 1539–1545.

45. Kato N, Hirano T, Kawaguchi *et al.* Aneurysmal degeneration of the aorta after stent-graft repair of acute aortic dissection. *J Vasc Surg* 2001; **34**: 513–518.
46. Bortone AS, Schena S, Mannatrizio G *et al.* Endovascular stent-graft treatment for diseases of the descending thoracic aorta. *Eur J Cardio-Thorac Surg* 2001; **20**: 514–519.
47. Lundbom J, Wesche J, Hatlinghus S *et al.* Endovascular treatment of type B aortic dissections. *Cardiovasc Surg* 2001; **9**: 266–271.

Thoracic aneurysms and type B dissections should be treated by stent-graft

Charing Cross Editorial Comments towards Consensus

The argument for stent-graft for these conditions is essentially that the natural history without intervention carries a high mortality and rupture of the aneurysm as a cause of death ranges from 42% to 70% in three series. Yet surgery for descending thoracic aneurysms carries an operative mortality of 11% as quoted by Dr Nienaber. Then there is also the risk of paraplegia. The quoted mortality of stent-graft for dissecting thoracic aneurysm at 9% with a 5% paraplegia rate is similar to the surgical paraplegia rate. There are no random control trials. For type B dissections comparisons between a conventional surgery and stent-graft are also based upon small experiences entirely because the condition is not common and no centres have enormous experiences. Both the proposer and the opposer of this motion stress the recent nature of the data, the shortage of data, and their own uncertainties. Opinions are argued and referenced very carefully. The other feature is the relative lack of company enthusiasm for these conditions compared with infrarenal abdominal aortic aneurysm. At the time of going to press, W L Gore have recently withdrawn their thoracic stent-graft device even though it was very popular in the hands of several enthusiasts. It seems that this subject has some distance to go before the answer is settled.

Roger M Greenhalgh
Editor

The main EVAR indication will be patients unfit for open repair

For the motion

Juan C Parodi, Mark C Bates, Pedro Puech-Leao

Introduction

Aneurysmal disease of the abdominal aorta is the tenth leading cause of death among men in the USA and the thirteenth leading cause of death overall in Western society.[1,2] There is evidence to suggest that the incidence of abdominal aneurysmal disease is increasing, with an estimated tripling of the number of patients diagnosed over the last three decades.[3] The increased frequency of disease may be related to heightened awareness and diagnostic acumen superimposed on the increase in life expectancy attributable to improvements in comfort and modern medicine.

The natural history of abdominal aortic aneurysmal disease is that of progressive remodelling, expansion and ultimately rupture. In fact, only 14% of patients with abdominal aneurysmal disease have symptoms.[4] The major health risk associated with this condition appears to be sudden rupture which accounts for approximately 15 000 deaths in the USA annually.[4]

Traditional surgery background

Since the pioneering work of Dubost, in surgical resection of aneurysmal disease via graft interposition, traditional surgery was until the early 1990s the only treatment proven to positively change patient outcomes. Unfortunately, patients with abdominal aortic aneurysmal disease often have significant associated co-morbidities increasing their risk for surgical intervention. A total of 67% of patients have coronary artery occlusive disease, 63% hypertension, 24% peripheral vascular disease, 22% chronic obstructive pulmonary disease, 10% diabetes and 7.3% renal failure.[5-11]

In population based studies, the mortality rate for abdominal aortic aneurysmal surgery is between 5 and 10%[12] and the morbidity ranges from 15 to 30%.[13] In fact, functional recovery of patients, who were fully ambulatory before surgical aneurysm resection, was achieved in only 60% of patients 2 years following the procedure.[14] The 5-year survival rate after abdominal aortic aneurysm traditional surgical resection is approximately 60%; in addition, even after successful surgical repair there is still the late risk of pseudoaneurysm rupture, suprarenal and iliac aneurysm formation, graft infection, aortoenteric fistula, and graft thrombosis.[14] In one large series of patients, followed for 5 years after abdominal aortic aneurysm resection, mortality from rupture of false or true aneurysm was 5%.[15]

EVAR background

Stent-grafting is an attractive alternative to surgery: The experiences with traditional surgery in these typically high-risk patients prompted us to develop a less aggressive treatment strategy for abdominal aortic aneurysmal disease. The principal was that of aneurysmal exclusion and flow restoration following the anatomical route.

Since our first report in 1991 of a patient who underwent endoluminal treatment for abdominal aortic aneurysmal disease (Fig. 1) there has been an exponential growth and expansion of this technology has dramatically changed how patients are treated internationally with abdominal aortic aneurysmal disease.

The pre-emptory challenge at this point is to define, in an evidence-based model, the advantage of endovascular aneurysm repair (EVAR) to traditional surgery.

The early vision from our team was to treat a subgroup of patients considered high-risk candidates for standard surgical treatment who have large abdominal aortic aneurysms. We found that in this series of patients, treated endoluminally compared with traditional surgery, there appeared to be advantages in the short- and mid-term with a lower incidence of complication and a much shorter length of stay in the hospital. There appeared to be a very rapid and complete recovery in the endoluminal group and systemic signs of inflammation were remarkably fewer. However, this was not randomized controlled data and we have now watched with interest the progress of randomized trials comparing traditional surgery with new endovascular stent-graft devices.[16]

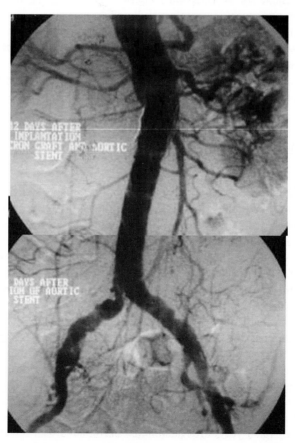

Figure 1. Angiogram of the patient in the first case.

It is difficult to define true evidence-based inference that EVAR is safer than traditional surgery. The Aneurex trial for example, studied 1192 patients in 12 sites and there was 2% mortality in those undergoing stent-grafting compared with 0% in those having open repair. However, 87% of the patients in this trial received stent-grafting and therefore statistical equivalence cannot be determined.[9,17] Similarly, the EVT trial looked at treatment in 870 patients in 22 centres. This trial showed a 2.7% operative mortality for those with open surgery compared with 1.7% with endovascular repair. However, again, 82% of these patients did receive a stent-graft in that trial.[18]

Although mortality could not be defined in these initial trials comparing endovascular repair with traditional surgery, many of the trials were powered significantly to show some clear benefits of stent-grafting including a statistically significant reduction in operative blood loss, lower transfusion requirements, decreased operative time, reduction of intensive care unit length of stay and hospital length of stay.[7,9,11,17–20]

Endoluminal treatment of aneurysms is an evolving field; one has to consider the learning curve and evolution of the devices as biases when the method is compared with open surgery. Abdominal aortic aneurysm correction through laparotomy has been performed with the same technique for the last three decades, with very few modifications in the grafts used; results have improved over time. Conversely, endovascular devices have changed constantly in the last 10 years. Most of the large series published were the results of the use of several types of devices in sequence, and every change in the graft design or delivery system requires a new learning curve. It is to be expected that, once a surgeon gets used to a given kind of device and acquires a prolonged experience with it, the results tend to improve.

Although EVAR appears to have some clear advantage over traditional surgery there is no current panacea for treating these patients. Sub-analysis of patients in Phase II of the Anurex trial matched to those of open surgical technique based on Medicare provider analysis review (MEDPAR) suggests the hospital costs of endovascular repair may be much higher than open repair. The EVAR higher cost were primarily driven by the cost of the stent-graft and in this analysis accounted for 52% of the total cost.[19] These findings were echoed by data published on cost evaluation of EVAR at the Cleveland Clinic Foundation by Dr Clair.[20] The higher cost of these devices is also amplified by the requirement for follow-up imaging and graft surveillance.

The second issue with stent-grafting has been concern regarding durability. Remodelling of the aneurysmal sac after its effective exclusion has been shown potentially to impact the inlaying endograft and could also participate in material fatigue of the different endograft components. This has resulted in a concern about late rupture and endotension.

Endoleaks resulting from migration, disconnection of modular segment, arterial dilatation, wearing of the fabric in the graft and back flow from open branches into the aneurysm represent a significant drawback of endoluminal treatment.[21] Thus far, there have been 30 reported late ruptures with the AneuRx stent graft system and one reported rupture with the Ancure system detailing the importance of initial visceral concern about durability. In fact, the EUROSTAR database reported an annual rupture rate of 1% in patients who have received EVAR.[22] The average size of the aneurysm in their series exceeded 5.5 cm. in diameter and the annual expected rupture for these patients would have been greater than 10%. This means that even the first- and second-generation endovascular devices have dramatically improved on the natural history of these advanced patients.

Conclusions

In summary, abdominal aortic aneurysmal disease is a common entity that has an unfavourable natural history. Surgical resection in some subset of patients is fraught with high morbidity and mortality perhaps related to the frequent associated co-morbidities in such patients. Natural outcome of patients not considered candidates for surgical treatment is only partially known. There are, however, series showing that even in patients suffering several and severe co-morbid conditions rupture is a significant cause of death when the aneurysm is larger than 5.5 cm in diameter.

In view of the discouraging results of non-resective technique to treat aneurysms, some colleagues advocate that patients unfit for abdominal aortic aneurysm surgery should be treated conservatively. In a series of 106 patients turned down for elective aneurysm surgery because of their high risk, Conway *et al.* reported that a ruptured aneurysm was the cause of death in 36% of patients with an aneurysm of 5.5–5.9 cm, 50% of patients with an abdominal aortic aneurysm of 6–6.9 cm and 55% of patients with an aneurysm of 7 cm or larger. Puesh-Lao following 36 patients considered unfit for surgery found a 40% rupture rate after 2 years in patients with aneurysms larger than 6 cm in diameter. This means that even in a high-risk group of patients rupture remains the main cause of death in patients with large aneurysms.

If a less aggressive but effective treatment becomes available, this is the group that will receive the greater benefits of the new approach. This seems to be the trend in small series of patients treated after an abdominal aortic aneurysm rupture and in patients with thoracic aneurysms and Stanford Type B aortic dissections.

The definitive therapeutic goal is to develop a minimally invasive, complication-free method that would allow a very rapid recovery and could be applied to high-risk patients harbouring a large aneurysm.

Endovascular aneurysm repair appears to be a safe alternative to traditional surgery and does appear to change favourably the natural history of these patients at least early after treatment. The limitation of EVAR is related to concerns about durability as well as cost. Both these issues can be resolved. It is through continuous improvement, that EVAR is becoming more reliable, easier to apply and ultimately may replace surgery in those patients who have appropriate anatomy.

At this point, one cannot argue that the technology applied to the development of endografting is still primitive and evolving. The potential application of adjuvant technology to EVAR may add to the effectiveness of this treatment. A combination with laparoscopic techniques, application of staples or fasteners are some resources that can eventually be incorporated into the field. Most cases of failures detailed above are technically solvable and can be compared with the early failures and understandings of metallurgy that came from work in cardiac valve replacement. This high stress environment could also produce failures and new developments in technology and valve design were needed for optimal performance; the same would be true for stent-grafting.

Potential design solution in response to specific problems

1. Limb occlusion is the cause of failure in 7% of our series of 136 consecutive patients after a mean follow-up of 3 years. It is obvious that the development of kink-resistant limbs able to accommodate remodelling of the aneurysm will solve this issue.

2. The second most common cause of late failure (2.2%) occurred typically after 2 years of initial treatment and included disarticulation or migration of modular segments. A locking mechanism is under study to prevent this type of disconnection between segments.
3. Wearing a fabric graft was responsible for 2.2% of failures in our series. New designs that prevent fabric abrasion of the metal exoskeleton as it is stressed within the graft may resolve the problem, as may the development of stronger fabrics or the use of different types of more malleable metals.
4. Fractures of sutures and metal components were seen in 20% of our cases after a mean follow-up of 3 years. In 0.7% of these cases, a modular second-generation endograft was used (Vanguard). Fracture of sutures and metal bars produced disconnection of the first two rows causing migration of the endograft. This problem of material fatigue is similar to that found with cardiac valves and is one of the main drawbacks of current technology; it could easily be treated with pre-clinical testing of different metals to optimize durability.
5. Persistent Type II endoleaks are rarely a cause of failures, but represent the last problem to be solved. This problem is being extensively studied with several solutions proposed.

In summary, the issues with EVAR have been analysed and solutions proposed. A reasonable small early complication rate and durability problem may be acceptable accounting for the great advantages of endoluminal treatment when compared with traditional open surgery. A myriad of possibilities that could eventually be added to this minimally invasive approach are still being explored and provide us with significant optimism about the future of this technology.

The main concern that we still have with the utilization of the EVAR is related to the atrophy of the wall of the aneurysm that occurs following stent-graft once the aneurysm has been completely excluded. If the patient subsequently develops an endoleak it will find an atrophic wall with no outflow since many of the side branches occlude over time. In the few cases in which we have observed this complication the aneurysm grows rapidly and ruptures. This last observation regarding the limitation of this technology indicates that devices should be designed to last for the life-span of the patient and rapid detection and treatment of endoleaks should be undertaken in patients who develop endoleaks.

Secondary endovascular procedures when needed after EVAR are usually simple and effective. Open conversion should be reserved for those patients not amenable to treatment using secondary endoluminal procedures.

Recently David Brewster gave his presidential address as president of the New England Vascular Society[21] in which he thoroughly analysed the EVAR alternative and said:

> If my father had an abdominal aortic aneurysm, the first thing I would tell him would be to seriously consider endovascular repair. It's a real treatment possibility, and not a fad likely to disappear like laser angioplasty … if he has suitable anatomy, he'll choose the endograft pathway and willingly accept the baggage this choice dictates that he must carry on this road …
>
> The parallels to coronary angioplasty are obvious. Even though it is well documented that up to 30–40% of patients treated with percutaneous transluminal coronary angioplasty may require additional catheter procedures during follow-up, this is generally well accepted by most patients if the ultimate outcome is competitive with major surgical revascularization and the much more invasive treatment can be avoided.

If human kind were able to develop the space station, it is unreasonable to think that it would not be possible to replace the old vascular suture to affix a sealed fabric graft to the ends of aneurysms.

Summary

- EVAR was introduced for this.

- EVAR is getting better.

- EVAR is here to stay.

- Improvements are being applied.

References

1. Gillum RF. Epidemiology of aortic aneurysms in the United States. *J Clin Epidemiol* 1995; **48**: 1289–1298.
2. Pleumeekers HJ, Hoes AW, van der Does E *et al.* Epidemiology of abdominal aortic aneurysms. *Eur J Vasc Surg* 1994; **8**: 119–128.
3. Melton LJ, Bickerstaff LK, Hollier LH *et al.* Changing incidence of abdominal aneurysm: a population-based study. *Am J Epidemiol* 1984; **120**: 379–386.
4. Greenfield LJ, Mulholland M, Oldham KT *et al. Surgery: Scientific Principles and Practice* 2nd edn. Philadelphia: Lippincott-Raven Publishers, 1997.
5. White RA, Donayre CA, Walot I *et al.* Modular bifurcation endoprosthesis for treatment of abdominal aortic aneurysms. *Annl of Surg* 1997; **3**: 381–391.
6. Makaroun M, Zajko A, Orons P *et al.* The experience of an academic medical center with endovascular treatment of abdominal aortic aneurysms. *Am J Surg* 1998; **176**: 198–202.
7. Brewster DC, Geller SC, Kaufman JA *et al.* Initial experience with endovascular aneurysm repair: comparison of early results with outcome of conventional open repair. *J Vasc Surg* 1998; **27**: 992–1005.
8. Quinones-Baldrick WJ, Garner C, Caswell D *et al.* Endovascular transperitoneal, and retroperitoneal abdominal aortic aneurysm repair. *J Vasc Surg* 1999; **30**: 59–67.
9. Zarins CK, White RA, Schwarten D *et al.* AneuRx stent graft versus open surgical repair of abdominal aortic aneurysms: multicenter prospective clinical trial. *J Vasc Surg* 1999; **29**: 292–308.
10. Howell MH, Zaqqa M, Villareal RP *et al.* Endovascular exclusion of abdominal aortic aneurysms. *Texas Heart Inst J* 2000; **27**: 136–145.
11. Moore WS, Kashyap VS, Vescera CL *et al.* Abdominal aortic aneurysm: a 6-year comparison of endovascular versus transabdominal repair. *Annl of Surg* 1999; **230**: 298–308.
12. Katz DJ, Stanley JC, Zelenok GB. Operative mortality rates for intact and ruptured aortic aneurysms in Michigan:an eleven year statewide experience. *J Vasc Surg* 1994; **19**: 804–817.
13. Johnston KW. Multicenter prospecyive study of nonruptured abdominal aortic aneurysms, part II: variables predicting morbidity and mortality. *J Vasc Surg* 1989; **9**: 437–440.
14. Kent Williamson W, Nicoloff AD, Taylor LM, Moneta GL, Landry GL, Porter JM. Functional outcome after open repair of abdominal aortic aneurysms. *J Vasc Surg* 2001; **33**: 5.
15. Parodi JC, Palmaz JC, Barone H. Transfemoral intraluminal graft implantation for abdominal aortic aneurysms. *Ann Vasc Surg* 1991; **5**: 491–499.
16. Zarins CK, White RA, Moll FL *et al.* The AneuRx stent-graft: four-year results and worldwide experience 2000. *J Vasc Surg* 2001; **33**: S135–S145.
17. Makaroun MS. The Ancure endografting system: an update. *J Vasc Surg* 2001; **33**: S129–S134.

18. Sternbergh WC, Money SR. Hospital cost of endovascular versus open repair of abdominal aortic aneurysms: a multicenter study. *J Vasc Surg* 2000; **31**: 237–244.
19. Clair DG, Gray B, OHara PJ *et al*. An evaluation of the costs to health care institutions of endovascular aortic aneurysm repair. *J Vasc Surg* 2000; **32**: 148–152.
20. Brewster DC. Presidential address: what would you do if it were your father? Reflections on endovascular abdominal aortic aneurysm repair. *J Vasc Surg* 2001; **33**: 6.

The main EVAR indication will be patients unfit for open repair • **For the motion** • J C Parodi *et al.*

The main EVAR indication will be patients unfit for open repair

Against the motion
Edward B Diethrich

Introduction

Agreement on this proposition might have been reached more easily a decade ago, when endoluminal exclusion of abdominal aortic aneurysms was in its early stages. Indeed, the initial stent-grafts were placed only in the patients considered to be at highest risk for the open procedure. Those with hostile abdomens, cutaneous fistulas such as colostomies and ureterostomies, critical cardiac and pulmonary pathologies, and severe co-morbidities were included in the group. Subsequently, as worldwide investigations were initiated, protocols were designed to include patients with less severe co-morbidities, smaller aneurysms, and even those with lesions <5 cm who would not normally have been considered for an open procedure.[1] Consequently, thousands of devices have been deployed, and a wealth of information accumulated and analysed. It is difficult to determine how many of these patients would have been declared 'unfit' for open repair given that no real definition of 'fitness' has achieved any sort of consensus agreement. Nevertheless, it remains clear that in the majority of cases in which stent-grafts were placed, the patient probably could have had an open resection instead – providing an experienced surgical team was available. It is, therefore, with that background in mind that we strongly advocate the use of endoluminal graft technology for abdominal aortic aneurysm exclusion in patients who are interested in the procedure and willing to participate in the long-term surveillance that is required following placement of these devices.

Technique and device comparisons

The technical aspects of endoluminal grafting have been well described and, to a great extent, standardized from centre to centre. In advocating universal use of stent-grafts, however, one must appreciate the fact that, at least at present, there are no long-term results available and that intermediate-term success must be evaluated separately for each specific device. Indeed, the two devices approved by the Food and Drug Administration (FDA) have distinctly different performance records. For example, the Ancure prosthetic (Guidant, Menlo Park, CA) has been associated with a high occlusion rate of the bifurcated limb, requiring either primary stenting or, in many instances, a secondary procedure to reopen or expand a limb in the iliac artery. Indeed, conversion rates with these stent-grafts have been higher than those associated with other devices.[2] Although late (2-year) type II endoleaks have been a problem and multicentre trials of the tube and bifurcated devices indicate evidence of proximal neck dilatation at 1–3 years,[3] there has not been a single reported case of aneurysm rupture following successful deployment of the prosthesis.[4] This one statistic alone provides evidence to support wider use of endoluminal devices – particularly if this trend holds true in long-term follow-up.

In contrast, a total of 1192 patients were treated with the AneuRx stent (Medtronic, Santa Rosa, CA) in a multicentre trial,[5] and there were 10 (0.8%) ruptures, with most ruptures (n=6) occurring in patients treated with an early bifurcation design (n=174). Since the new device – which has a flexible, segmented bifurcation design – was introduced, four (0.4%) ruptures have occurred among 1018 patients in follow-up. More recent information about device rupture, however, indicates the total number of device ruptures is closer to 25, encouraging the FDA to issue a Public Health Notification in April 2001.[6] Migration of the devices has also been reported, with rates as high as 6% in one study.[7] Overall, these are clearly problems inconsistent with the technical features of the AneuRx modular design, and they will have to be addressed.

Newer grafts that have yet to receive FDA approval include the Zenith (Cook, Bloomington, IN), Excluder (WL Gore, Flagstaff, AZ), and Endologix graft (Endologix, Irvine, CA) (Fig. 1a), which is a bifurcated unibody design. These devices are exhibiting lower complication rates in clinical trials than those seen with earlier prostheses. One can anticipate that the new devices may well earn higher marks than the earliest

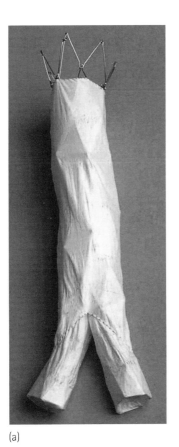
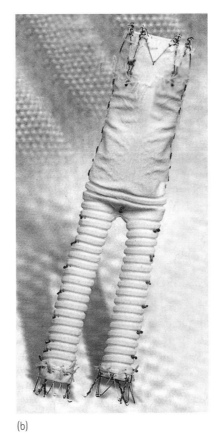

(a)   (b)

Figure 1. The (a) Endologix and (b) Ancure endoluminal grafts. These are bifurcated, unibody designs, which have not, to date, been associated with late migration or rupture. The design features of these grafts may be superior to those of modular grafts; however, as yet, there are insufficient long-term follow-up data to make a firm determination regarding their superiority.

devices, many of which are no longer even available. Interestingly enough, the Endologix and the Ancure devices (Fig. 1b), which incorporate a unibody design that rests on the aortic bifurcation, have very low migration rates, and there have been no reported ruptures to date with either device. The Ancure device was recalled in March 2001 because of device malfunctions associated with the delivery system but is now back on the market.

Proponents of the movement to vastly limit the application of endoluminal grafting technology for abdominal aortic aneurysms exclusion will be glad to emphasize the negative aspects of the discussion presented above. They will argue that presently the long-term durability of the prosthesis has not been determined. We admit the lack of long-term data but believe the weakness in their arguments is in suggesting that these devices should be used only in patients considered to be at high risk with the open procedure. Such patients possess severe co-morbidities, including cardiac and pulmonary pathologies. Data already show the limited lifespan of these patients, even following successful exclusion of the abdominal aortic aneurysms. In general, their deaths are not related to the treated aneurysm or to endoluminal exclusion of the lesion, but rather to underlying systemic disease. The fact is that long-term data regarding the performance of endoluminal grafting will never be available from this particular group of patients.

Evidence

The value of patient selection

The success of the endovascular procedure depends on a variety of factors. Thorough clinical assessment and imaging are key in determining which patients are best suited to the procedure. It appears that men and those patients with less tortuous arteries are often the best candidates. In a study of Ancure (Guidant) and Talent (World Medical/Medtronic Corporation, Sunrise, FL) grafts, 144 patients were evaluated (19 women and 122 men).[8] Unsuitable anatomy caused investigators to reject 63.2% of the women vs only 33.6% of the men (p = 0.026). Our position is clear. Patients should be selected for endoluminal grafting procedures on the basis of favourable anatomy. If this is carried out accordingly, outcomes will favour wider implementation of the technology. Conversely, selecting patients for the procedure based on surgical risk status alone is a recipe for disaster.

Comparisons of endoluminal and open surgical repair

There are some data to suggest that morbidity may be reduced in elective endoluminal graft repair of abdominal aortic aneurysms compared with elective open surgical repair. In one study,[9] 250 patients with infrarenal abdominal aortic aneurysms were treated with the AneuRx stent graft (Medtronic) (n=190) or with open repair (n=60), and those who received endovascular treatment had significant reductions in blood loss, time to extubation, and days in the Intensive Care Unit and hospital. Major morbidity was reduced from 23% in the surgical group to 12% in the stent-graft group (p < 0.05).

In another study comparing use of a low-profile, fully supported, modular, second-generation endoprostheses (n=148) with open repair (n=135) during the same period, the difference in perioperative mortality rates between the endoluminal graft group (2.7%) and the open repair group (5.9%) was not statistically significant.[10] However, survival curves did favour the endoluminal graft group (p = 0.004), and a Kaplan–Meier curve for graft failure revealed 3-year success probabilities were similar between the two groups (82% vs 85% in the endoluminal graft and open repair group, respectively).

In another study,[11] following elective repair of infrarenal abdominal aortic aneurysm, significantly more patients went home (rather than to a rehabilitation facility) after an endovascular procedure than after open surgery. Indeed, procedure type was a significant predictor of discharge destination. Following open procedures in a second study,[12] patients undergoing surgical abdominal aortic aneurysm repair had substantial functional impairment. One-third of these patients stated they had not fully recovered at a mean follow-up of 34 months, and nearly 20% of patients said they would not undergo abdominal aortic aneurysm repair again given the required recovery.

While these and other studies do not yet provide conclusive data of the superiority of the of the endoluminal grafting procedure over open resection, they also do not support the concept that the procedure should be reserved only for patients considered to be at 'high risk' for surgical intervention. Indeed, the opposite conclusion can be reached in that all the positive features of endoluminal grafting, such as high technical success rates and significant reductions in operating time, blood transfusions, infection rates, and Intensive Care Unit and hospital stays are even more likely in patients who fall into the 'low-risk' category.

Complications

One must ask the question, if patients are screened correctly, the operator is skilled in device deployment, and the patient and physician are committed to long-term surveillance, what valid reason is there to curtail the use of endoluminal graft technology in the 'low-risk' patient? Certainly, the current complications do not support limiting use. It is clear, however, that the propensity for endoleak is the Achilles' heel of current endoluminal graft technology. Anatomic variations, the type of graft used, and the method of insertion all influence the endoleak rate.[13]

A meta-analysis of clinical studies describing endoleak after endoluminal grafting of abdominal aortic aneurysms was compiled from reports published since 1995.[14] Results from a total of 23 papers and 1189 patients were included. There were 1118 patients with successfully inserted transfemoral endoluminal grafts, and 270 (24%) of these patients developed endoleaks. In all, 36% of the endoleaks involved the distal stent attachment; 66% of these were present immediately after the procedure, and 37% of them persisted over time. Tube grafts were more frequently affected by endoleaks than bifurcated grafts (p = 0.004). Self-expandable grafts were associated with more endoleaks than balloon expandable grafts (p = 0.037). The problem with these studies is clear; the data represent a majority of experience with first-generation devices, and the outcomes are not applicable to current experience with more advanced endoluminal graft technology.

Research indicates that the potential for endoleaks may be predicted in some cases. In a group of patients treated with AneuRx grafts, Cox proportional hazards regression analysis demonstrated that both patent internal mesenteric arteries (p < 0.01) and patent lumbar arteries (p < 0.0001) were independent risk factors for persistent endoleaks.[15] The researchers also concluded that persistent type II endoleaks were associated with an increase in abdominal aortic aneurysm size and no significant change in the infrarenal neck diameter.

Endoleaks are treated by a variety of means, including conversion to surgical repair, or insertion of a new stent or graft. Unfortunately, both primary and secondary conversion carry a high operative mortality rate.[16] Recently, type II endoleaks have been treated with a liquid embolic agent containing an ethylene-vinyl-alcohol co-polymer.[17] The liquid is injected in the endoleak sac, and early experience indicates it may be a viable treatment alternative. While further study is required, injecting the co-polymer may reduce procedure time and achieve a complete, durable occlusion in many cases.

In spite of these data, we are experiencing a significant decline in the incidence of endoleaks now that newer endoluminal graft designs are in use. In a study from our centre, we treated 115 patients who were not candidates for placement of FDA-approved grafts with the Endologix graft (Endologix). Nearly half of these patients had level III aneurysm morphology, but the endoleak rates at discharge and 30 days were 4.3% and 2.3%, respectively. These data suggest that improvements in device design may indeed increase safety and efficacy of the endoluminal procedure, perhaps eventually resulting in wider acceptance of endoluminal grafting for abdominal aortic aneurysm exclusion.

Quality of life

There is currently a paucity of quality-of-life data to support the use of endovascular surgery over the open procedure. However, in one study, quality-adjusted life expectancy rates were calculated after endovascular and open abdominal aortic aneurysm repair, and results indicated that the benefit of endovascular repair (although small) was consistently greater than that of that of open repair.[18] In another evaluation, patients treated with endovascular procedures exhibited better physical and functional scores as early as 1 week after discharge and also returned to baseline status significantly earlier than patients who had open procedures.[19]

Economics

The cost of the endoluminal graft itself currently nearly exceeds the total reimbursement allotted for the procedure in the US Medicare system. Still, some comparisons of endovascular and open procedures indicate overall costs of these interventions are similar.[20] In one study, the cost of endovascular therapy was about 14% less than the open procedure; the higher cost of open surgery was explained by longer Intensive Care Unit and hospital stays.[21] Recent reports suggest that overall costs are greater with bifurcated than with tube stent-grafts.[22] We are hopeful that as competition increases among device manufacturers, the price of all graft devices will eventually decrease.

Conclusion

Data can be presented to prove any point – even when information is scarce or, worse yet, inaccurate. Physicians incapable of accepting the premise that we have achieved clinical equipoise with endoluminal grafting for abdominal aortic aneurysms will argue that only patients considered to be at 'high-risk' for open procedures are appropriate candidates – even though there are no data to support such a conclusion. These same clinicians will attempt to limit the treatment options of patients who might otherwise be excellent candidates for the less invasive endoluminal procedure. Unfortunately, the patients who might benefit most from a minimally invasive procedure that reduces operating time, blood transfusions, infection rates, and Intensive Care Unit and hospital stays may not even be allowed the option of considering it.

Patients with aneurysmal disease are being referred for treatment by clinicians in a number of different specialties. As such, all of us have an obligation to present these patients with as much information about procedural choices as we possibly can. Assuming that a patient's vascular anatomy supports the endoluminal option, the patient should be informed to a degree that he can choose the procedure he believes is most in concert with his wishes. There is no reason to exclude patients from the decision process. Rather, our role is to inform, advise, and ultimately, facilitate the selected course of therapy. Clearly, at this moment in the development of endoluminal grafting technology, the idea of offering this promising technology only to 'high-risk' patients is untenable.

Summary

- Endoluminal grafting for abdominal aortic aneurysms has achieved clinical equipoise with the open surgical procedure.

- The minimally invasive procedure compared with surgical intervention reduces operating time, blood transfusions, infection rates, and Intensive Care Unit and hospital stays.

- There are no data to support the conclusion that endoluminal grafting should be offered only to patients considered to be at 'high-risk' for open abdominal aortic aneurysms procedures.

- All clinicians have an obligation to present patients with as much information about procedural choices as possible, and ultimately, facilitate the patient's selected course of therapy.

- At this moment in the development of endoluminal grafting technology, the idea of offering this promising technology only to 'high-risk' patients is untenable.

References

1. May J, White G, Yu W, Waugh R, Stephen MS, Harris J. Concurrent comparison of endoluminal repair versus no treatment for small abdominal aortic aneurysms. *Eur J Vasc Endovasc Surg* 1997; 13: 472–476.
2. Cuypers PW, Laheij RJ, Buth J. Which factors increase the risk of conversion to open surgery following endovascular abdominal aortic aneurysm repair? The EUROSTAR collaborators. *Eur J Vasc Endovasc Surg* 2000; 20: 183–189.
3. Makaroun MS, Deaton DH for the Endovascular Technologies Investigators. Is proximal aortic neck dilatation after endovascular aneurysm exclusion a cause for concern? *J Vasc Surg* 2001; 33: S39–45.
4. Makaroun MS. The Ancure endografting system: An update. *J Vasc Surg* 2001; 33: S129–134.
5. Zarins CK, White RA, Moll FL *et al.* The AneuRx stent graft: Four-year results and worldwide experience 2000. *J Vasc Surg* 2001; 33: S135–145.
6. Feigal DW. FDA Public Health Notification: Problems with Endovascular Grafts for Treatment of Abdominal Aortic Aneurysm (abdominal aortic aneurysm). http://www.fdagov/cdrh/safety.html

7. Tutein Nolthenius RP, van Herwaarden JA, van den Berg JC *et al.* Three-year single centre experience with the AneuRx aortic stent graft. *Eur J Vasc Endovasc Surg* 2001; 22: 257–264.

8. Velazquez OC, Larson RA, Baum RA *et al.* Gender-related differences in infrarenal aortic aneurysm morphologic features: Issues relevant to Ancure and Talent endografts. *J Vasc Surg* 2001; 33: S77–84.

9. Treiman GS, Lawrence PF, Edwards WH *et al.* An assessment of the current applicability of the EVT endograft for the treatment of patients with an infrarenal abdominal aortic aneurysm. *J Vasc Surg* 1999; 30: 68–75.

10. May J, White GH, Waugh R *et al.* Improved survival after endoluminal repair with second-generation prostheses compared with open repair in the treatment of abdominal aortic aneurysms: A 5-year concurrent comparison using life table method. *J Vasc Surg* 2001; 33: S21–26.

11. Bosch JL, Beinfeld MT, Halpern EF, Lester JS, Gazelle GS. Endovascular versus open surgical elective repair of infrarenal abdominal aortic aneurysm: predictors of patient discharge destination. *Radiology* 2001; 220: 576–580.

12. Williamson WK, Nicoloff AD, Taylor LM Jr *et al.* Functional outcome after open repair of abdominal aortic aneurysm. *J Vasc Surg* 2001; 33: 913–920.

13. White GH, May J, Waigh RC, Chaufour X, Yu W. Type III and type IV endoleak: toward a complete definition of blood flow in the sac after endoluminal AAA repair. *J Endovasc Surg* 1998; 5: 305–309.

14. Schurink GW, Aarts NJ, van Bockel JH. Endoleak after stent-graft treatment of abdominal aortic aneurysm: a meta-analysis of clinical studies. *Br J Surg* 1999; 86: 581–587.

15. Arko FR, Rubin GD, Johnson BL *et al.* Type II endoleaks following endovascular repair: preoperative predictors and long-term effects. Presentation at the International Congress XIV on Endovascular Interventions, Scottsdale AZ, 11–15 February 2001.

16. Cuypers P, van Marrewijk C, Buth J for the EUROSTAR collaborators. Conversion to open surgery following endovascular abdominal aortic aneurysm repair: risk factors and outcome. Presentation at the International Congress XIV on Endovascular Interventions, Scottsdale AZ, 11–15 February 2001.

17. Martin ML, Dolmatch BL, Fry PD, Machan LS. Treatment of type II endoleaks with Onyx. *J Vasc Interv Radiol* 2001; 12: 629–632.

18. Finlayson SR, Birkmeyer JD, Fillinger MF, Cronenwett JL. Should endovascular surgery lower the threshold for repair of abdominal aortic aneurysms? *J Vasc Surg* 1999; 29: 973–985.

19. Aquino RV, Jones M, Makaroun MS. Quality of life assessment in patients with endovascular or conventional abdominal aortic aneurysm repair. Presentation at the International Congress XIV on Endovascular Interventions, Scottsdale AZ, 11–15 February 2001.

20. Berman SS, Gentile AT, Berens ES, Haskell J. Institutional economic losses associated with abdominal aortic aneurysm repair are independent of technique. Presentation at the International Congress XIV on Endovascular Interventions, Scottsdale AZ, 11–15 February 2001.

21. Polterauer P, Hoelzenbein T, Kretschmer G *et al.* Economic aspects of endovascular abdominal aortic aneurysm treatment. Presentation at the International Congress XIV on Endovascular Interventions, Scottsdale AZ, 11–15 February 2001.

22. Lester JS, Bosch JL, Kaufman JA, Halpern EF, Gazelle GS. Inpatient costs of routine endovascular repair of abdominal aortic aneurysm. *Acad Radiol* 2001; 8: 639–646.

The main EVAR indication will be patients unfit for open repair

For the motion

James May, Geoffrey H White, John P Harris

Introduction

Endovascular treatment of patients with aortic aneurysm is not new. As early as 1864, Moore is credited by Keen with the introduction of large masses of intraluminal wire into an aneurysm in an attempt to precipitate thrombosis.[1] In pre-antibiotic days the majority of aneurysms were syphilitic in origin and sacular in morphology which made them more amendable to treatment by wiring than the fusiform variety seen today. In 1915, Colt, while working as a house surgeon in London, developed a self-expanding wire umbrella that could be introduced via a trocar into an aneurysm.[2] The loading capsule and delivery system had many similarities with current endovascular systems. Electrothermic coagulation of aortic aneurysm by wiring was used up until 1953, when graft replacement of aneurysms was introduced. The relatively high morbidity and mortality rates for graft replacement of aortic aneurysm, particularly in high risk patients, maintained the interest of researchers in developing an endovascular method of repair. It was not, however, until 1991 that Parodi *et al.*[3] reported the clinical use in humans of transfemoral, endovascular grafting to exclude aortic aneurysms. Their concept was the use of balloon expandable, vascular stents to replace sutures and secure the proximal and distal ends of a fabric graft within the lumen of the aorta.

Because it avoids the need for laparatomy, cross-clamping of the aorta and the obligatory blood loss associated with opening the aneurysm sac required with open repair, the endovascular technique has much to recommend it. It has the potential to reduce the morbidity and mortality rates associated with conventional open abdominal aortic aneurysm repair.[4,5] Despite the attractions there are two major areas of concern with the endovascular method. One is the unknown long-term outcome and specifically whether the deployment for an endograft in the proximal neck of the abdominal aortic aneurysm will arrest a natural history of progressive aneurysm degeneration in that segment of the aorta. Similarly the durability of the prostheses in the long term is unknown, with structural failure already having been reported in most types of device.

Technique and illustration

Following the early use of improvised, non-commercial endovascular grafts for abdominal aortic aneurysms, a number of commercially produced endovascular grafts became available (Table 1). These endografts may be classified as first- or second-

Table 1. Endovascular grafts for abdominal aortic aneurysms

Manufacturer	Device composition				Delivery system		
	Graft material	Stent material	Stent pattern	French size (OD)	Method of expansion	Method of fixation
Endovascular Technologies	Polyester	Elgiloy	Stent at proximal and distal ends only	27F	Self-expanding + balloon	Hooks
Guidant	Polyester	Elgiloy	Stent at proximal and distal ends only	22F	Self-expanding + balloon	Hooks
Boston Scientific	Polyester thinwall	Nitinol	Continuous mesh (internal)	22F	Self-expanding	Small hooks + friction
Medtronic	Polyester thinwall	Nitinol	Intermittent Continuous mesh (external)	22F	Self-expanding	Friction + compression fit
Cook	Polyester	Stainless steel (Gianturco type)	Repetitive (total cover)	22F	Self-expanding	Friction + hooks
Baxter	Polyester	Elgiloy	Intermittent	22F	Balloon expandable	Friction + crimps
Gore	PTFE	Nitinol	Continuous	20F	Self-expanding	Friction + small hooks
Endologix	PTFE	Stainless steel	Continuous	20F	Self-expanding	Friction

OD = Outside diameter. PTFE = Polytetrafluoroethylene.
Modified from Ref 15, with permission.

generation devices. First-generation devices were characterized by large (24 French internal diameter) delivery systems, one-piece construction, and a lack of metallic support throughout their length. Second-generation devices had smaller (21 French or smaller internal diameter) delivery systems, modular construction and metallic frame support throughout the length of the prosthesis. The technique of delivering and deploying these devices varies but the principles of endovascular aneurysm repair (EVAR) are the same. These principles include gaining access to an artery at a superficial site in the body remote from the aneurysm. This is usually the common femoral artery in the lower half of the body and either the axillary or common carotid artery in the upper half of the body. The access artery is used to pass the endovascular prosthesis within its delivery catheter to the site of the aneurysm using radiological screening for guidance. The majority of devices are self-expanding and these are deployed by withdrawal of a restraining sheath or corset. Modular devices require access from the contralateral groin to deliver the contralateral limb of the device. This is deployed within the contralateral stump in an overlapping manner to obtain a haemostatic seal. Some devices are in three parts to allow greater flexibility in sizing with regard to the diameter and length of the limbs of the bifurcated endograft (Fig. 1).

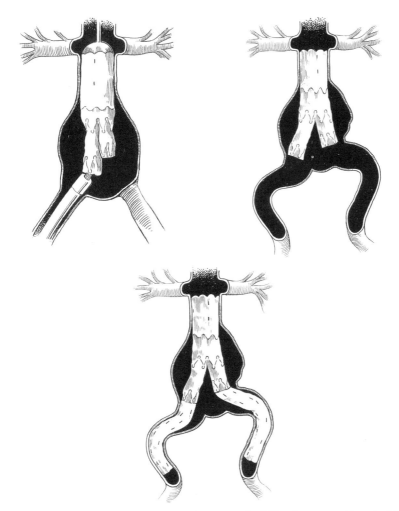

Figure 1. Three part modular endograft allowing greater flexibility diameter and length of the component limbs. Reproduced from Ref 15, with permission.

Evidence

The conventional method of abdominal aortic aneurysm repair by open operation produces excellent long-term results and this is the standard by which the endovascular technique will be judged. Endovascular repair of abdominal aortic aneurysm found its place originally in those patients who were unfit for open repair. The endovascular procedure is indeed a blessing for those high-risk patients who were previously denied treatment for their aneurysm. Before the endovascular method, however, can be recommended for those patients who are fit enough to undergo either endovascular or open repair, a comparison of these two methods must be made. There are currently no reports of a prospective randomized concurrent comparison of these two methods in the literature although such a trial is currently being conducted in the United Kingdom. There are three reports of concurrent comparison of the two methods.[4,5,6] In all three reports, failure to cure the aneurysm was significantly higher in the endovascular group than in the open group (Table 2, Fig. 2). In addition there are also complications which are unique to endovascular aneurysm repair.[7] These include iatrogenic injury to the arteries of access, endoleak, migration of the endograft, ischaemia resulting from side-branch occlusion and conversion from endovascular to open repair.

Table 2. Graft failure

	Endoluminal	Open	Total
Successful repair	126	135	261
Failed repair	22	0	22
Total	148	135	183

Fisher exact test, p <0.0001.
Reproduced from Ref 5, with permission.

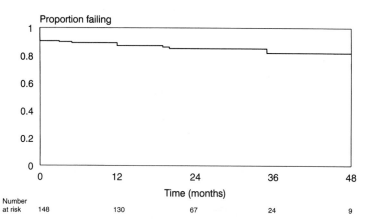

Figure 2. Kaplan Meier curve for graft failure in 148 patients treated with second-generation (endoluminal) prostheses. Probability of failure at 3 years is 18%. Reproduced from Ref 5, with permission.

The higher failure rate and complications unique to endovascular repair, of themselves are sufficient reason to advise open repair for those patients fit to undergo this procedure, thus leaving the main EVAR indication to patients unfit for open repair.

Other downside aspects to endovascular abdominal aortic aneurysm repair reinforce the admonition above. One is the previously mentioned unknown long-term outcome, and specifically whether the deployment of an endograft in the proximal neck will prevent progression of aneurysm degeneration in that segment of the aorta. In a 3-year longitudinal study, Prinssen et al.[8] using state of the art imaging demonstrated an increase in diameter of 1mm per year in the proximal neck. Similarly the durability of prostheses in the long term is unknown. Structural failure has already been reported in the majority of devices within 4 years of implantation (Table 3).

Table 3. Device failure

Prosthesis	Manufacturer	Failure mode
EVT	Endovascular Technologies	Hook fractures
Stentor	Mintec	Fabric defects Seam failure
Vanguard	Boston Scientific Corporation	Fabric defects Tie breaks Disintegration of metal frame
AneuRx	Medtronic	Modular dislocation Microleaks
Lifepath	Baxter	Wireform fracture
Talent	Medtronic	Lateral bar and proximal spring fractures
Ancure	Guidant	Delivery catheter

Other negative aspects of endovascular abdominal aortic aneurysm repair include the need for a life-long surveillance and the likelihood that repeated intervention will be required. Holzenbein et al.[9] have reported that 27% of 166 patients required reintervention for graft failure at a median follow up of 18 months. One of the corollaries of this high rate of reintervention is the risk of infection. Schlensak et al.[10] in Freiburg have recently reported an increase in serious complications requiring surgical explantation in 17 of 150 patients originally reported in the *New England Journal of Medicine* by Blum et al.[11] The indication for explantation in five of these was graft infection occurring between 6 months and 4.5 years after endovascular repair.

Of greatest concern, however, is the risk of rupture following endovascular abdominal aortic aneurysm repair. Reports in the literature of this occurrence are listed in Table 4. Although the overall incidence of rupture is small, the unpredictable nature of it is a cause of anxiety for both patient and surgeon. Of the seven late ruptures reported by Zarins et al.[12] two were predictable, having endoleak together with an increase in diameter of the sac, but five had no endoleak and no increase in size during regular follow-up.

A further worry is the recognition that aneurysms that have been successfully excluded from the circulation for a period of time and then subjected again to systemic pressure may be at greater risk of rupture than if nothing had been done to the aneurysm in the first place, because of collapse and atrophy of the sac wall that occurs after successful exclusion (Fig. 3).

Table 4. Reports of late rupture following endovascular abdominal aortic aneurysm repair

Lumsden AB *et al.*	*Am J Surg*	1995; **170**: 174–178
Parodi JC	*J Vasc Surg*	1995; **21**: 549–557
Alimi YS *et al.*	*J Vasc Surg*	1998; **28**: 178–183
Torsello *et al.*	*J Vasc Surg*	1998; **28**: 184–187
Matsumura JS *et al.*	*J Vasc Surg*	1998; **27**: 606–613
Wain A *et al.*	*J Vasc Surg*	1998; **27**: 69–80
Walker SR *et al.*	*J Endovasc Surg*	1999; **6**: 233–238
Krohg-Sorenson K *et al.*	*J Vasc Surg*	1999; **29**: 1152–1158
May J *et al.*	*J Vasc Surg*	1999; **29**: 32–39
Becquemin JP *et al.*	*J Vasc Surg*	1999; **30**: 209–218
Politz JK *et al.*	*J Vasc Surg*	2000; **31**: 599–606
Zarins C *et al.*	*J Vasc Surg*	2000; **31**: 960–970

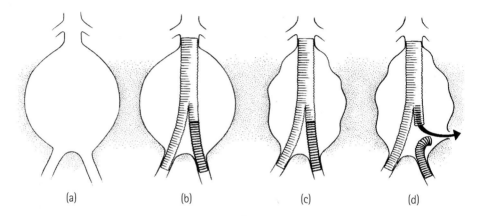

(a)　　　　　(b)　　　　　(c)　　　　　(d)

Figure 3. Diagram illustrating (a) abdominal aortic aneurysm; (b) Aneurysm following endovascular repair; (c) Isolation and depressurization of aneurysm sac, resulting in diminished size; (d) repressurization of collapsed and atrophied sac resulting in rupture. Reproduced from Ref 7, with permission.

Further arguments in favour of ensuring that the main EVAR indication will be patients unfit for open repair relate to the widespread application of the method in inexperienced hands. In 1999 the Food and Drug Administration approved the AneuRx and Ancure devices for general use in the USA. Prior to this, all patients undergoing EVAR in that country did so under protocol in specialized medical centres. The success rate and complication rates from these experienced centres cannot be extrapolated to provincial centres, making it imperative that patients who are fit enough to undergo open repair are protected from the initial and continuing risks of endovascular repair. The skills required to perform EVAR may be taught and acquired but it must be recognized that the complications of EVAR are more difficult and dangerous to treat than the primary operation. In particular the procedures of primary and secondary conversion from endovascular to open repair, secondary endovascular abdominal aortic aneurysm repair and the management of rupture following EVAR are particularly dangerous.[13,14]

The complications and downside aspects of EVAR will ensure that its main indication will continue to be patients unfit for open repair.

Summary

Patients unfit for open repair will be the <u>main</u> but not <u>the only</u> indication for EVAR.

Patients fit for open operation will not be the main indication for EVAR because:

- In concurrent trials of open vs endovascular repair that had been reported, the graft failure rate has been significantly greater in the endovascular group.

- One-quarter of patients undergoing EVAR require reintervention at a medium follow up of 18 months.

- The diameter of the proximal neck following EVAR has been shown to enlarge at a rate of 1mm per year in a 3-year longitudinal study.

- The durability of endoprostheses is unknown with failure modes being reported for most types.

- The unpredictable risk of rupture following EVAR is an unacceptable burden for fit patients to carry throughout their life.

- The complications of EVAR, particularly conversion, secondary repair and rupture are more difficult and dangerous to treat than the primary operation.

References

1. Keen WW. *Surgery: Its Principles and Practice*. Philadelphia: WB Saunders, 1921: 216–349.
2. Power D'A Sir. The palliative treatment of aneurysms by wiring with Colt's apparatus. *Br J Surg* 1921; **9**: 27.
3. Parodi JC, Palmaz JC, Barone HD. Transfemoral intraluminal graft implantation for abdominal aortic aneurysm. *Ann Vasc Surg* 1991; **5**: 491–499.
4. May J, White GH, Yu W *et al.* Concurrent comparison of endoluminal versus open repair in the treatment of abdominal aortic aneurysms: Analysis of 303 patients by life table method. *J Vasc Surg* 1998; **27**: 213–222.
5. May J, White GH, Waugh R *et al.* Improved survival following endoluminal repair with second-generation prostheses compared with open repair in the treatment of abdominal aortic aneurysm: A five-year concurrent comparison by life table method. *J Vasc Surg* 2001; **33**: 21S–26S.
6. Brewster DC, Geller SC, Kaufman JA *et al.* Initial experience with endovascular aneurysm repair: Comparison of early results with outcome of conventional open repair. *J Vasc Surg* 1998; **27**: 992–1005.
7. May J, White GH, Harris P. The complications and downside of endovascular therapies In *Advances in Surgery* Vol. 35. Cameron J (ed). London: Mosby Inc., 2001: 153–172.
8. Prinssen M, Wever JJ, Mali WP *et al.* Concerns for the durability of proximal AAA endograft fixation from a 2-year and 3-year longitudinal CT angiography study. *J Vasc Surg* 2001; **33**: 64S.
9. Holzenbein TJ, Kretschmer G, Thurnher S *et al.* Midterm durability of abdominal aortic aneurysm endograft repair: A word of caution. *J Vasc Surg* 2001; **33**: 46S–54S.
10. Schlensak C, Doenst T, Moreno JB *et al.* Serious complications requiring surgical interventions after endoluminal stent graft placement for the treatment of infrarenal aortic aneurysms. *J Vasc Surg* 2001; **34**: 198–203.
11. Blum U, Voschage G, Lammer J *et al.* Endoluminal stent-grafts for infrarenal abdominal aortic aneurysms. *N Engl J Med* 1997; **336**: 13–20.
12. Zarins CK, White RA, Fogarty TJ. Aneurysm rupture after endovascular repair using the AneuRx stent graft. *J Vasc Surg* 2000; **31**: 960–970.
13. May J, White GH, Yu W *et al.* Conversion from endoluminal to open repair of abdominal aortic aneurysms: a hazardous procedure. *Eur J Vasc Endovasc Surg* 1997; **14**: 4–11.

14. Politz JK, Newman VS, Stewart MT. Late abdominal aortic aneurysm rupture after AneuRx repair: A report of three cases. *J Vasc Surg* 2000; **31**: 599–606.
15. White G, May J. Endovascular grafts. In *Vascular Surgery* 5th edn. Rutherford R (ed). Philadelphia: WB Saunders, 1999.
16. White GH, Yu W, May J. LifePath abdominal aortic aneurysm graft system: the only balloon-expandable type. In *Vascular and Endovascular Surgical Techniques* 4th edn. Greenhalgh RM (ed). London: WB Saunders, 2001: 251–254.

The main EVAR indication will be patients unfit for open repair

Against the motion
Piergiorgio Cao, Fabio Verzini,
Simona Zannetti

Introduction

Abdominal aortic aneurysm represents a clinically relevant and frequent disease: about 5% of men over 65 years of age have an abdominal aortic aneurysm.[1] Ageing of the population, increasing frequency of imaging studies performed for other causes, and a growing prevalence of the disease itself, will all probably contribute to a further increase of the disease in the future.[2]

Surgical treatment of an asymptomatic abdominal aortic aneurysm is a well established procedure to prevent death from rupture in patients with abdominal aortic aneurysm diameter exceeding 5.5 cm. Open repair with laparotomy and abdominal aortic aneurysm endoaneurysmorraphy is the gold standard treatment, it involves general anaesthesia, aortic cross-clamping, significant blood losses and major haemodynamic charges. Although elective mortality rates as good as 1% are reported in high volume single institutional studies, population-based reports show mortality rates in the range of 5–10%.[3-7] Major morbidity rates are reported as high as 30%, principally related to cardiac, pulmonary and renal complications.[8-10] Mortality and morbidity obviously increase in patients with significant co-morbidities and in the elderly population, while some high-risk patients are denied treatment because they are unlike to survive the procedure.

The possibility of having a less invasive treatment choice, such as endovascular aortic repair (EVAR), has been favourably accepted by the medical community and it is gaining growing consensus since its introduction. EVAR might in fact be undertaken under local anaesthesia; it can reduce perioperative risk, shorten recovery time and extend indication to patients unfit for open repair.

It is generally accepted that EVAR represents a suitable treatment strategy for patients unfit for surgery. On the other hand, there are fewer certainties in proposing endovascular treatment to good risk patients. To examine whether EVAR may represent a valid option also in patients fit for surgery, we reviewed the available literature, with a specific attention to studies in which comparison between endovascular and open surgical treatment was made.

Evidence

Evidence-based comparison between EVAR and open repair is not available at present. Prospective randomized trials are ongoing in the United Kingdom (EVAR Trial), in France (ACE Trial) and in The Netherlands (DREAM Trial).

Comparative studies have been carried out in single centres in the form of case control studies, concurrent single or multicentric prospective non-randomized comparisons. In some instances these studies have been used for safety and efficacy evaluation of specific endografts.[11-13] Early published series reported similar peroperative mortality rates after EVAR and open repair. EVAR was associated with reduced blood loss, Intensive Care Unit and hospital stay, and quicker recovery. These advantages came at a cost of higher local complication rates due essentially to graft limb and access artery problems.

In the phase 2 Endovascular Technologies (EVT) trial, mortality and morbidity were the same in the open and endovascular groups; the open repair group showed a greater incidence of postoperative pulmonary complications while the EVAR group had more episodes of transient renal insufficiency as a result of medium contrast load.[11]

In the AneuRx trial, major morbidity of the EVAR group was significantly lower than that of the open repair group (12% vs 23%), while in the case control study by Brewster *et al.* total complication rate was similar (50% with EVAR and 46% with open repair). In this case a predominance of general complications in the open repair group (18/28 vs 4/28) and a prevalence of local complications in the EVAR group (16/28 vs 2/28) were recorded.[12,14]

The most significant outcome measure of endoluminal repair is represented by absence of abdominal aortic aneurysm rupture. Prevention of rupture is indeed the reason for which repair is undertaken. In this regard, recently published large series of patients treated with endovascular repair reported late rupture rates up to 1.5% per year, raising concern about durability of the procedure. A number of the reported ruptures occurred in compassionate cases in patients treated with first-generation devices.[15-16] A recent revision of a series of 1192 patients treated with Medtronic AneuRx endograft showed a more encouraging actuarial abdominal aortic aneurysm rupture rate of 0.5% at 3 years after operation.[17] Makaroun *et al.* reported no abdominal aortic aneurysm ruptures in follow-up of 352 patients treated with the Ancure device.[18] On the basis of this trend, it may reasonable to hypothesize that with new

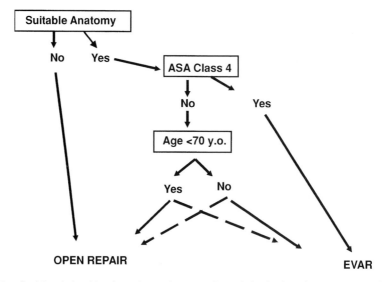

Figure 1. Decisional algorithm in patients who necessitate abdominal aortic aneurysm repair (interrupted lines indicate alternative patient choices).

Table 1. Comparative results after open repair and endovascular repair (EVAR)

Author (year)	Open repair postoperative mortality	EVAR postoperative mortality	p	Open repair postoperative morbidity	EVAR postoperative morbidity	p	Open repair survival (years)	EVAR survival	p
Goldstone (1998)[11]	3.8	1.1	NS						
May (1998)[26]	5.6	5.6	NS	43	29	NA	83 (5)	88	0.14
Zarins (1999)[12]	0	2.6	NS	23	12	<0.05	3 (1)	4	NA
Brewster (1998)[14]	0	0	NS	50	46	NS			
De Virgilio (1999)[27]	4.7	3.6	NS	4[a]	6[a]	NS			
Beebe (2001)[13]	3.1	1.5	NS				80 (2)	85	NS
May (2001)[19]	5.9	2.7	NS	19	39	NA	85 (3)	96	0.004
Zarins (2001)[20]	3.5	0.5	<0.05				74 (3)	74	NS

NS, not significant.
[a]Only cardiac morbidity reported.

generation devices and meticulous follow-up sessions, concerns of rupture may become less onerous than previously thought.

May *et al.* and Zarins *et al.*, provided the most recent and substantial available data.[19-20] May *et al.* reported on a consecutive series of 283 patients, 135 undergoing open repair and 148 EVAR. Perioperative mortality rates were not statistically different (5.9% in the open repair group and 2.7% in the EVAR group) while late survival differed significantly: 96% for EVAR vs 85% for open repair at 3 years.

With respect to graft failure, defined in the EVAR group as exclusion of the aneurysmal sac, stability or reduction in abdominal aortic aneurysm maximum transverse diameter, and persistent endoleak, the open repair group showed better outcome (0 vs 14%). We are not so convinced that endoleak *per se* should be considered as a marker of failure. Several reports failed to show a correlation between the presence of endoleaks and aneurysm growth or rupture.[21-23]

The comparative report by Zarins *et al.*[20] analysed outcome of 441 consecutive patients, 264 undergoing open repair and 177 EVAR. Perioperative mortality was 3.5% and 0.5% (p>0.05) for the open repair and endovascular groups, respectively. In the open repair group 4-year freedom from abdominal aortic aneurysm related death was 89% and 95% in EVAR group. Interestingly, incidence of secondary procedures was not different (13% for open repair vs 15% for EVAR) but magnitude, morbidity and mortality of secondary procedures after open repair were significantly higher. Survival curves showed similar 3-years estimates (74%).

Personal experience

From October 1996 to October 2001 383 patients underwent EVAR. A total of 358 (93%) of these patients were male, mean age was 70 years. Mean abdominal aortic aneurysm diameter (measured as the smallest diagonal in the biggest section at axial CT slices) was 51 mm. There were five perioperative deaths (1.3%) one of which was aneurysm-related. Eight patients required immediate conversion to open repair, with a resulting conversion rate of 2.3%. The average postoperative stay was 3.4 days. During follow-up, secondary conversion to open repair was carried out in eight patients (2.1%), one of them due to abdominal aortic aneurysm rupture in a patient with separation between the main body and a proximal cuff of a modular device. Late abdominal aortic aneurysm rupture rate of 0.27% at a mean follow up of 19 months was recorded. Thirty-one secondary re-interventions were performed in 28 patients (8%) to treat persistent endoleak or correct graft migrations.

Abdominal aortic aneurysm diameter decreased of a mean of 4.3 mm; 56% of patients showed a diameter reduction (>2 mm), while 39% had a diameter unchanged and 5% showed a diameter increase.

In our experience EVAR showed a good feasibility and efficacy in the mid-term. Only 5% of the treated abdominal aortic aneurysms showed increase in diameter and only one ruptured, resulting in late treatment failure rate of 5.3%. These results support the use of EVAR in patients anatomically fitted for the procedure.

Discussion

Indication for EVAR is the result of balancing anatomical features and co-morbidities that may affect open surgical outcome. The only unquestionable issue is represented by anatomical characteristics, crucial in determining short- and long-term success.

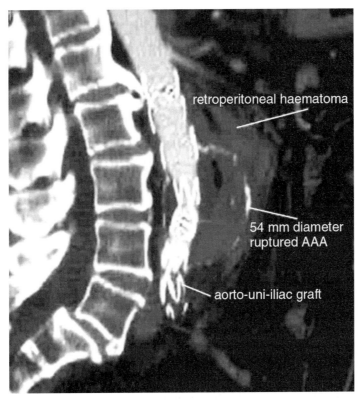

Figure 2. Postoperative computed tomography scan of a patient treated with aorto-uni-iliac endografting for ruptured abdominal aortic aneurysm.

Other variables i.e. patient age and general conditions, need to be individualized. In our view, it is reductive, at least in centres with considerable experience, to consider EVAR a procedure for patients unfit for surgery. As illustrated by our results and reports from experienced centres, EVAR is now a well-established technique, with a satisfactory outcome.

In nearly all reports on endoluminal repair there is the same claim, that there is insufficient follow-up to determine its performance in the long-term. This lack is considered by some as a good reason for excluding patients fit for surgery from endovascular treatment. In this regard, several issues need to be taken into account. 'Unfit for surgery' is a strict definition. It means that the patient is very sick and cannot tolerate surgery. Of course, everybody would agree that if this patient has to be treated for an abdominal aortic aneurysm, he should undergo endoluminal treatment. On the other hand 'fit for surgery' is a very broad definition. This includes patients in excellent health and eventually patients in poor clinical conditions, although expected to survive an operation.

It is our opinion, that a significant proportion of patients 'fit for surgery' may represent good candidates for the endovascular procedure. In the case, for example, of a 70-year-old man, with a 5.5 cm abdominal aortic aneurysm, suitable anatomy and no significant risk factors, if he is willing to attend follow-up sessions, why not attempt endovascular repair? He will most likely have a satisfactory technical outcome, a quick recovery, and no sexual dysfunction. In the worse case scenario, he might need to undergo a secondary procedure, yet, if he is followed by a reliable centre, there are very good chances that the secondary procedure will be carried out successfully before devastating complications occur. Some would argue that data in the long-term are not available, so this patient would be at risk of a scarce durability of the procedure. In our opinion the issue of durability, although certainly very important, should not be overemphasized.

We usually do not suggest EVAR in young patients. Mean age of our EVAR patients is 70 years. However, patients with abdominal aortic aneurysm have reduced life-expectancy: in the UK small aneurysm trial the 6-year survival rate of patients with abdominal aortic aneurysm between 40 and 55 mm was 64%, similar to the one reported by Hallett et al. (60% 5 years after repair for abdominal aortic aneurysm larger than 5 cm).[6,24] Surgery for abdominal aortic aneurysm is carried out in the majority of cases in old patients, and with careful follow-up, shortcomings related to durability of the graft can be avoided.

Another central issue, when recommending EVAR, is to make sure that the patient is treated by a surgeon and centre with sufficient experience. This is a good advice in all cases, but it is a mandatory condition for patients with good chances to survive the open operation. Despite the apparent simplicity of the procedure, it is now well known that these can become very complex and that problems are more likely to arise in the first stages of a learning curve. A recent report from the EUROSTAR registry shows that complications more likely to compromise technical success of EVAR and patient outcome (type I and type III endoleaks) are more frequent in centres where less than 30 implants have been performed.[25]

In summary, we believe that the available evidence is competitive enough that there is a justification to offer at least the possibility of endoluminal repair to low-risk patients. These should be informed of advantages and limitations of the technique and then decide which risks they would like to take.

Summary

- Published comparative studies between open repair and EVAR do not show any significant difference in mortality and morbidity rates in the early postoperative period.

- Reported mortality rates after EVAR in experienced centres range between 0.5 and 2%.

- Long-term reports are not available, but mid-term follow-up of EVAR showed incidence of reinterventions ranging between 10 and 20% and a rate of abdominal aortic aneurysms ruptures of 0.5–1.5%/year.

- In few studies do newer generation endografts show mid-term results better than open repair, but longer observations are needed.

- Based on the available evidence, endovascular treatment may be offered, with an individualized approach, to patients fit for surgery.

References

1. Scott RAP, Wilson NM, Ashton HA, Kay DN. Influence of screening on the incidence of ruptured abdominal aortic aneurysm: 5-year result of a randomized controlled study. *Br J Surg* 1995; 82: 1066-1070.

2. Hollier LH, Taylor LM, Ochsner J. Recommended indications for operative treatment of abdominal aortic aneurysms. Report of a subcommittee of the joint Council of the Society for Vascular Surgery and the North American Chapter of the International Society for Cardiovascular Surgery.

3. Ernst CB. Abdominal aortic aneurysms. *N Engl J Med* 1993; 328: 1167-1172.

4. Katz DJ, Stanley JC, Zelenock GB. Operative mortality rates for intact and ruptured aortic aneurysms in Michigan: an eleven-year statewide experience. *J Vasc Surg* 1994; 19: 804-817.

5. Kazmiers A, Jacobs L, Perkins A, Lindenauer SM, Bates E. Abdominal aortic aneurysm repair in Veterans Affairs medical centers. *J Vasc Surg* 1996; 23: 191-200.

6. The UK Small Aneurysm Trial Participants. Mortality results for randomized controlled trial of early elective surgery or ultrasonographic surveillance for small abdominal aortic aneurysm. *Lancet* 1998; 352: 1649-1655.

7. Lawrence PF, Gozak C, Bhirangi L *et al*. The epidemiology of surgically repaired aneurysms in the United States. *J Vasc Surg* 1999; 30: 632-640.

8. Johnston KW. Multicenter prospective study of nonruptured abdominal aortic aneurysm, part II: variables predicting morbidity and mortality. *J Vasc Surg* 1989; 9: 437-447.

9. Cambria RP, Brewster DC, Abbott WM *et al*. The impact of selective use of dipyridamole thallium scans and surgical factors on the current morbidity of aortic surgery. *J Vasc Surg* 1992; 15: 43-50.

10. Steyerberg EW, Kievit J, de Mol Van Otterloo JCA *et al*. Perioperative mortality of elective abdominal aortic aneurysm surgery: a clinical prediction rule based on literature and individual patient data. *Arch Intern Med* 1995; 155: 1998-2004.

11. Goldstone J, Brewster DC, Chaikof EL *et al*. for the EVT Investigators. Endoluminal repair versus standard open repair of abdominal aortic aneurysms: early results of a prospective clinical comparison trial. Proceedings of the 46th Scientific Meeting of the NA Chapter of the International Society for Cardiovascular Surgery; 1998 June; San Diego, Calif.

12. Zarins CK, White RA, Schwarten D *et al*. For the Investigators of the Medtronic AneuRx Multicenter Clinical Trial. AneuRx stent graft versus open surgical repair of abdominal aortic aneurysms: multicenter prospective clinical trial. *J Vasc Surg* 1999; 29: 292-308.

13. Beebe HG, Cronewett JL, Katzen BT, Brewster DC, Green RM for the Vanguard Endograft Trial Investigators. Results of an aortic endograft trial: impact of device failure beyond 12 months. *J Vasc Surg* 2001; 33: S55-63.

14. Brewster DC, Geller SC, Kaufman JA *et al*. Initial experience with endovascular aneurysm repair: comparison of early results with outcome of conventional open repair. *J Vasc Surg* 1998; 27: 992-1003.

15. Zarins CK, White RA, Fogarty TJ. Aneurysm rupture after endovascular repair using the AneuRx stent graft. *J Vasc Surg* 2000; 31: 960-970.

16. Harris PL, Vallabhaneni SR, Desgranges P *et al*. Incidence and risk factors of late rupture, conversion, and death after endovascular repair of infrarenal aortic aneurysms: the EUROSTAR experience. *J Vasc Surg* 2000; 32: 739-749.

17. Zarins CK, White RA, Moll FL *et al*. The AneuRx stent graft: four-year results and worldwide experience 2000. *J Vasc Surg* 2001; 33: S135-145.

18. Makaroun MS. The Ancure endografting system: an update. *J Vasc Surg* 2001; 33: S129-134.

19. May J, White GH, Waugh R *et al*. Improved survival after endoluminal repair with second generation prostheses compared with open repair in the treatment of abdominal aortic aneurysms: a 5-year concurrent comparison using life table method. *J Vasc Surg* 2001; 33: S21-26.

20. Zarins CK, Arko FR, Lee WA *et al*. Effectiveness of endovascular versus open repair in prevention of aneurysm related death. Proceedings of the 49th Scientific Meeting of the American Association for Vascular Surgery; 2001, June, Baltimore.

21. Zarins CK, White RA, Hodgson KJ, Schwarten D, Fogarty TJ for the AneuRx Clinical Investigators. Endoleak as a predictor of outcome following endovascular aneurysm repair: AneuRx multicenter clinical trial. *J Vasc Surg* 2000; 32: 90-107.

22. Schurink GWH, Aarts NJM, van Bockel JH. Endoleak after stent graft treatment of abdominal aortic aneurysm: a meta-analysis of clinical studies. *Br J Surg* 1999; 86: 581-587.

23. Resch T, Ivancev K, Lindh M *et al*. Persistent collateral perfusion of the abdominal aneurysm after endovascular repair does not lead to progressive change in aneurysm diameter. *J Vasc Surg* 1998; 28: 242-249.

24. Hallett JW Jr, Naessens JM, Ballard DJ. Early and late outcome of surgical repair for small abdominal aortic aneurysms: a population-based analysis. *J Vasc Surg* 1993; **18**: 684–691.
25. Van Marrewijk C, Buth J, Harris PL *et al.* Significance of endoleaks after endovascular repair of abdominal aortic aneurysms: the EUROSTAR experience. *J Vasc Surg* (in press).
26. May J, White GH, Yu W, Ly CN *et al.* Concurrent comparison of endoluminal versus open repair in the treatment of abdominal aortic aneurysms: Analysis of 303 patients by life table method. *J Vasc Surg* 1998; **27**: 213–221.
27. De Virgilio C, Bui H, Donayre C *et al.* Endovascular vs open abdominal aortic aneurysm repair. *Arch Surg* 1999; **134**: 947–951.

The main EVAR indication will be patients unfit for open repair

For the motion

Peter L Harris, Jacob Buth, Corine van Marrewijk, Robert Laheij

Introduction

The availability of endovascular aneurysm repair (EVAR) has altered the balance of risks for patients with abdominal aortic aneurysms. Minimal anaesthesia together with much reduced surgical trauma and, therefore, physiological stress has rendered patients operable who were previously considered inoperable due to serious co-morbidities.[1,2]

Concerns about the durability of endovascular repair are a justifiable cause for doubt about the appropriateness of EVAR for relatively fit patients with a long life expectancy but these concerns are of less relevance to many high-risk patients.

Clearly there is a case to be made for offering EVAR preferentially to those for whom major abdominal surgery or general anaesthesia are considered to carry excessive risk. The critical issues upon which this case depends are; a) does limited durability and the need for secondary intervention render EVAR less efficacious than open repair, in the long term, for good-risk patients? and b) can EVAR be expected to confer worthwhile prolongation of life in high-risk patients? These questions will be examined in this chapter.

Source of evidence

The EUROSTAR Registry Database

Details on the organization of the EUROSTAR Registry have been published previously.[3,4] The objective of this registry is to collect and analyse data from patients treated by EVAR in European centres of vascular surgery. The analyses in this chapter are based upon a cohort of 3075 patients operated upon between June 1996 and March 2001. In all, 101 centres were involved in treatment of the patients and procurement of the data. The type and number of different devices used are listed in Table 1. A standardized protocol for follow-up included contrast-enhanced computed tomography (CT) examinations at regular intervals in addition to clinical assessment. The mean duration of follow-up for the whole cohort of patients was 13 months with a range from 0 to 57 months.

Table 1. Devices used in patients registered on the EUROSTAR database

Vanguard (Boston Scientific)	910
AneuRx (Medtronic AVE)	794
Talent (World Medical & Medtronic AVE)	525
Zenith (Cook)	464
Excluder (Gore)	216
EVT/Ancure (Guidant)	65
Other	101

Evidence
Durability of EVAR

So far all devices intended for endovascular repair of aortic aneurysms have been constructed from fabric and metal stents in various combinations. While some types of construction have proved to be more robust than others, the potential for materials fatigue and frictional wear has been observed in most with a frequency that increases with time. Modular devices have shown a propensity for disengagement of the constituent parts. Furthermore, changing morphology of the aneurysm and the fixation sites in the neck and iliac arteries after operation tend to undermine fixation and seal progressively with time.

Figure 1, derived from EUROSTAR data, shows the cumulative rupture rate of aneurysms following EVAR.[4] Although much lower than the rate of rupture observed in untreated patients[5] there is a progressive increase with time after operation.

Multivariate analysis of the risk factors for rupture identifies only three that are statistically significant; 1) the last diameter measurement of the aneurysm (RR: 1.057), 2) mid-graft endoleak (RR: 7.5) and 3) stent/graft migration (RR: 5.3). Fixation site (type I) endoleak is a significant risk factor for rupture on univariate analysis but drops out on multivariate analysis indicating that late type I endoleaks are usually secondary to migration. Therefore, it can be seen that disintegration and migration of stent-grafts are the primary and as yet unresolved causes of treatment failure following EVAR.

The number of secondary interventions after EVAR (Fig. 2) gives a guide to the

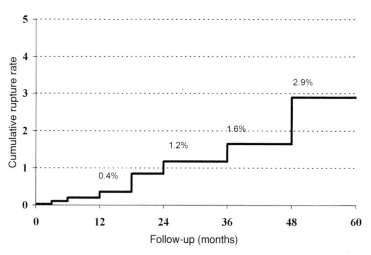

Figure 1. Cumulative aneurysm rupture rate following EVAR. EUROSTAR data.

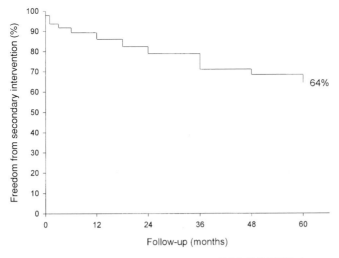

Figure 2. Cumulative rate of secondary intervention after EVAR. EUROSTAR data.

frequency of occurrence of adverse events that are considered to threaten the durability of EVAR. The annual rate in the EUROSTAR series is approximately 10% without any sign of reduction with time to date.

Figure 3 shows the classification of endoleaks after EVAR.

Classification of endoleak
Type Ia: proximal fixation site
Type Ib: distal fixation site
Type Ic: iliac occluder
Type IIa: inferior mesentric artery
Type IIb: lumbar artery
Type IIIa: disjunction of modular parts
Type IIIb: fabric tear
Type IV: fabric porosity (up to 30 days post-op only)

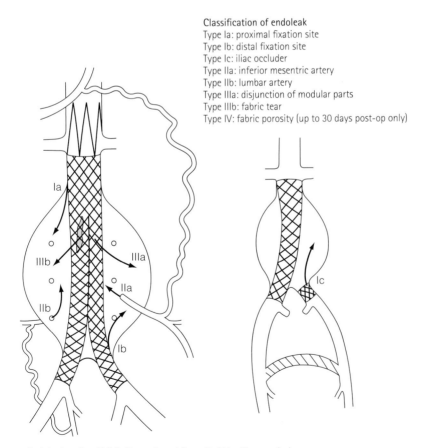

Figure 3. Endoleaks after EVAR. Reproduced from Ref 7 with permission.

The UK EVAR I randomized trial will, in due course, provide data comparing the outcome of open and endovascular repair of aortic aneurysms. Until the results of this trial are known it would be rational to conclude that open repair is a better option than EVAR for fit patients.

Survival of high–risk patients after EVAR[6]

If the risk of death from other causes far outweighs the risk of death from rupture of the aneurysm treatment of the aneurysm, by any method, could not be justified in the absence of symptoms. Probability of survival with or without treatment is the issue that will be addressed primarily in this section.

Risk stratification
Three groups of patients were identified for the purpose of analysis:

Group A (2525 patients)   Fit for major surgery and general anaesthesia.
Group B (399 patients)   Unfit for major surgery.
Group C (151 patients)   Unfit for general anaesthesia.

Fitness for surgery and anaesthesia was determined locally by criteria in current application in each centre. Comparison of age, gender, American Stroke Association (ASA) class and preoperative aneurysm diameter is shown in Table 2.

Table 2.   Comparison of age, gender, ASA class and aneurysm diameter in fit and unfit patients

	Fit	Unfit	
	Group A (2525 patients)	Surgery Group B (399 patients)	Anaesthesia Group C (151 patients)
Age (years)	71	72	73*
Male gender (%)	93	92	94
ASA class 3/4 (%)	50	82**	91***
AAA Diam. (mm)	56	58****	60*****

ASA: American Stroke Association. AAA: Abdominal aortic aneurysm.
*p=0.005; **p=0.001; ***p=0.001; ****p=0.002; *****p=0.0015.

Co-morbid conditions that were cited as reasons for patients being classified as 'high-risk' are listed, in order of frequency, in Table 3.

Table 3.   Co-morbid conditions cited as reasons for classification of patients as high-risk in order of frequency

Cardiovascular conditions
(Including cerebrovascular and heart transplant)
Pulmonary disease
Combined cardiac and pulmonary disease
Malignancies
'Hostile' abdomen and local anatomical factors
Specified general disorders
(e.g. chronic renal failure, rheumatoid arthritis)
Poor condition – non-specified general disorders
(e.g. ASA 4, old age)

ASA: American Stroke Association.

Perioperative risk of morbidity and mortality (Table 4)

There were significantly more device-related complications encountered during the operative procedure in groups B/C than in group A. Cardiac complications also occurred significantly more often in these groups than in group A. There were no differences between the groups with respect to early conversion.

The 30-day mortality rates were; 2.0% for group A, 4.8% for group B and 5.3% for group C (p=0.001). Significant variables correlating with death within 30 days were; groups B/C (open repair: 1.8), ASA 3/4 (open repair: 1.9), renal failure (open repair: 2.5) and age (open repair: 3.0).

Table 4. Perioperative risk of morbidity and mortality in fit and unfit patients

	Fit	Unfit	
	Group A (2525 patients)	Surgery Group B (399 patients)	Anaesthesia Group C (151 patients)
Device-related complications	7%	10%*	11%*
Cardiac complications	3%	8%**	10%**
Conversion	1.7%	1.5%	1.3%
Mortality	2.0%	4.8%***	5.3%***

*p=0.02; **p=0.001; ***p=0.001.

Late morbidity and mortality (Table 5)

There was no difference in the rates of late rupture and conversion between the three groups. However the cumulative rate of systemic complications in groups B/C was 25% at 3 years compared with 19% for group A (p=0.009).

Table 5. Late morbidity and mortality after EVAR in fit and unfit patients

	Fit	Unfit
	Group A (2525 patients)	Groups B/C (550 patients)
Conversions (%)	81(3.2)	13(1.5)
Rupture (%)	17(0.67)	3(0.54)
Systemic complication (%) (3-year cumulative rate)	19	25*
Survival (%) (3-year cumulative rate)	82.6	68.3**

*p=0.009; **p=0.0001.

The 3-year cumulative survival (Fig. 4) of patients in groups B/C was significantly lower than that of patients in group A at 68.3% compared with 82.6% (p=0.0001). Significant variables correlating with late death were; groups B/C (RR: 1.7), age (RR: 1.5), pulmonary disease (RR: 1.5), renal disease (RR: 1.6) and preoperative aneurysm diameter (RR: 1.7).

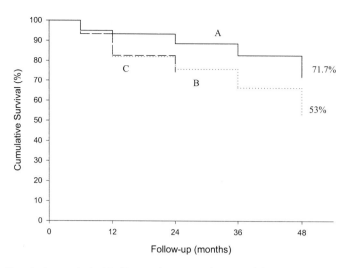

Figure 4. Cumulative survival of fit (Group A) and unfit (Groups B/C) patients after EVAR. EUROSTAR data.

Data–based analysis of mortality after EVAR

These data confirm expectations that both early and late mortality after EVAR are higher in high-risk patients than in those at 'normal' risk. At 3 years after operation the mortality rate for patients in the high-risk groups was 31.7% compared with 17.4% in the others.

It is hardly surprising that high-risk patients fare relatively badly after EVAR compared with patients who are considered to be 'good risk'. But this is not the critical issue. In this context, what matters is whether high-risk patients fare better with or without EVAR.

Four of a total of 83 deaths (4.8%) in groups B/C were aneurysm-related. The other causes of death were, in order of frequency; cardiac diseases 28, malignancy 10, stroke 7, pulmonary disease 8, miscellaneous causes 19 and unknown 7. What the EUROSTAR data do not tell us is how many aneurysm-related deaths were prevented by EVAR and whether this number was sufficient to make a significant difference to the prospects for survival of these groups of patients. The UK EVAR II randomized trial is expected to provide this information in time. Until the results of this trial are available it is necessary to rely to other methods of analysis to assess the likely impact of EVAR upon survival. The device we have employed is to compare the actual outcome following EVAR in high-patients registered with EUROSTAR with the predicted outcome theoretical group of comparable untreated patients.[6]

Theoretical model for prediction of survival in untreated high-risk patients: Comparison with observed survival of high-risk EUROSTAR patients

Taking the observed survival of high-risk EUROSTAR patients as a basis, the survival of a comparable group of untreated patients has been calculated by adding a correction for additional aneurysm-related deaths. An annual rupture rate of 11% for untreated aneurysms with a diameter >5mm was derived from the literature[5] and it was assumed that all patients who experienced rupture would have died from this rupture.

For details of the mathematical formula used to model the survival curve of this theoretical cohort of patients and the results of this study the reader is referred to our article published in the *Journal of Vascular Surgery.*[6]

Actual cumulative survival curves for the 550 EUROSTAR patients in groups B/C and the calculated survival curves in a theoretical comparable cohort of untreated patients are shown in Fig. 5. It can be seen that, in the early postoperative period any potential benefit associated with EVAR is outweighed by deaths related to the procedure. However, beyond 12 months after operation there is an increasing difference in survival in favour of the treated patients. After 2 years survival in the treated group was 75% compared with 63% in the untreated group.

From these data it can be concluded that EVAR can be expected to confer a significant survival advantage for high-risk patients with a life expectancy greater than 1 year. Review of the EUROSTAR database indicates that a substantial number of patients with abdominal aortic aneurysms and serious co-morbidities are able to benefit.

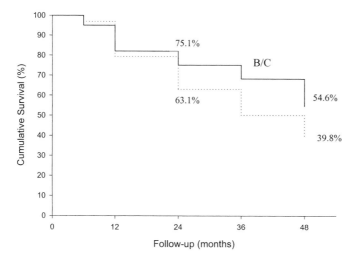

Figure 5. Cumulative survival curves of unfit patients treated by EVAR (Groups B/C) and of a theoretical comparable cohort of untreated patients.

Conclusions

1. Because the durability of endovascular aneurysm repair is limited open surgery is a better option for fit patients. EVAR is mainly indicated for high-risk patients.
2. Comparison between observed survival of EVAR treated high-risk patients and predicted survival of a theoretical comparable cohort of untreated patients demonstrates a significant survival advantage associated with treatment in patients with a life expectancy of 1 year or more.
3. The main indication for EVAR will be patients unfit for open repair.

Summary

- Durability of EVAR is a legitimate cause of concern in relation to the treatment of fit patients with a long life-expectancy.

- EUROSTAR data indicates that midgraft endoleaks and stent migration are the principle independent risk factors for rupture after EVAR. These events increase with time after operation.

- The rate of secondary intervention after EVAR exceeds 10% per annum and does not diminish with time.

- Improved performance of stent-graft must be demonstrated before EVAR can be considered the treatment of choice for fit patients.

- The 3-year cumulative survival rates of high and low-risk patients after EVAR are 68% and 83% respectively.

- The observed 2-year cumulative survival rate of high-risk patients afer EVAR is 63%.

- The predicted 2-year cumulative survival rate of a theoretical comparable cohort of untreated high-risk patients is 75%.

- EVAR confers a survival benefit in high-risk patients with a life expectancy of more than 1 year.

References

1. Chuter TAM, Reilly RM, Faruqi RM *et al.* Endovascular aneurysm repair in high-risk patients. *J Vasc Surg* 2000; **31**: 122–133.
2. Zanetti S, DeRango P, Parlani G *et al.* Endovascularabdominal aortic aneurysm repair in high risk patients: a single centre experience. *Eur J Vasc Endovasc Surg* 2001; **21**: 334–338.
3. Buth J, Laheij RJF. Early complications and endoleaks after endovascular abdominal aortic aneurysm repair: report of a multicentre study. *J Vasc Surg* 2000; **31**: 134–146.
4. Harris PL, Vallabhaneni SR, Desgranges P *et al.* Incidence and risk factors of late rupture, conversion and death after endovascular repair of infrarenal aortic aneurysms: the EUROSTAR experience. *J Vasc Surg* 2000; **32**: 739–749.
5. Reed WW, Hallett JW, Damiano MA, Ballard DJ. Learning from the last ultrasound. A population-based study of patients with abdominal aortic aneurysm. *Arch Int Med* 1997; **157**: 2064–2068.
6. Buth J, van Marrewijk C, Harris PL, Riambau V, Laheij RJK, on behalf of the EUROSTAR Collaborators. Outcome of endovascular abdominal aortic aneurysm repair in patients considered unfit for an open procedure: a report on the EUROSTAR experience. *J Vasc Surg* 2002 (in press).
7. Harris PL. Management of endoleaks and endotension. In *Vascular and Endovascular Surgical Techniques* 4th edn. Greenhalgh RM (ed). London: WB Saunders, 2001: 265–270.

The main EVAR indication will be patients unfit for open repair

Against the motion

Krassi Ivancev, Timothy Resch, Martin Malina,
Bjorn Sonesson, Bengt Lindblad

Introduction

The primary reason for treating aortic aneurysm is to prevent rupture and death from aneurysm rupture.[1] Open aneurysm repair with aneurysmorraphy and inlay graft placement (open repair) has been the gold standard of care since its introduction some 50 years ago. Endovascular aneurysm repair (EVAR) was introduced as a treatment alternative in 1991. As with all new treatment modalities, EVAR was used initially mainly for high risk patients deemed unsuitable for open repair.[2] However, encouraging results soon led to widening of criteria to include normal risk patients. At present no prospective, randomized study has been published comparing open repair and EVAR but such studies are underway in the United Kingdom. The following is a comparison based on published series comparing concurrent open repair and EVAR as well as data from non-comparative studies.

Evidence

Short-term results

Several studies have shown EVAR to lead to less blood loss, shorter intensive care as well as total hospital stay,[3-6] faster resumption of daily activities and speedier improvement of life quality postoperatively.[7] In most studies, no difference is seen in operative time or total cost. Treatments are similar with regard to operative 30-day mortality ranging from 2 to 8% (Table 1).

Table 1.   Studies comparing open repair (OR) and EVAR (all data are percentages)

	30 days		1 year		2 years		3 years		5 years	
	OR	EVAR	OR	EVAR	OR	EVAR	OR	EVAR	OR	EVAR
Moore[6]	3	2							72	65
May[8]	6	3					85	96		
Zarins[1]	0	2.6	97	96						
Beebe[4]	1.5	3.1	96	94	80	85				
Becquemin[3]	2.8	2.7	96	82						
Makaroun[5]	2.7	1.7	95	95			90	86		

EVAR: Endovascular aneurysm repair, OR: conventional open repair; 30-day presented as mortality, later follow-up presented as survival.

Mid– and long–term results

Since EVAR is a fairly new treatment option which has gone through rapid technical development, data on mid- and long-term results are largely lacking. As seen in Table 1,[1,3–6,8] results on survival seem to be comparative between EVAR and open repair in the range of 1–3 years. Scarce results from longer follow-up point in the same direction but are hard to interpret. The often rigorous follow-up that patients treated with EVAR are subjected to has led to the discovery of several procedure-specific complications: endoleaks, migration of endografts and endotension. These complications lead to secondary interventional or open procedures in many cases (Table 2)[1,3,4,6,8–11] subjecting patients to the risks that these interventions incur. However, as most secondary interventions are endovascular, the associated risks are low. Furthermore, the majority of these interventions are performed because of a perceived risk of subsequent stent-graft failure leading to thrombosis or aneurysm rupture. The actual clinical significance of most of these complications is unclear at the present time. Some cases of late aneurysm rupture after EVAR have been reported and there is a general agreement that an expanding aneurysm is at risk of rupture and should be treated endovascularly or by open conversion. By comparison, open repair also carries risk of late complications such as, anastomotic pseudoaneurysm, thrombosis, and infection in the range of 7%.[12] These complications are of a serious nature and often require major surgery.

Table 2.   Secondary interventions after EVAR

	Percent subjected to secondary procedure or conversion
Moore[6]	16%
May[9]	15–33% (2 years)
May[8]	18% (3 years)
Zarins[1]	12% (3 years)
Bequemin[3]	21% (1 year)
Beebe[4]	60% (2 years)
Hölzenbein[10]	22% (1.5 years)
Resch[11]	20% (2.5 years)

Numbers within parenthesis in right column indicate length of follow-up

Conclusions

Presently, most short- and mid-term results indicate that EVAR is a viable alternative to open repair in normal risk patients with suitable aneurysm anatomy. Many EVAR patients are subjected to secondary interventions during follow-up. However, in our experience, the number of such interventions seems to be diminishing with the introduction of new endografts, adequate patient selection and improved technical skills.[11] Long-term results are still lacking and therefore younger patients (life expectancy >20 years) should still primarily be considered for open repair. Given this exception, there is increasing evidence that EVAR should be the primary treatment alternative in patients with normal operative risk and suitable anatomy.

Summary

- EVAR has equally good or better short-term results than open repair of abdominal aortic aneurysms in normal surgical risk patients.

- Mid- and long-term results following EVAR show that the frequency of secondary interventions is higher than after open repair of abdominal aortic aneurysms.

- With improving technology and growing experience, EVAR has become a viable alternative to open repair in normal risk patients with suitable aneurysm anatomy.

- Randomized trial studies are needed to prove the superiority of EVAR over open repair.

References

1. Zarins CK, White RA *et al*. The AneuRx stent graft: four-year results and worldwide experience 2000. *J Vasc Surg* 2001; **33**(2 Suppl): S135–145.
2. Chuter TA, Reilly LM *et al*. Endovascular aneurysm repair in high-risk patients. *J Vasc Surg* 2000; **31**: 122–133.
3. Becquemin J, Bourriez A *et al*. Mid-term results of endovascular versus open repair for abdominal aortic aneurysm in patients anatomically suitable for endovascular repair. *Eur J Vasc Endovasc Surg* 2000; **19**: 656–661.
4. Beebe HG, Cronenwett JL *et al*. Results of an aortic endograft trial: impact of device failure beyond 12 months. *J Vasc Surg* 2001; **33**(2 Suppl): S55–63.
5. Makaroun MS. The Ancure endografting system: an update. *J Vasc Surg* 2001; **33**(2 Suppl): S129–134.
6. Moore WS, Kashyap VS *et al*. Abdominal aortic aneurysm: a 6-year comparison of endovascular versus transabdominal repair. *Ann Surg* 1999; **230**: 298–308.
7. Aquino RV, Jones MA *et al*. Quality of life assessment in patients undergoing endovascular or conventional abdominal aortic aneurysm repair. *J Endovasc Ther* 2001; **8**: 521–528.
8. May J, White GH *et al*. Improved survival after endoluminal repair with second-generation prostheses compared with open repair in the treatment of abdominal aortic aneurysms: a 5-year concurrent comparison using life table method. *J Vasc Surg* 2001; **33**(2 Suppl): S21–26.
9. May J, White GH *et al*. Comparison of first- and second-generation prostheses for endoluminal repair of abdominal aortic aneurysms: a 6-year study with life table analysis. *J Vasc Surg* 2000; **32**: 124–129.
10. Hölzenbein TJ, Kretschmer G *et al*. Midterm durability of abdominal aortic aneurysm endograft repair: a word of caution. *J Vasc Surg* 2001; **33**(2 Suppl): S46–54.
11. Resch T, Malina M *et al*. The impact of stent-graft development on outcome of abdominal aortic aneurysm repair – a 7 year experience. *Eur J Vasc Endovasc Surg* 2001; **22**: 233–238.
12. Hallett J, Marshall DM *et al*. Graft-related complications after abdominal aortic aneurysm repair: reassurance from a 36-year population-based experience. *J Vasc Surg* 1997; **25**: 277–284.

The main EVAR indication will be patients unfit for open repair

Charing Cross Editorial Comments towards Consensus

What a tremendous privilege to have Juan Parodi commence the argument supported by such able world leading experts as Jim May and Peter Harris. Then, an opposition by Ted Diethrich, Piergiogio Cao and Krassi Ivancev is awsome. Do we know where endovascular aneurysm repair will end up? Will it find a place eventually and prove to be durable and satisfactory? Will it be shown to be preferable to open repair? Will it be preferred for patients unfit for open repair? Will it be used for patients with rupture?

At the time of writing EVAR is struggling to find its place. It is likely, however, that the proof of its benefit will first emerge for ruptured aneurysm and the next possible proof is likely to come for patients unfit for open repair. The last area of certainty will be the alternative to open repair because open repair results are well established. In the UK Small Aneurysm Trial 50% of patients unfit for open repair were dead within 2 years. The question is whether EVAR can alter this mortality. Over a relatively short period of time it should be possible to answer the question. The EVAR trials in the UK are set up precisely for that purpose. EVAR I compares open repair with EVAR in fit patients whereas EVAR II compares best medical and EVAR against best medical alone. Vascular surgeons across Europe seem to prefer to use EVAR in the patients as an alternative to open repair. This is unlikely to be the area where proof of benefit of the procedure emerges first.

Will EVAR be shown to be of benefit in unfit patients? By now many of us have had the opportunity of performing endovascular repair under local anaesthetic and some have even performed the procedure percutaneously outside an operating theatre. The advances of the 1990s have been overwhelming. The question simply is whether endovascular repair significantly reduces death from rupture. Patients who are unfit for open repair are already old, fragile and at high risk of death as we have stated. We cannot assume that they are going to die of a ruptured aneurysm because many have a bad heart, bad chest and bad kidneys. Only if the death from ruptured aneurysm reduces all cause mortality sufficiently will EVAR be shown to be of value in this group. Time alone and the EVAR II trial will give us the answer.

Roger M Greenhalgh
Editor

EVAR will take over emergency abdominal aortic aneurysm rupture

For the motion

Jaap Buth, Neval Yilmaz,
Philippe WM Cuypers, Alexander V Tielbeek,
Luciën EM Duijm

Introduction

Rupture of an abdominal aortic aneurysm remains lethal despite rapid prehospital transport, early diagnosis, and resuscitations, expeditious surgical repair and progress in anaesthesia and intensive care. Mortality rates remain between 32% and 70% with significant associated morbidity.[1-5] Most centres quote rates near 50%.[6-8]

These high operative mortality rates reflect the magnitude of the physiological stress of patients following rupture. Haemorrhage, prolonged hypotension, laparotomy and prolonged lower limb ischaemia because of aortic clamping, all contribute to the risk of cardiac complications, multiple organ failure, and death. In addition, the patients are usually elderly and often have pre-existing co-morbidities.

Hypotension following rupture is often controlled at first by tamponade within the retroperitoneum, but the relaxation of the abdominal tone at induction of general anaesthesia often precipitates cardiovascular collapse. Exposure of the neck of the aneurysm together with the dissection through the haematoma causes disruption of retroperitoneal veins and small arteries, resulting in further haemorrhage that is often difficult to control in coagulopathic patients. In the presence of large retroperitoneal haematoma, the aorta is frequently clamped at the supracoeliac segment. This renders the viscera and lower extremities ischaemic, which contributes to the establishment of a fibrinolytic state,[9,10] and has a dramatic effect on cardiac afterload and lactic acid production. Subsequent reperfusion of the lower limbs add further physiologic injury. Secondary bleeding episodes and other complications, such as renal failure, adult respiratory distress syndrome, colonic and gall-bladder ischaemia are ultimately responsible for most of the deaths.

The excessive operative mortality also has important resource implications since most patients will spend many days in the intensive care unit before finally succumbing to the complications of rupture and emergency surgery.[11] In general patients who undergo open surgery represent a relatively favourable subset as a considerable number are not operated on at all because of significant co-morbid factors. These patients inevitably will die without a surgical option.[12]

Endovascular approach

Endovascular repair of ruptured abdominal aortic aneurysm offers the possibility of a significant reduction in operative mortality. This approach relies on the intravascular deployment of an aortic stent-graft, introduced via the femoral arteries to exclude the aneurysm from the circulation.[13,14] Laparotomy is avoided and the procedure can be performed under local anaesthesia. It is likely that the risk of turning a contained rupture into intraperitoneal haemorrhage by the induction of general anaesthesia would be significantly reduced. Additional blood loss due to opening of the retroperitoneal haematoma is avoided, while prolonged infra- or suprarenal aortic clamping is not necessary. Additionally, cardiac stress and duration of lower limb ischaemia will be minimized.

There is now ample evidence, that endovascular aortic repair (EVAR) is technically feasible and safe in patients scheduled for elective abdominal aortic aneurysm-repair.[15-18] In this chapter the organization of a programme to use EVAR for the treatment of patients with ruptured abdominal aortic aneurysm will be described and the initial clinical results reported.

Management protocol of EVAR in patients with ruptured abdominal aortic aneurysm in the Catharina Hospital

The Catharina Hospital in Eindhoven, The Netherlands, has considerable experience over the last 6 years with EVAR in elective abdominal aortic aneurysms. It was one of the first centers in The Netherlands, where the technique came into use and currently, this institution is a key contributor to the Dutch DREAM trial, in which elective EVAR is compared with open aneurysma repair.

The protocol of the management of ruptured abdominal aortic aneurysms allows for patients to be treated by a technique that is modified from the endovascular method used in elective abdominal aortic aneurysm. Under this protocol endovascular repair of ruptured abdominal aortic aneurysm is attempted on an 'intention-to-treat by EVAR' basis. An aorto-uni-iliac endograft system manufactured according to our specifications by Medtronic AVE-Talent, is used. There is a choice of four proximal and four distal device components to provide a 'few-grafts'fit-all system' (Fig. 1). This protocol came into effect in May 2001 after a number of patients with ruptured abdominal aortic aneurysm were treated with similar techniques as elective treated cases.

The management team comprises a vascular surgeon, and/or an interventional radiologist, an endovascular trained open repair-nurse, and a radiological technician. In addition, the full range of personnel is involved (e.g. anaesthesiologist, anaesthesiology nurses, Emergency Department personnel), as appropriate for the standard management of a ruptured abdominal aortic aneurysm.

The protocol involves all steps of the patient's management starting at arrival in the emergency ward. Once the diagnosis of ruptured abdominal aortic aneurysm is considered, fluid resuscitation is halted, allowing the systolic blood pressure of the patient to fall to below 100 or even 70 mmHg. Only systolic blood pressures below

70 mmHg or severe cardiac arrhythmia are indications to resume fluid and/or blood resuscitation. A computed tomography (CT)-scan using 30 ml contrast is swiftly made, the responsible surgeon being present during this examination. Immediate assessment of the aorto-iliac anatomy is made during the CT-examination (Fig. 2a). If the infrarenal neck appears suitable for EVAR and access via one of the iliac arteries seems possible, the operating room team is notified whether either open surgical or endovascular repair will be performed. Our aim is that the entire procedure of CT-scanning will take at most 15 minutes. This is the time that normally is needed to prepare an operating room for conventional emergency surgery from the time the initial diagnosis of ruptured abdominal aortic embolism has been made. Standard initial steps involve: establishment of high calibre peripheral venous accesses, blood samples for routine laboratory studies, cross-matching of blood group, urethral catheterization, and arranging 6 units of cross-matched blood.

All patients with symptomatic and ruptured abdominal aortic aneurysm are now managed by this schedule. Only patients, who would have been eligible for open emergency conventional surgery will be treated by this schedule. A previous decision not to operate electively is a contra-indication, as was the rule with conventional emergency surgery.

The procedure

The patient is transferred to the operating room. The operating table is to have its longest free-floating segment by the side of the head of the patient. Radial artery canulation for continuous blood pressure monitoring is performed by the anaesthesiologist. For fluid management in ruptured abdominal aortic aneurysm the rule of 'as little infusion as possible' is applicable. Increasing the circulating volume before aortic control is obtained can be detrimental by increasing the aneurysmal leak. Nitroprussid intravenously is often used to treat systolic blood pressures higher than 100 mgHg and Ketansin may be used to treat pain and anxiety.

One of the femoral arteries is exposed under local anaesthesia. An introducer sheath is used for canulation of the artery, and a Terumo-guidewire is introduced under fluoroscopic control, followed by a straight angiography catheter with multiple sideholes at the tip segment. Angiography is performed to visualize the level of the renal arteries (Fig. 2b). When no preoperative CT-scan is made, confirmation of the suitability of EVAR is obtained at this point on the basis of the angiogram. In the case of an inappropriate infrarenal neck a decision is taken to proceed with open surgical repair and general anaesthesia is induced. If the infrarenal neck is suitable for endograft sealing, a delivery system containing an appropriate proximal component of the aorto-uni-iliac device, is forwarded and deployed at the infrarenal position. The second component of the endovascular graft is then selected, introduced into the distal part of the first endograft, and deployed with its distal portion in a suitable segment of either the common or the external iliac artery. A completion angiogram is performed to confirm adequate sealing at the proximal and distal landing zones, and to check on the occurrence of endoleaks (Fig. 2c,d,e).

As in all patients who receive an aorto-uni-iliac-system, a femorofemoral bypass is performed. Before this final step general anaesthesia is induced. To obliterate the contralateral common iliac artery an 'occluder' (a closed stent-graft) is deployed. The operation is completed by closing the anastomoses and groin wounds. All patients are admitted to the intensive care unit, and are on artificial ventilation for at least 12 hours.

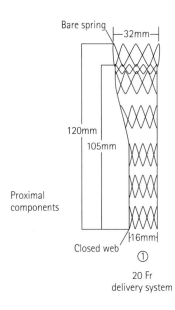

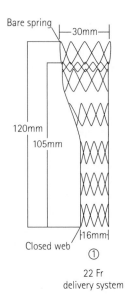

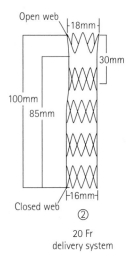

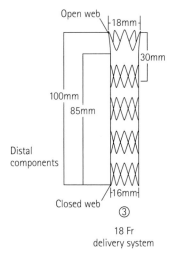

Figure 1.

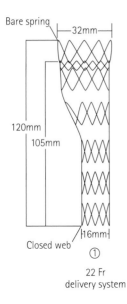

Bare spring
32mm
120mm
105mm
16mm
Closed web
①
22 Fr
delivery system

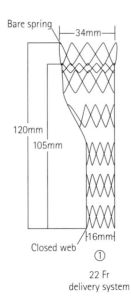

Bare spring
34mm
120mm
105mm
16mm
Closed web
①
22 Fr
delivery system

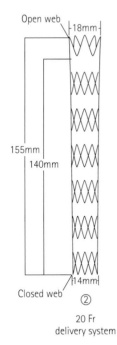

Open web
18mm
155mm
140mm
14mm
Closed web
②
20 Fr
delivery system

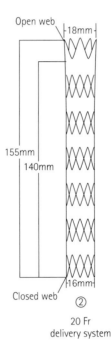

Open web
18mm
155mm
140mm
16mm
Closed web
②
20 Fr
delivery system

Figure 1 (*continued*). Endografts used for emergency treatment of ruptured abdominal aortic aneurysm. Upper row indicates proximal device components, and lower row distal device components. The two longer distal device limbs can be used in patients with associated common iliac aneurysms, as these will reach the external iliac artery for sealing.

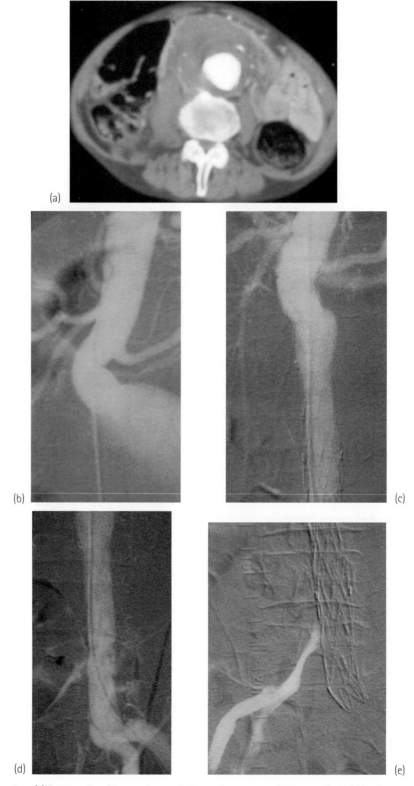

Figure 2. (a) Preoperative CT-scan demonstrates peri-aneurysmal extravasation of blood. (b) Intraoperative angiogram. (c, d and e) Completion angiogram demonstrates aorto-uni-iliac endograft to the left iliac artery and 'occluder' in the right common iliac artery.

Results in patients treated by emergency EVAR

A total of 16 patients with an acute presentation of their abdominal aortic aneurysm underwent EVAR between May 1999 and October 2001. The mean age of these patients was 73 years (range 56–89) 14 were male, and two were female. The diagnosis of ruptured abdominal aortic aneurysm was made on the basis of immediate CT-scanning, ultrasound, or the severity of clinical symptoms in 11 patients. Five patients were diagnosed as having a symptomatic but not ruptured abdominal aortic aneurysm. Ten of the patients were treated under the management protocol including intent-to-treat by EVAR, whereas six patients, treated before May 2001, were selected on the basis of availability of devices and the presence of a surgeon or radiologist experienced in EVAR. In seven patients the first part of the EVAR procedure was performed under local anaesthesia. These patients were treated under the management protocol. In three patients spinal anaesthesia was used and in the other patients general anaesthesia was used for the entire procedure. The endograft consisted of an aorto-uni-iliac device in five patients, a bifurcated endograft in nine, and a straight tube graft in two.

The Intensive Care Unit admission time was 2 days, and the total hospital stay was 14 days. There were three deaths during the first month, which equals 19% of the patient group with emergency EVAR, and 27% of the patients with rupture of their aneurysm. The causes of death were colon ischaemia in one patient, colon and small bowel ischaemia in another patient, and a myocardial infarction in the third patient. Other complications consisted of a large proximal endoleak in the first patient of this series. Treatment consisted of proximal banding by laparotomy. A second patient developed a cholecystitis requiring open cholecystectomy. A third patient required prolonged artificial ventilation because of a pneumonia due to aspiration.

Emergency EVAR compared with open repair

From January 1999 until October 2001 38 patients underwent open surgery for acute abdominal aortic aneurysm. The annual numbers of patients, treated by open surgery and by EVAR, are indicated in Fig. 3a. Of the patients with open surgery, 27 had rupture of their aneurysm, as documented at operation and in nine the aneurysm was symptomatic but not ruptured. Baseline characteristics of patients with open surgical treatment were comparable with patients who underwent emergency EVAR (Table 1). Significant differences were observed with regard to admission times in the Intensive Care Unit and in the hospital. The mortality rate was lower in patients treated by endovascular technique. However, limited group size precluded statistical comparison.

Table 1. Patients treated for acute abdominal aortic aneurysm (AAA) during a 3-year period.

	Endovascular AAA-repair 16 patients	Open AAA-repair 38 patients
Mean age (years)	73	73
Female	2 (12%)	6 (16%)
Preoperative shock	8 (50%)	20 (53%)
Aneurysm ruptured	11 (69%)	27 (71%)
Deaths within the first month	3 (19%)	10 (26%)
Mean operative blood loss (ml – range)	660 (100–1300)	3550 (300–>12 000)
Mean duration of operation (minutes – range)	176 (60–385)	237 (110–300)
Mean hospital stay (days)	14	18[a]
Mean Intensive Care Unit stay (days)	1	6[a]

Figures indicate patient numbers unless stated otherwise.
[a]Excluding values in patients with death within 3 days.

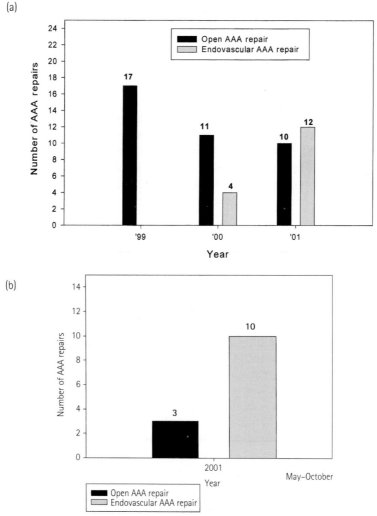

Figure 3. (a) Annual number of patients treated by open surgery and by EVAR. (b) Patients treated by open surgery and by EVAR during the recent 6 months under the management protocol. AAA: abdominal aortic aneurysm.

Emergency EVAR performed under 'management protocol'

The management protocol as described in the **Management Protocol** section (p. 182) was adopted and came into effect on 1 May 2001. During the 6 months period in which the management protocol was followed, 10 of 13 patients presenting with acute abdominal aortic aneurysm actually underwent emergency EVAR and three underwent open surgery (Fig. 3b). The reasons for open surgery in these three patients included unavailability of a matching device in two, and a short infrarenal neck filled with thrombus in one patient. Thus during a 6-month period 92% of our patients presenting with acute symptoms of an abdominal aortic aneurysm were suitable candidates for EVAR and this treatment was actually provided in 77%. During this period two patients died postoperatively (20% of patients with EVAR and 15% of the entire group).

Evidence

Endovascular repair of acute symptomatic or ruptured abdominal aortic aneurysm has received little attention compared with the immense interest in EVAR for elective abdominal aortic aneurysm. This is surprising, as the gain in overall survival and reduction of costs compared with open surgery might be relatively larger than in elective EVAR. The first report consisting of a case history appeared in 1994,[19] and more recently a couple of small patient series were described.[13,14] These studies had in common that prototype aorto-uni-iliac endografts, manufactured from standard arterial stents and conventional prosthetic materials were used. Aortic occlusion balloons introduced from the axillary artery were used to treat haemodynamic unstable patients. The early mortality was 16% in one series,[13] and in the other all three patients survived.[14]

In contrast, in the recent part of our series we have used commercially manufactured aorto-uni-iliac endografts, consisting of two components, one proximal and one distal device. The advantage compared with prototype endografts include technical ease and immediate availability without the need for preparation or sterilization. Compared with the use of the more elaborate bifurcated endograft system only one groin needs local infiltration anaesthesia. Perhaps most importantly, a rapid lowering of the intra-aneurysmal blood pressure and control of the intra-abdominal bleeding is achieved as the introduction of these aorto-uni-iliac devices can be performed quickly.

We have not used intra-aortic occlusion balloons in any of our patients. The introduction via an axillary cutdown and positioning in the suprarenal aorta consumes precious time, delaying the introduction and deployment of the aorto-uni-iliac device.

Preoperative CT-scanning appears quite useful for the preoperative decision whether endovascular treatment is feasible and for the assessment of anatomic dimensions. Prompt availability of CT facilities for emergency cases is essential for a successful management programme of emergency aneurysm repair. When CT examination cannot be performed because of hemodynamic instability of the patient the decision making is based on an initial intraoperative arteriogram using fluoroscopy.

The organization of a programme for management of acute abdominal aortic aneurysm by EVAR is not an easy undertaking. The general approach differs considerably from the customary care with conventional treatment. Important aims are to maintain a systolic blood pressure below 100 mmHg, to avoid general anaesthesia, and to relieve pain and anxiety. All medical and paramedical personal involved need to be instructed and supported. Perhaps the most complicated aspect is to arrange a permanent on rota call of specialists with experience in EVAR. We have been able to make this arrangement by including vascular surgeons and interventional radiologists and devising a scheme in which one of these specialists is always available for emergency treatment of abdominal aortic aneurysms.

Conclusion

Endovascular treatment of ruptured and acute symptomatic abdominal aortic aneurysms is a feasible option in most of the presenting patients. Initial experience with this approach was encouraging in that the operative mortality appeared lower than in patients treated in the same unit in the recent years with conventional surgical management. Organizational efforts are considerable, nevertheless essential for a successful set-up of a structured programme for the management of this disorder. If sufficient initial experience is obtained in a number of specialized centres, a randomized trial comparing open and endovascular repair of ruptured abdominal aortic aneurysms should be organized.

Summary

- Poor results of conventional open abdominal aortic aneurysm repair are the general experience since the beginning of operative treatment of ruptured aneurysms.

- EVAR has been quite successful in the elective management of non-symptomatic abdominal aortic aneurysm.

- The technique of EVAR can and should be adapted to emergency repair of acute symptomatic abdominal aortic aneurysm.

- Initial results have demonstrated markedly reduced early mortality rates.

- It is quite likely that open surgery for emergency abdominal aortic aneurysm will soon be replaced by EVAR.

References

1. Johansson G, Swedenborg J. Ruptured abdominal aortic aneurysms: a study of incidence and mortality. *Br J Surg* 1986; **73**: 101–103.
2. Johansen K, Kohler TR, Nicholls SC, Zierler RE, Clowes AW, Kazmers A. Ruptured abdominal aortic aneurysm: the Harbor view experience. *J Vasc Surg* 1991; **13**: 240–245.
3. Gloviczki P, Pairolero PC, Mucha PJ *et al*. Ruptured abdominal aortic aneurysms: repair should not be denied. *J Vasc Surg* 1992; **15**: 851–857.
4. Kniemeyer HW, Kessler T, Reber PU, Ris HB, Hakki H, Widmer MK. Treatment of ruptured abdominal aortic aneurysm, a permanent challenge or waste of resources? Prediction of outcome using a multi-organ disfunction score. *Eur J Vasc Endovasc Surg* 2000; **19**: 190–196.
5. Noel AA, Gloviczki P, Cherry KJ *et al*. Ruptured abdominal aortic aneurysms: the excessive mortality rate of conventional repair. *J Vasc Surg* 2001; **34**: 41–46.

6. Katz DJ, Stanley JC, Zelenock GB. Operative mortality rates for intact and ruptured abdominal aortic aneurysms in Michigan: An eleven-year state-wide experience. *J Vasc Surg* 1994; **19**: 804–817.

7. Kantonen I, Lepäntalo M, Brommels M *et al*. and the Finnvasc Study Group. Mortality in ruptured abdominal aortic aneurysms. *Eur J Vasc Endovasc Surg* 1999; **17**: 208–212.

8. Prance SE, Wilson YG, Cosgrove CM, Walker AJ, Wilkins DC, Ashley S. Ruptured abdominal aortic aneurysms: Selecting patients for surgery. *Eur J Vasc Endovasc Surg* 1999; **17**: 129–132.

9. Green RM, Ricotta JJ, Ouriel K *et al*. Results of supraceliac clamping in the difficult elective resection of infrarenal aortic aneurysms. *J Vasc Surg* 1989; **9**: 124–134.

10. Illig KA, Green RM, Ouriel K *et al*. Primary fibrinolysis during supraceliac aortic clamping. *J Vasc Surg* 1997; **25**: 244–251.

11. Van Ramshorst B, Van der Griend R, Eikelboom BC. Survival and quality of life after surgery for ruptured abdominal aneurysm. In *The Cause and Management of Aneurysms*. Greenhalgh RM, Mannick JA (eds). London: WB Saunders, 1990.

12. Bradbury AW, Makhdoomi KR, Adam DJ, Murie JA, Jenkins AMCL, Ruckley CV. Twelve-year experience of the management of ruptured abdominal aortic aneurysm. *BJS* 1997; **84**: 1705–1707.

13. Ohki T, Veith FJ, Sanchez LA, Cynamon J, Lipsitz EC, Wain RA *et al*. Endovascular graft repair of ruptured aortoiliac aneurysms. *J Am Coll Surg* 1999; **189**: 102–112.

14. Greenberg RK, Srivastava SD, Ouriel K *et al*. An endoluminal method of hemorrhage control and repair of ruptured abdominal aortic aneurysms. *J Endovasc Ther* 2000; **7**: 1–7.

15. Matsumara JS, Pearce WH. Early clinical results and studies of aortic aneurysm morphology after endovascular repair. *Surg Clin North Am* 1999; **79**: 529–540.

16. Zarins CK, White RA, Schwarten D, Kinney E, Diethrich EB, Hodgson KJ, Fogarty TH for the investigators of the Medtronic AneuRx Multicenter Clinical trial. *J Vasc Surg* 1999; **29**: 292–308.

17. Becquemin J-P, Lapie V, Favre J-P, Rousseau H for the French Vanguard Study Group. Mid-term results of a second generation bifurcated endovascular graft for abdominal aortic aneurysm repair: the French Vanguard trial. *J Vasc Surg* 1999; **30**: 209–218.

18. Cuypers Ph, Buth J, Harris PL, Gevers E, Laheij R. Realistic expectations for patients with stent-graft treatment of abdominal aortic aneurysms. Results of a European multicentre registry. *Eur J Vasc Endovasc Surg* 1999; **17**: 507–516.

19. Yusuf SW, Whitaker SC, Chuter TA *et al*. Emergency endovascular repair of leaking aortic aneurysm. *Lancet* 1994; **344**: 1645.

EVAR will take over emergency abdominal aortic aneurysm rupture

Against the motion

Wilhelm Sandmann, Tomas Pfeiffer

Introduction

The EUROSTAR Registry (European Collaborators on Stent-Graft Techniques for Aneurysm Repair), which was established in 1996 collects today in a prospective manner data to evaluate the technical success, the failure rates, the early and late complications of endovascular stent-graft repair of abdominal aortic aneurysm and analyses the type of complication with regard to the type of aneurysm treated and the type of graft being inserted. By November 2001, 3658 patients had been enrolled in the data base from over 100 centres.[1] Failure to treat was 7.2%, early mortality 2.5%, 12% of all deaths were abdominal aortic aneurysm-related and the risk of rupture showed not a linear but an exponential line amounting to 12.4% after 72 months. The same type of increasing risk over time appeared to be true for the conversion rate to open repair, amounting to 24% after 72 months. As all these patients were not treated on an emergency basis because of rupture, it can be expected, that endovascular aneurysm repair (EVAR) in the emergency case treated for rupture may produce results which are much inferior to the elective situation. The mortality for conversion procedures, which were performed for proximal type I endoleak, midgraft endoleak, type II endoleak, distal type I endoleak, stent-graft migration, kinked endograft, thrombosed/stenosed endograft was found to be 18% perioperatively in an earlier series of EUROSTAR.[2] The freedom from death and secondary intervention after 60 months was below 50%. These figures have led to a recent publication in the *British Journal of Surgery*, which resulted in the conclusion, that endovascular repair for abdominal aortic aneurysm (based on data from elective cases!) has been a failed experiment.[3]

In contrast, the perioperative mortality after conventional open repair in the elective case can be lowered to 1.2–1.54%[4,5] and in most of the series does not exceed 3% in publications from major centres, although the published series report on patients being treated at or before the time endovascular repair was initiated. Even in patients undergoing simultaneous renal artery reconstruction for renal artery occlusive disease and conventional treatment of abdominal aortic aneurysm perioperative mortality was kept below 1.5%.[6] In a report summarizing the experiences of veterans administration medical affair centres, which are not supposed to be centres of excellence, hospital mortality rates were 4.86% after repair of non-ruptured abdominal aortic aneurysm.[7]

One has to admit, that in teaching hospitals, in which conventional abdominal aortic aneurysm repair is not exclusively performed by vascular surgeons, mortality rates can be substantially higher, especially if historical series of patients are evaluated and reach nearly 7% for non-ruptured cases. However, subsequent operative procedures were required in only 8%, which is far below endovascular series.[8] Graft-related complications in a 36-year population-based series occurred in only 9.4% of the patients, although not only intact but also ruptured types of aneurysms were included.[9] An argument often used by the promotors of endovascular stent-graft management relates to the general health status of the patients. However, the annual report 2000 of the Committee for Quality Assurance of the German Society for Vascular Surgery[10] showed, that the percentage of patients belonging to the various groups of American Stroke Association (ASA) classification does not show evidence, that the sicker patients are managed by the endovascular route and there seems to be a strong tendency to treat more patients with smaller aneurysms with a stent-graft, obviously because in smaller aneurysms endografts have a lesser tendency to migrate, kink or leak, due to longer and less dilated proximal necks.[11] It is noteworthy, that conventional surgery replaces only the diseased segment of the aorta in patients with abdominal aortic aneurysm while endovascular treatment needs to be carried out either with a bifurcated graft or an aorto-monoiliac graft combined with conventional crossover femorofemoral graft. Not unfrequently the internal iliac arteries become occluded accidentally or are intentionally overstented, thus leading to buttock claudication, erectile impotence and large bowel ischaemia.

The ruptured case

A great number of publications exist concerning conventional open repair for ruptured cases. The leading cause of death is haemodynamic shock from bleeding.[12-15] The presence of iliac artery aneurysms requiring a bifurcation graft seems to increase operative mortality as well, although from the publications it cannot be concluded, whether an aorto-bi-iliac interposition graft maintaining hypogastric circulation or

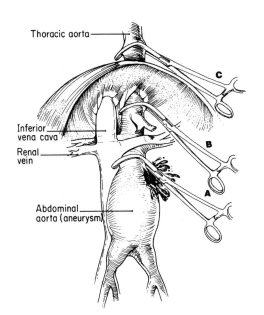

Thoracic aorta

Inferior vena cava

Renal vein

Abdominal aorta (aneurysm)

Figure 1. Diagram depicting a ruptured abdominal aortic aneurysm below the renal arteries. The bleeding from the ruptured aneurysm can be controlled at three levels : (A) just below the renal vessels, which is the most common site of control; (B) below the diaphragm and just above the coeliac axis; and (C) in the lower portion of the thoracic aorta through a thoracotomy.

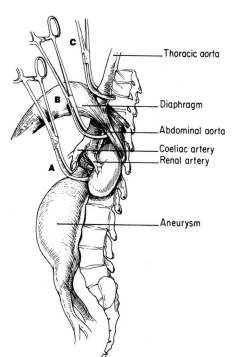

Thoracic aorta

Diaphragm

Abdominal aorta

Coeliac artery

Renal artery

Aneurysm

Figure 2. Lateral view of the abdominal aneurysm, indicating three clamps in position similar to those described in Fig. 1: (A) below the renal vessels, (B) below the diaphragm and above the coeliac artery, and (C) at the distal end of the thoracic aorta.

an aorto-bifemoral graft combined with ligation of the iliac arteries and often compromising blood flow to the hypogastric area has been performed. The 30-day mortality rates vary substantially (24%[9] to 57%[15]) and are reported to be as high as 80% in countries with necessity of long-distance transportation to the next centre.[16,17] However, in major centres with long-standing experienced, vascular surgeons performing the operation exclusively and a well organized transportation system, 30-day mortality rates near to 33% seem to be normally achievable.[5,13,18]

The treatment of ruptured abdominal aortic aneurysm by the endovascular method has evolved only recently. There are only a few publications, which report with one exception only on single cases.[19–22] Especially the group from the Montefiore Hospital in New York has obtained convincing results leading to only two deaths out of 25 patients treated and the mean hospital stay lasted only 6 days.

Evidence

Open repair of abdominal aortic aneurysm is a well mastered technique, but requires an experienced team in the presence of rupture, because operative techniques may very substantially. Blood volume replacement has to be carefully avoided before the surgeon has gained control over the aorta. Especially if the surgeon is hasty and nervous, control of bleeding is not always easy. The levels of clamp position can be near to the diaphragm, above the renal arteries or juxtarenal.[22,23] All preparations of the patient should be performed in the operating room and the surgical team must be ready whether scrubbed or wearing two pairs of gloves while anaesthesia is commenced. The moment medication for muscle relaxation is injected intravenously the abdomen must be entered quickly and in case of instability from continuous

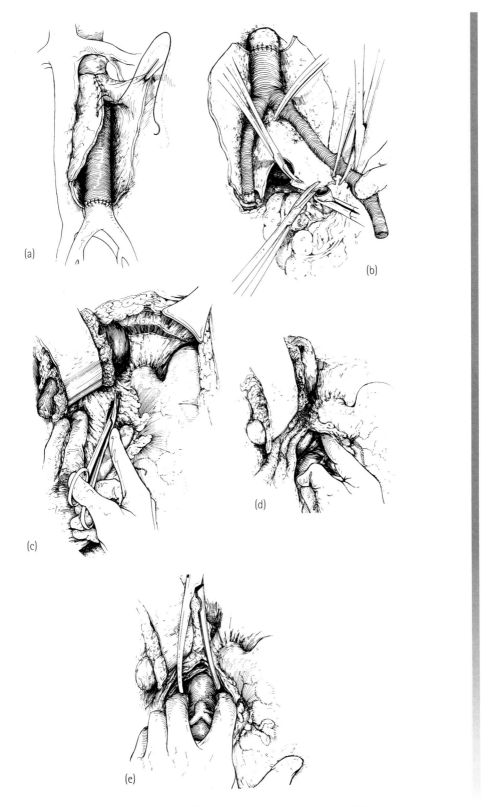

(a)

(b)

(c)

(d)

(e)

Figure 3a–e. Operative techniques for repairing abdominal aortic aneurysm and iliac aneurysm. Reproduced with permission from Ref. 24.

bleeding, immediate control of the aorta is obtained by occluding the subdiaphragmatic aorta with the surgeon's hand. Once this has been established the next steps can follow without rush. The haematoma is only evacuated as much as sight or touch control of the aorta is concerned to place the aortic clamp as far distally as possible. After entering the aneurysm sack, back-bleeding from the iliac arteries can be controlled by the use of balloon catheter. Except in cases with rupture into adjacent organs (inferior vena cava, duodenum, urinary bladder) the technique is pretty much the same as in non-ruptured cases.

Volume is replaced while the graft is attached by running sutures. Heparine is given intravenously in smaller doses and should be partially reversed after the clamp is taken off to release blood flow. As those patients are very sensitive concerning myocardial function blood flow should be released gradually and separately in each iliac artery. There should be no cosmetic replacement of the iliac arteries. Only in cases with significant iliac aneurysms, which if left unreconstructed would leave the patient in substantial danger for another impending rupture, should a bifurcation interposition graft be implanted. The coagulopathy is managed with fresh frozen plasma, red cells and platelets. Urine output must be monitored and stimulated by furosemid and cristalloides. Finally the circulation of the distal colon, sigmoid and rectum is checked and if in doubt, the inferior mesenteric artery is reimplanted quite liberally. In experienced hands the operating time can be much shorter than in the elective case, because the haematoma has prepared the route for surgical dissection already. Even in patients developing profound shock, while in the hospital and on the way to the operating theatre, surgical results can be astonishingly good. The role of the anaesthesiologist in the ruptured case is much more important for the outcome than in elective cases and not only must the vascular surgeon be readily available but also the experienced anaesthesiologist. In close collaboration and by frequent control of electrolytes, blood gases and coagulation the mortality rate can be reduced to 10–20%. However, unofficial critical remarks concerning superior results often express doubt that the aneurysm has really ruptured and assume a selection bias either caused by the referring physician or by the distance the patient had to be transported. In other words, only the stable patients might have reached the hospital and therefore survived. There is no doubt, that on one side the percentage of patients developing a ruptured abdominal aortic aneurysm has decreased during the last 10 years, because elective surgery is performed much more frequently and on the other side, experience in performing surgery for abdominal aortic aneurysm has increased leading to better results in emergency cases.[22,23]

Good experience in ruptured abdominal aortic aneurysm patients emphasizes that the more one is able to simplify the operative steps, the more one concentrates on what is really necessary and the better will be the results. It has to be pointed out, that the diagnosis in most cases can be established by clinical means. Sometimes, a duplex scan performed near to or in the operating theatre may be necessary and computed tomography (CT)-scanning may be not only unnecessary but will also put the patient in danger because it is usually located far away from the surgical area. Intravenous injection of contrast material in patients with hypoperfusion of the kidneys impairs renal function.

The above described procedures have never been evaluated in modern terms of evidence, but are evident in themselves.

The endovascular treatment seems to be very elegant at first view. Control of bleeding and rebleeding can be obtained by a simple balloon catheter guided by fluoroscopic control. When the balloon catheter is in place, time is gained to prepare the endovascular equipment, because the patient is safe. There must be either a large variety of stent-grafts, catheters and guidewires readily available to allow immediate placement of the stent-graft or a one-fits-most type of graft can be used. The decision-making process requires CT-scanning and other imaging methods using contrast material to find out whether the patient's anatomy and the type of aneurysm allow endovascular grafting, while open repair is promptly feasible. Only in centres where large numbers of stent-grafts are placed, may endovascular stent-graft repair for ruptured abdominal aortic aneurysm be considered an option.

In the recent report of Ohki and Veith[21] it remains uncertain, how many patients were attempted for endovascular stent-graft repair and how many died while in the preparation process. The decision-making process as to which patient can undergo endovascular graft repair and who should immediately being brought to the operating theatre remains unclear. Just as superior results of open repair have been criticized by selection bias, it may be questioned, how much instability and leaking really occurs in the individual patient treated with stent-graft repair. The surgeon performing open surgery experiences from time to time on patients who have developed rupture several hours or even days earlier and remain very stable unless some overactive conservative treatment for anaemia was initiated. So in order to assess the value of the endovascular approach for ruptured abdominal aortic aneurysm we must know more details of the patient material. This will give us the possibility of putting the exciting news in the right perspective. As the results of endovascular stent-graft repair for elective treatment of abdominal aortic aneurysm have been worse than has been advertised by enthusiasts in the past a healthy scepticism may be justified for patients with ruptured abdominal aortic aneurysm as well. But if the principle of endovascular stent-graft repair continues to produce good results for the majority of patients and if it is primarily understood as a bridging procedure, then it will save several patients' lives. It should, however, be made public, what is the financial interest of the advocators, because many of the promoters of the endovascular stent-grafting have either fruitful contracts with the companies, which produce the stent-grafts and the adjuncts, or are co-owners themselves.

Summary

- EUROSTAR data illustrate that more patients with abdominal aortic aneurysm are technically inoperable compared with open conventional repair.

- Early and late complication rates after EVAR for abdominal aortic aneurysm are substantially higher than after open conventional repair.

- Durability of EVAR and freedom from death and secondary intervention is substantially smaller than with open conventional repair.

- The treatment of ruptured abdominal aortic aneurysm by the conventional open method has made substantial progress in recent years although even in very experienced centres mortality could not be reduced below 20% and shock from bleeding and the presence of iliac artery aneurysms requiring a bifurcation graft remain the major determinants for postoperative deaths.

- The few publications on endovascular stent-graft repair for ruptured abdominal aortic aneurysm are fascinating but at the moment it remains undefined, which patients can undergo this type of treatment.

- One suspects that ruptured abdominal aortic aneurysm patients must be very carefully selected to be good candidates for EVAR.

- Only in centres with a high volume of EVAR for abdominal aortic aneurysm would a patient with a ruptured aneurysm of this type have a chance to survive by this technique.

- At the moment the routine treatment for ruptured abdominal aortic aneurysm remains open conventional repair in experienced hands and EVAR is at best a clinical experiment in the selected patient with stable haemodynamic conditions.

References

1. Harris P. Incidence of early and late complications in aortic endovascular grafts presented at the Northwestern University of Illinois Symposium. *Adv Vasc Surg*, 12–14 Nov. 2001.
2. Cypers PW, Lahej RJ, Buth J. Which factors increase the risk of conversion to open surgery following endovascular abdominal aortic aneurysm repair? EUROSTAR Collaborators. *Eur J Vasc Endovasc Surg* 2000; **20**: 183–189.
3. Collin J, Murie JA. Endovascular treatment of abdominal aortic aneurysm: a failed experiment. *Br J Surg* 2001; **88**: 1281–1281.
4. Pfeiffer T, Reiher L, Grabitz K, Sandmann W. Results of conventional surgical therapy for abdominal aortic aneurysms since the beginning of the 'endovascular era'. *Chirurg* 2000; **71**: 72–79.
5. Stühmeier KD, Mainzer B, van Poppelen R, Rossaint R, Kniemeyer HW. Abdominal aortic aneurysm – is a conservative attitude still justified? Experiences with 56 emergency and 128 elective surgical patients from the anesthesiological and vascular surgery viewpoints. *Dtsch Med Wochenschr* 1987; **122**: 1930–1935.
6. Sandmann W, Grabitz K, Pfeiffer T, Ritter R. Extrathoracic reconstruction of aortic arch branches. In *Long-Term Results of Arterial Interventions*. Brancherau A, Jacobs M (eds). New York: Futura Publishing, 1997; 89–96.
7. Kazmers A, Jacobs L, Perkins A, Lindenauer SM, Bates E. Abdominal aortic aneurysm repair in Veterans Affair Medical centres. *J Vasc Surg* 1996; **23**: 191–200.
8. Sayors RD, Thompson MM, Nasim A *et al*. Surgical management of 671 abdominal aortic aneurysms: a 13-year review from a single centre. *Eur J Vasc Endovasc Surg* 1997; **13**: 322–327.
9. Hallett JW, Marshall DM, Petterson TM *et al*. Graft related complications after abdominal aortic repair: reassurance from a 36-year population – based experience. *J Vasc Surg* 1997; **25**: 277–284.
10. Umscheid T, Eckstein HH, Noppeney T, Weber H, Niedermeier, HP. Quality management 'infrarenal aortic aneurysms' of the German Society of Vascular Surgery – results 2000. *Gefäßchirurgie* 2001; **6**: 194–200.
11. Sasaki S, Sakuma M, Samjima M *et al*. Ruptured abdominal aortic aneurysms: analyses of factors influencing surgical results in 184 patients. *J Cardiovasc Surg* 1999; **40**: 401–405.
12. van Dongen HP, Leusink JA, Moll FL, Brons FM, de Boer A. Ruptured abdominal aortic aneurysms: factors influencing postoperative mortality and large term survival. *Eur J Vasc Endovasc Surg* 1998; **15**: 62–66.
13. Dardik A, Burleysan GP, Bowman H *et al*. Surgical repair of ruptured abdominal aortic aneurysms in the State of Maryland: factors influencing ourcome among 527 recent cases. *J Vasc Surg* 1998; **28**: 413–420.
14. Koskas F, Kieffer E. Surgery for ruptured abdominal aortic aneurysm: early and late results of a prospective study by the AURCIN 1989. *Ann Vasc Surg* 1997; **11**: 90–99.
15. Semmens JB, Norman PE, Lawrence-Brown MM, Holman CD. Influence of gender on outcome from ruptured abdominal aortic aneurysm. *Br J Surg* 2000; **87**: 191–194.
16. Kantonen I, Lepantalo M, Brommels M *et al*. Mortality in ruptured abdominal aortic aneurysms. The Finn Vasc Study Group. *Eur J Vasc Endovasc Surg* 1999; **17**: 208–212.
17. Kniemeyer HW, Kessler T, Reber PU, Ris HB, Widmer MK. Treatment of ruptured abdominal aortic aneurysm, a permanent challenge or a waste of resources? Prediction of outcome using a multiorgan dysfunction score. *Eur J Vasc Endovasc Surg* 2000; **19**: 190–196.
18. Greenberg RK, Srivasta SD, Ouriel K, Waldman D, Ivancev K, Illig KA *et al*. An endoluminal method control and repair of ruptured abdominal aortic aneurysms. *J Endovasc Ther* 2000; **7**: 1–7.

19. Lachat M, Pfammatter T, Bernhard E *et al*. Successful endovascular repair of a leaking abdominal aortic aneurysm under local anaesthesia. *Swiss Surg* 2001; 7: 86–89.
20. Umscheid T, Stelter WJ. Endovascular treatment of an aortic aneurysm ruptured into the inferior vena cava. *J Endovasc Ther* 2000; 7: 31–35.
21. Ohki T, Veith FJ. Endovascular grafts and other catheter based adjuncts to improve the treatment of ruptured aorto-iliac aneurysms. *Ann Surg* 2000; 232: 466–479.
22. Chen JC, Hildebrand HD, Salvian AJ, Hsiang YN, Taylor DC. Progress in abdominal aortic aneurysm surgery: four decades of experience at a teaching center. *Cardiovasc Surg* 1997; 5: 150–156.
23. O'Dwyer ST, McCollum CN. A policy for ruptured abdominal aortic aneurysms. In *Emergency Vascular Surgery*. Greenhalgh RM, Hollier LH (eds). London: WB Saunders 1992; 183–191.
24. Mannick JA, Whittemore AD. Abdominal aortic aneurysms. In *Vascular and Endovascular Surgical Techniques* 4th edn. Greenhalgh RM (ed). London: WB Saunders, 2001; 131–138.

EVAR will take over emergency abdominal aortic aneurysm rupture

For the motion
BR Hopkinson, RJ Hinchliffe

Introduction

Time for a new approach

The incidence of ruptured abdominal aortic aneurysms is increasing.[1] In the UK they account for 10 000 deaths per year.[2]

Mortality from elective repair of abdominal aortic aneurysm has improved significantly in the past two decades in line with advances in anaesthetic and critical care. These improvements have not been mirrored in ruptured aneurysms where the mortality remains excessive (in the region of 50%).[3] Similarly the surgical technique has remained essentially unaltered from that which was described by Creech in the 1950s.[4]

A national screening programme would appear appropriate and has been shown to reduce mortality in observational studies.[5] At present screening appears unlikely to be adopted on a national basis. Consequently any improvements in outcome need to be met by altered surgical activity.

Endovascular aneurysm repair (EVAR) was introduced over a decade ago. There have been a number of criticisms of this technique, in particular its durability. However, in cases of ruptured abdominal aortic aneurysm perioperative mortality is the salient outcome. The reduced physiological stress associated with the endovascular method would appear to be a desirable component in critically ill patients. The questions of durability are to be regarded of lesser importance.

The feasibility of endovascular repair of ruptured abdominal aortic aneurysm was first reported in 1994.[6] Since then the technique has been used in an estimated 50

Table 1. Published and presented results of endovascular repair of ruptured abdominal aortic aneurysm

Centre	Numbers treated	High risk for open repair	Perioperative mortality
New York[19]	12	12	2 (16%)
Cleveland[20]	3	3	0 (0%)
Zurich[21]	17	N/A	1 (6%)
Nottingham[22]	20	8	9 (45%)

centres in Europe and elsewhere. Published reports have been restricted to a number of highly selected patients with rupture but have also included aorto-caval and enteric fistula.

Consequently the evidence for endovascular repair of ruptured abdominal aortic aneurysm is limited. Lessons learned from feasibility studies, similarities in patients with thoracic aneurysm rupture and parallels drawn from elective repair constitute the horizons of our knowledge and understanding.

Preoperative factors

Concerns have been expressed regarding the delay involved in preparing patients for endovascular repair in the emergency setting. These concerns must, however, be taken in context.

1. Patients who are unstable, hypotensive or are rushed to theatre for open repair are widely regarded to have a poor prognosis.
2. It is known that 80% of patients will survive 6 hours following onset of symptoms.[7]
3. Mean time of survival on reaching hospital with ruptured abdominal aortic aneurysm is 8 hours.[8]
4. The centralization of vascular services in the UK, along with the realization that specialist units have improved outcome is likely to increase the preoperative delay for the majority of patients.
5. UK surgeons overwhelmingly prefer patients to undergo a period of observation when the decision to operate has been taken. Only one-third of surgeons pursue a policy of immediate patient transfer to the operating theatre.[9]

The reasons for preoperative delay

Accurate imaging
Computerized tomography (CT) is a useful investigation in all patients with suspected ruptured abdominal aortic aneurysm (confirms diagnosis, shows extent of aneurysm and excludes a number of other causes of the acute abdomen). A proportion of patients with suspected ruptured abdominal aortic aneurysm already undergoes CT. Accurate assessment of aneurysm morphology is vital.

Graft manufacture
Grafts must be rapidly available, ideally as an 'off-the-shelf' item. Initial experiences were a 'luck of the draw' scenario. Patients happened to fit an available endovascular graft.

Endograft design has progressed to suturing a variety of top and bottom ends of a uni-iliac endograft on table to create some customization.

Alternatively pre-expanded polytetrafluoroethylene (PTFE) grafts with balloon expandable stents allowing intraoperative length accommodation have been used.

Factors which reduce preoperative delay

1. Increased availability of CT (in Accident and Emergency Departments).
2. The use of pre-expanded PTFE grafts and balloon expandable stents may obviate the need for preoperative imaging.

3. Improved intraoperative imaging (combined angiography/intravascular ultrasound).
4. Availability of 'off-the-shelf' grafts or 'home-made' devices.

Does preoperative delay really affect outcome?

Preoperative delay does not necessarily prejudice outcome.[10] Transfer of more stable patients to theatre is associated with improved outcome. Whether the morbidity related to the endovascular technique and its time delay ('a trial by CT') outweigh open repair and its sequelae remains to be seen.

Patient selection

Medical fitness

In the UK vascular surgeons operate on ruptured abdominal aortic aneurysm selectively.[9] In Wales 43% of patients reaching hospital alive do not receive an operation.[11]

Our ability to predict those patients who will survive ruptured abdominal aortic aneurysm is limited. Current evidence is based on physiological parameters and investigations (which may not be available in patients who are transferred rapidly to the operating theatre) on patients undergoing open repair.[12] These scoring systems remain unproven in patients undergoing endovascular repair.

The majority of the feasibility studies of endovascular repair of ruptured abdominal aortic aneurysm have been performed in patients who were declared as being at high risk of open repair; or in whom endovascular repair was undertaken on compassionate grounds (there have been successes in both these patient groups).

Endovascular repair may offer some hope for medically high-risk patients, including those turned down for open repair. There are even reports of success where open repair has failed.

Aneurysm morphology

Around 60% of aneurysms are ideally suited for endovascular stent-grafts in the elective setting. This figure varies slightly, dependent upon the type of graft used and the experience of the surgeon.

Whether the proportion of ruptured abdominal aortic aneurysms treatable by the endovascular method will differ significantly from those seen electively is unknown. Importantly there is no clear relationship between size of aneurysm and suitability for endovascular repair.[13]

Increasing the applicability – recent advances

It is now possible to treat aneurysms previously thought untreatable by the endovascular method (due to experience, improved graft carriers, improved stents and ancillary techniques such as Palmaz stents).

Unilateral internal iliac artery occlusion to incorporate common iliac artery aneurysms can be performed with relative impunity.

Successful exclusion of ruptured abdominal aortic aneurysms has been achieved in patients who do not have 'ideal' morphology. Immediate seal to prevent on-going haemorrhage is imperative but durability of the exclusion is of lesser importance.

Current endovascular graft options

Graft configuration

1. Aorto–aortic: rapidly deployed, low applicability.
2. Bifurcated: more 'physiological'; delay to haemorrhage control.
3. Aorto-uni-iliac: the most accommodating; rapid deployment.

Uni-iliac endografts accommodate a wide range of iliac artery morphology and allow rapid control of haemorrhage. They are currently the 'best buy'.

An estimated 750 grafts would be required to cover most eventualities.[14] This problem is circumnavigated by:

1. Manufacture of 'home-made' stent-grafts.
2. Expeditious delivery of commercially available stent-grafts.
3. Expanded PTFE graft with a proximal balloon expandable stent. Balloon inflation allows intraoperative customization to required neck diameter. Length accommodation is dealt with by suturing the graft distally in to the external iliac artery or the common femoral artery.
4. Modular uni-iliac endograft. A variety of proximal and distal sizes to accommodate the landing zones (aortic neck and iliac arteries). 'Tromboning' of the modular components facilitates length accommodation (BiFab system, Cook Europe: Fig. 1).

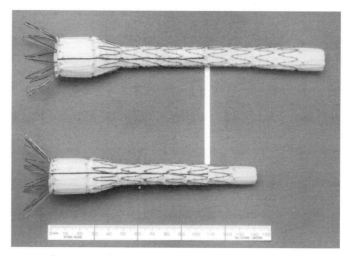

Figure 1. The BiFab (Cook Europe) aorto-uni-iliac modular endovascular stent-graft.

Intraoperative factors

Physiological

Ruptured abdominal aortic aneurysm occurs in an elderly population. Many patients have co-morbid disease including ischaemic heart disease, chronic respiratory disease and renal impairment.

Table 2. The ideal endograft for ruptured abdominal aortic aneurysm

Available 'off the shelf'
Easy introduction (small sheath, compliant graft carrier)
Rapid, precise deployment and haemorrhage control
Applicable to a wide variety of aneurysm morphology
Allows intraoperative customization (especially with reference to length)

Patients undergoing open repair frequently suffer intraoperative myocardial infarction and major postoperative morbidity, including organ failure.

Recently endovascular repair of ruptured abdominal aortic aneurysms under local anaesthesia has been reported.[21] This technique may negate some of the adverse cardiovascular and respiratory features of general anaesthesia. The loss of abdominal wall tamponade associated with general anaesthesia and laparotomy potentially increases haemorrhage. Furthermore, induction of general anaesthesia is frequently associated with hypotension.

Reduced bleeding is expected following endovascular repair. Laparotomy is associated with haemorrhage due to the loss of tamponade and collateral damage during surgical dissection. Exposure of the bowel and peritoneum to ambient temperature frequently results in hypothermia, further exacerbating bleeding due to coagulopathy.

Elective endovascular procedures are associated with less physiological stress than open procedures. Haemodynamic changes are reduced and there is a lower incidence of myocardial ischaemia.[15] Renal and respiratory functions have also been shown to be less upset by EVAR as has splanchnic perfusion.

Multiple organ-failure is the biggest killer in those patients surviving 48 hours.[16] Cytokines have been implicated in the development of multiple organ failure. An attenuated cytokine response is seen following elective EVAR due to a reduction in the reperfusion injury. By extrapolation, EVAR may be expected to make an impact on the incidence of multiple organ failure following ruptured abdominal aortic aneurysms.

Technical

Open repair of ruptured abdominal aortic aneurysms are difficult operations due to haemorrhage and anatomical distortion. Iatrogenic injury of surrounding structures such as the duodenum, left renal vein and inferior vena cava carries a very high mortality due to prolonged haemorrhage and increased operative time.[17] Conversely EVAR is no more technically demanding than elective repair.

'Cross-clamping' of the aorta is not generally necessary during EVAR. Haemorrhage control is best managed by rapid deployment of the endovascular graft. A selective approach to aortic occlusion can be taken. The deleterious effects of aortic clamping (ischaemia-reperfusion injury and hypotension most notably) are therefore obviated in the majority. Intra-aortic occlusion devices are efficacious but should be reserved for those cases where haemorrhage is rapid and the endovascular graft cannot be deployed swiftly. Aortic occlusion may be secured by balloons inserted either via the femoral or brachial routes. Arterial sheaths and stiff guidewires prevent migration due to aortic pulsatile blood flow.

Adverse aneurysm morphology poses problems for open surgery in the same way as it does for the endovascular surgeon. Short necks are difficult to clamp (and may require supra-coeliac clamping); calcified iliac arteries may be incompressible and aneurysms of the iliac arteries require more complex and time-consuming reconstruction and are associated with worse outcome.[18] Similarly iliac aneurysm rupture and thoracoabdominal aneurysms carry a very high mortality, in part related to problems created by access difficulty. Conversely preliminary reports have shown that adverse anatomical features do not necessarily preclude successful endovascular aneurysm exclusion. Particularly, iliac aneurysms and hostile abdomens may lend themselves to the endovascular technique.

Recent improvements in EVAR have reduced intraoperative complications (e.g. embolization and conversion to open repair) and have brought about a reduction in operative time. Improving graft designs has allowed patients with more difficult anatomy to be treated. Ancillary endovascular techniques such as the use of Palmaz stents can deal with operational complications such as type I endoleak, reducing primary conversion rates.

Postoperative

Efficacy

1. Successful aneurysm exclusion is possible.
2. Aneurysm sac reduction has been documented during follow-up (see Figs 2 and 3).
3. Type I and III endoleak can be avoided.

Patients with type II endoleaks do not necessarily continue to bleed (Fig. 4).

Secondary procedures

1. Concerns regarding the long-term durability of endovascular grafts are much less relevant in ruptured abdominal aortic aneurysm, where the major outcome is perioperative mortality.

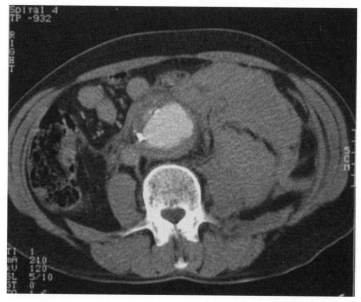

Figure 2. Ruptured abdominal aortic aneurysm (prior to endovascular exclusion).

2. Secondary procedures, if necessary can be carried out in an elective setting.
3. The majority of secondary procedures are endovascular.

The future

Preoperative imaging may not be required because of:

1. Improved intraoperative imaging (intravascular ultrasound?).
2. Pre-expanded PTFE grafts with balloon expandable stents.

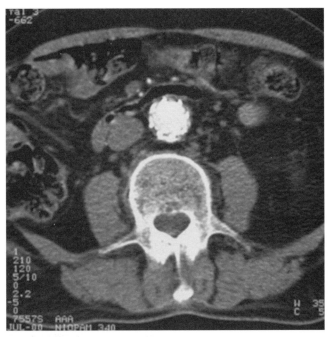

Figure 3. Successful aneurysm sac reduction following endovascular repair of the ruptured abdominal aortic aneurysm in Fig. 2.

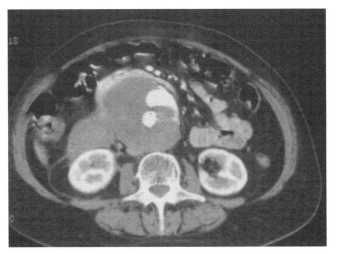

Figure 4. Type II endoleak post-EVAR of ruptured abdominal aortic aneurysm.

Conclusions

There is a sound theoretical basis as to why endovascular repair of ruptured abdominal aortic aneurysm may be a better option for some patients than open repair. The endovascular technique has been shown to be feasible and recent advances have allowed a greater number of patients to be treated by this method. A number of patients have survived endovascular repair where open techniques have been considered inappropriate.

Whether the necessary time delay and the morbidity associated with this technique outweigh that of open repair is unknown. Clearly further investigation of endovascular repair of ruptured abdominal aortic aneurysm is warranted.

Summary

- New technology is required to improve the outcome of ruptured abdominal aortic aneurysm.

- Endovascular repair of ruptured abdominal aortic aneurysm is feasible.

- Uni-iliac endograft configuration offers rapid aneurysm exclusion and increased applicability.

- Questions over the long-term durability of endovascular repair are of less relevance in ruptured abdominal aortic aneurysm if the perioperative mortality can be significantly reduced.

- More experience is required in the endovascular management of ruptured abdominal aortic aneurysm.

- The endovascular management of ruptured abdominal aortic aneurysm requires a different approach to open repair and may require the inclusion of interventional radiologists.

- Endovascular repair of ruptured abdominal aortic aneurysm is technically similar to elective repair.

- Properly stratified trials will be necessary in future to identify the place of endovascular repair in the managment of ruptured abdominal aortic aneurysm.

References

1. Fowkes FG, MacIntyre CC, Ruckley CV. Increasing incidence of aortic aneurysms in England and Wales. *Br Med J* 1989; **298**: 33–35.
2. Greenhalgh RM. Prognosis of abdominal aortic aneurysm. *Br Med J* 1990; **301**: 306.
3. Heller JA, Weinberg A, Aarons R *et al.* Two decades of abdominal aortic aneurysm repair: have we made any progress? *J Vasc Surg* 2000; **32**: 1091–1101.
4. Darling RC, Cordero JA, Chang BB. Advances in the surgical repair of ruptured abdominal aortic aneurysms. *Cardiovasc Surg* 1996; **4**: 720–723.
5. Heather BP, Poskitt KR, Earnshaw JJ *et al.* Population screening reduces mortality rate from aortic aneurysm in men. *Br J Surg* 2000; **87**: 750–753.
6. Yusuf SW, Whitaker SC, Chuter TA *et al.* Emergency endovascular repair of leaking aortic aneurysm. *Lancet* 1994; **344**: 1645.

7. Vohra R, Reid D, Groome J *et al*. Long-term survival in patients undergoing resection of abdominal aortic aneurysm. *Ann Vasc Surg* 1990; **4**: 460–465.

8. Walker EM, Hopkinson BR, Makin GS. Unoperated abdominal aortic aneurysm: presentation and natural history. *Ann R Coll Surg Engl* 1983; **65**: 311–315.

9. Hewin DF, Campbell WB. Ruptured aortic aneurysm: the decision not to operate. *Ann R Coll Surg Engl* 1998; **80**: 221–225.

10. Adam DJ, Mohan IV, Stuart WP *et al*. Transferring patients with ruptured abdominal aortic aneurysm to a regional vascular surgery unit does not prejudice outcome. Presented to the 31st Annual Conference of the Vascular Surgical Society of Great Britain and Ireland, London 1997.

11. Basnyat PS, Biffin A, Moseley L *et al*. Deaths from ruptured abdominal aortic aneurysm in Wales. *Br J Surg* 1999; **86**: 690–711.

12. Hardman DTA, Fisher CM, Patel MI *et al*. Ruptured abdominal aortic aneurysms: Who should be offered surgery? *J Vasc Surg* 1996; **23**: 123–129.

13. Armon MP, Yusuf SW, Whitaker SC *et al*. Influence of abdominal aortic aneurysm size on the feasibility of endovascular repair. *J Endovasc Surg* 1997; **4**: 284–285.

14. Armon MP, Yusuf SW, Whitaker SC *et al*. Anatomy of abdominal aortic aneurysms. *Eur J Vasc Endovasc Surg* 1997; **13**: 398–402.

15. Cuypers PWM, Gardien M, Buth J *et al*. Randomized study comparing cardiac response in endovascular and open abdominal aortic aneurysm repair. *Br J Surg* 2001; **88**: 1059–1065.

16. Roumen RMH, Hendriks T, van der Ven-Jongekrijg J *et al*. Cytokine patterns in patients after major vascular surgery, haemorrhagics shock and severe blunt trauma. Relation with subsequent adult respiratory distress syndrome and multiple organ failure. *Ann Surg* 1993; **218**: 769–776.

17. Donaldson MC, Rosenberg JM, Bucknam CA. Factors affecting survival after ruptured abdominal aortic aneurysms. *J Vasc Surg* 1985; **2**: 564–570.

18. van Dongen HPA, Leusink KA, Moll FL *et al*. Ruptured abdominal aortic aneurysms: factors influencing postoperative mortality and long-term survival. *Eur J Vasc Endovasc Surg* 1998; **15**: 62–66.

19. Ohki T, Veith F, Sanchez LA *et al*. Endovascular graft repair of ruptured aortoiliac aneurysms. *J Am Coll Surg* 1999; **189**: 102–113.

20. Greenberg RK, Srivastava SD, Ouriel K *et al*. An endoluminal method of haemorrhage control and repair of ruptured abdominal aortic aneurysms. *J Endovasc Ther* 2000; **7**: 1–7.

21. Lachat ML. Endovascular repair under local anaesthesia to improve outcome of ruptured aortoiliac aneurysms. Presented to the European Society for Vascular Surgery, Lucerne, September 2001.

22. Hinchliffe RJ, Yusuf SW, Maceriewicz JA *et al*. Endovascular repair of ruptured abdominal aortic aneurysm: A single centre experience in 20 patients. *Eur J Vasc Endovasc Surg* 2001; **22**: 528–534.

EVAR will take over emergency abdominal aortic aneurysm rupture

Against the motion
Dieter Raithel, Dittmar Boeckler

Introduction

Since Parodi's introduction of endovascular abdominal aortic aneurysm repair, great enthusiasm has developed for less invasive methods of treating even ruptured aortic aneurysms.

Despite aggressive elective screening programmes, 50% of patients whose aneurysms rupture die before reaching a medical facility, and another 24% arrive at a hospital alive but die before an operation can be performed. Average operative mortality of ruptured abdominal aortic aneurysms is 50–60%.

Endovascular repair in thoracic aortic aneurysms, electively or under emergency conditions, is well established and an accepted treatment First publications by Ohki and Veith predict also better outcome in treating abdominal aortic aneurysm-patients with endovascular endografts.[1] In this series the author showed a success rate of 29% for endovascular emergency abdominal aortic aneurysm repair, which compares with around 60% success rate for open emergency procedures.

Increasingly centres in Europe and the USA are looking at the endovascular route for repairing ruptured aneurysms.

Evidence

Endovascular repair of abdominal aortic aneurysms was celebrating its tenth anniversary and application of stents and endoluminal grafts in the aorta and the iliac arteries began to show encouraging mid and 'long'-term results. Operative and interventionals techniques have been fairly established and further developed over the years (Fig. 1).

Endoleak, migration, material problems (metalframe fracture, suture leaks, fabric tears) have been observed.[2] Despite many advances in diagnostic screening, operative techniques and postoperative intensive care treatment of elective abdominal aortic aneurysm patients, the morbidity and mortality for the treatment of ruptured aortolilac aneurysmy remain high. What will be the role of endovascular approach to ruptured abdominal aortic aneurysms? Is EVAR now taking over emergency abdominal aortic aneurysm rupture? What are the arguments against this approach?

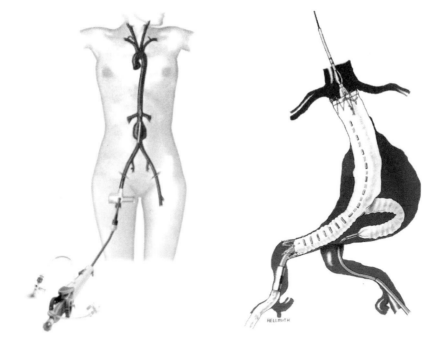

Figure 1. Implantation technique of an aortic endograft (e.g. Ancure).

Arguments against endovascular abdominal aortic aneurysm repair in ruptured aneurysms are:

1. Mainly logistical problems and lack of equipment and trained staff as well (mainly at night) make emergency endograft implantations extremely difficult.
2. For ruptured abdominal aortic aneurysm endografting, endografts with different sizes need to be available in a vascular department. Most centres do not have such devices or custom-made devices. Monoiliacal stentgraft designs with consecutive fem-fem crossover bypass are an alternative option but not ideal ('one size fits most').
3. The technical feasibility of endoluminal abdominal aortic aneurysm repair decreases with increasing aneurysm diameter. Most (~90%) ruptured abdominal aortic aneurysm's have large (>5.5cm) diameters. These large aneurysms often lack a proximal neck. Hardly ever is there a proximal infra-aortic neck available for a good sealing of the graft.
4. Most of the abdominal aortic aneurysm ruptures are located to the left side in **pararenal position**. In these patients endovascular treatment is not possible with a definite sealing of the rupture.
5. In haemodynamically unstable patients there is no time to perform exact preoperative measurement by computed tomography (CT)-scans (Fig. 2). The need for an abdominal CT scan may delay treatment. Abdominal aortic aneurysm rupture which is not treated immediately can end up in free and deadly rupture if prolonged preoperative diagnostics are performed, especially in hemodynamically unstable patients. The morphology, especially of the aortic neck, can be obtained by 'on table angiography', but may include faults in sizing the abdominal aortic aneurysm. Possible aortic endoleaks type I may result.
6. Renal artery occlusion may be an unpredicatable complication due to juxtarenal stentgraft deployment.

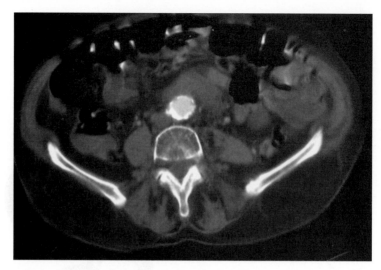

Figure 2. CT-Scan of a small (38mm) ruptured aortic aneurysm.

Discussion

As long as elective EVAR is associated with high endoleakage- and secondary intervention rates, emergency EVAR remains also uncertain. But, 90% primary success rate with low perioperative mortality is a good argument to change the critics' opinions regarding the use of EVAR.[1] Veith and Ohki reported of 26 patients with ruptured aorto-iliac aneurysms, 21 were treated endovascularly, five patients required open surgery, two deaths occurred in endovascularly treated patients with serious co-morbidities.[3]

Some authors argue not to be able to remove the retroperitoneal haematoma, mainly left-sided and pararenal, in EVAR as they do in conventional surgery. We never perform decompression of the retroperitoneal haematoma in ruptured abdominal aortic aneurysm. Therefore we do not consider this to be an argument against ruptured abdominal aortic aneurysm endografting.

Woodburn et al. analysed their patients assessed for abdominal aortic aneurysm repair: Only 30% of unselected abdominal aortic aneurysms are entirely suitable for EVAR.[4] The data suggest that increased use is only possible by deploying devices in suboptimal morphology and in patients who would not normally be considered for open abdominal aortic aneurysm repair.

Our own experience is very small due to the logistic reasons mentioned above. In a 6-year experience (August 1994–September 2001) six of 643 patients (1%) underwent endovascular treatment due to a ruptured aortic aneurysm (mostly contained rupture).

Endovascular experts are confident in ruptured endovascular abdominal aortic aneurysm grafting with good results in the future. The long-term-follow up will prove these findings. Surely only teams with high experience in elective EVAR will also obtain good results in such emergency cases.

Summary

- Mortality in ruptured abdominal aortic aneurysm remains high.

- Not technical but logistical reasons make emergent EVAR difficult to perform.

- The ideal graft has yet to be found; monoiliac systems are compromises.

- Practical experience in elective EVAR is essential to obtain good results in emergency.

- Endovascular treatment of ruptured aneurysms appears to improve treatment outcomes.

References

1. Ohki T, Veith FJ, Sanchez LA *et al.* Endovascular graft repair of ruptured aortoiliac aneurysms. *J Am Coll Surg* 1999; **189**: 102–112.
2. Diethrich EB. What is the future of aortic surgery? What will be the roles of endovascular, open and laparascopic procedures? 27th Veith Symposium, New York 15–18 November, 2001.
3. Veith F, Ohki T. Endovascular approach to ruptured AAAs. 27th Veith Symposium, New York 15–18 November, 2001.
4. Woodburn KR, Chant H, Davies JN, Blanshard KS, Travis SJ. Suitability for endovascular aneurysm repair in an unselect population. *Br J Surg* 2001; **88**: 77–81.

EVAR will take over emergency abdominal aortic aneurysm rupture

Charing Cross Editorial Comments towards Consensus

Will it or will it not? Already we know that it is possible. At the time of writing patients with ruptured aortic aneurysms go to a large number of hospitals. Will these be concentrated into larger groups in the future? Will these larger groups be ready for CT scan and off the shelf application of an endovascular graft under local anaesthetic through the femoral artery? The advantages are obvious. If it is possible to deploy a stent-graft system below the renal arteries and down to at least one iliac artery then the pressure on the rupturing aorta is controlled and the opposite iliac artery can be blocked and a femorofemoral crossover performed even under local anaesthetic. It can be done but is it feasible to do it on a large scale? It would require teams of surgeons and radiologists to be available on a rota to be able to work through a carefully designed protocol. This would take some organization. It is all very well doing it once but can you do it every night of the week? Is it going to happen? Certainly it will not happen in every hospital and only if there is a tendency towards centralization of arterial services can the concept be applied. It is likely that such a system would dramatically reduce aortic aneurysm deaths. When the size of this reduction of mortality is known and when the reduction of use of Intensive Therapy Unit beds and costs is calculated, it is likely that funders of health care will be in favour of starting to set up such an emergency service.

Roger M Greenhalgh
Editor

Renal artery lesions should be treated by angioplasty and stent

For the motion
Jon G Moss

Introduction

Renal artery stenosis is caused by either atherosclerosis (by far the largest group in the West) or a group of disparate disease processes, which include fibromuscular dysplasia and the various arteritides. There is a general consensus that fibromuscular dysplasia should be treated by an endovascular approach (usually percutaneous transluminal angioplasty (PTA)) and the rest of this chapter will focus exclusively on atherosclerotic renal artery stenosis.

Atherosclerotic renal artery stenosis is a common disorder prevalent in the population of patients encountered with coronary, carotid, and peripheral vascular disease. Although often clinically silent atherosclerotic renal artery stenosis may lead to renin-driven secondary hypertension and or progressive renal failure. Renovascular disease is now the most common cause of end-stage renal disease in dialysis patients aged over 60 years, accounting for at least 25% of this group.[1] It is a progressive disorder culminating in a cumulative incidence of progression to arterial occlusion of 5% per annum in stenoses >60%.[2]

There are two separate issues crucial to this debate.

1. Is there an evidence base to support revascularization of atherosclerotic renal artery stenosis?
2. If a renal artery lesion is to be revascularized, how should this be accomplished: angioplasty, stenting or open surgical methods?

Technique and illustration

The technique is fairly standardized and well established. Most operators would use PTA alone for non-ostial lesions (>10mm from the aortic wall) reserving stents for an unsatisfactory immediate outcome such as flow-limiting dissection, >30–50% recoil or complete vessel occlusion. In the far more common ostial lesion, however, primary stenting has become the norm (Fig. 1A–D). The choice of vascular access is best made on the pre-procedural imaging, e.g. magnetic resonance angiography. The lesion is crossed conventionally and dilated following the administration of heparin and antispasmodics. A balloon expandable stent is then deployed taking care to cover the lesion in its entirety to the aortic lumen. Accurate placement is best accomplished by using a guiding catheter. A C-arm fluoroscopy is essential to project the origin of the renal artery tangential to the X-ray beam to allow accurate stent positioning.

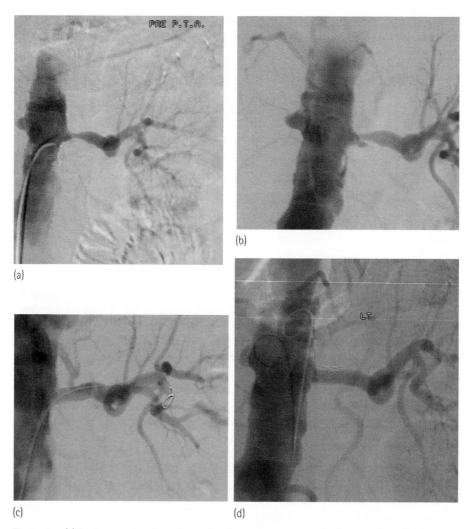

Figure 1. (a) Angiogram showing atherosclerotic renal artery stenosis; the contralateral kidney is occluded. (b) Post-angioplasty showing dissection and no appreciable improvement in lumen diameter. (c) Angiogram following stent placement shows an excellent morphological result. (d) Angiogram 6 months post-stent shows a minimal restenosis.

Complications

The complication rate following renal PTA with or without stenting varies from 0 to 25% and illustrates the problem when there are no agreed reporting standards and the literature is largely retrospective. There are some recent advances, which may help lower the morbidity rate.

1. Small platform 3F 0.014 balloon systems. These use coronary technology and there is some unpublished data from carotid stenting using transcranial Doppler that the embolic burden is reduced.
2. Protection devices. Again the largely unpublished data to support this technology comes from carotid stenting where the embolic burden caused by PTA/stenting is reduced.

These systems have been used in the renal artery and apart from the increase in complexity that they incur there is at yet insufficient evidence to support their routine use.

1. Closure devices. These together with the small platform 3F systems almost certainly reduce the incidence of local groin complications.
2. Use of alternative contrast media (carbon dioxide and gadolinium). There is little doubt that conventional iodinated contrast media is toxic to kidneys and more so in those already damaged. Provided the equipment is available CO_2 can provide adequate imaging to allow PTA/stenting without any or a minimum of iodinated contrast media. Gadolinium offers similar advantages but is far more expensive.
3. Minimization of contrast nephrotoxicity. This is more common than originally thought and occurs in up to 50% of patients with pre-existing renal impairment. There is evidence that this can be reduced by avoiding dehydration and maintaining a good diuresis with intravenous fluids given for 12 hours pre- and post-procedure (0.45% saline at 100–150 ml/h). In addition the volume of iodinated contrast media should be kept to a minimum and low osmolar agents used. There is some research in progress investigating the possible reno-protective potential of dopamine 1 receptor agonists (fenoldopam), which work by inducing vasodilatation countering the vasospasm of contrast media.

Evidence

There are five published recent clinical trials (see Table 1), no systematic or Cochrane reviews and one unpublished meta-analysis by the Clinical Trials Unit, University of Birmingham.

Only one recent clinical trial attempts to compare surgery with PTA.[3] This Swedish study randomized 58 hypertensive patients with unilateral atherosclerotic renal artery stenosis to either surgery or PTA. Technical success was higher in the surgical group (97%) than the PTA group (83%). Patency was assessed by angiography carried out for up to 2 years. Primary patency was higher in the surgical group (96%) than the PTA group (75%) but secondary patency was similar, surgical group (97%) PTA group (90%). Clinical results were similar and the trial recommended PTA as the first line of treatment provided there was intensive follow-up and aggressive reintervention.

This trial pre-dated the stent era and one would expect far superior technical and patency results had stents been available.

Table 1.

Trial and Ref	Year	Number	Arms	Result
Malmo[3]	1993	58	Surgery/PTA	PTA first choice
Scottish and Newcastle[4]	1998	55	Medical results/ PTA (BP)	Modest systolic BP improvement only in bilateral ARAS with PTA
EMMA[5]	1998	49	Medical results/ PTA (BP)	Reduction in drug requirement with PTA
Van de ven[6]	1999	85	Stent / PTA	Primary stent better technical success and patency
DRASTIC[7]	2000	106	Medical results/ PTA (BP)	No differences

BP: Blood pressure. ARAS: atherosclerotic renal artery stenosis. PTA: Percutaneous transluminal angioplasty.

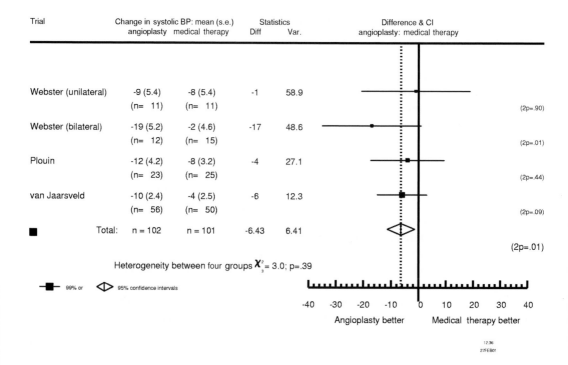

Figure 2. Change in systolic blood pressure (between baseline and 6 months): angioplasty vs medical therapy.

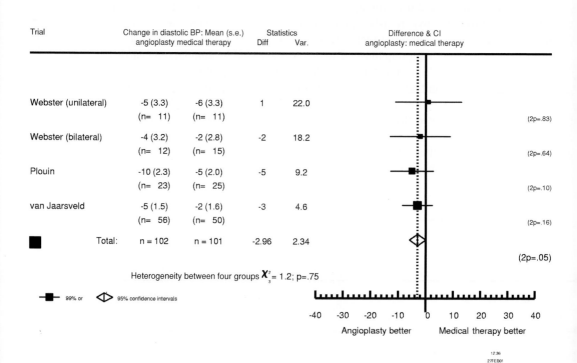

Figure 3. Change in diastolic blood pressure (between baseline and 6 months): angioplasty vs medical therapy.

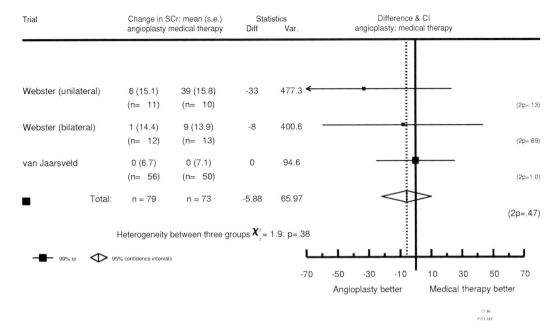

Figure 4. Change in SCr (between baseline and 6 months): angioplasty vs medical therapy.

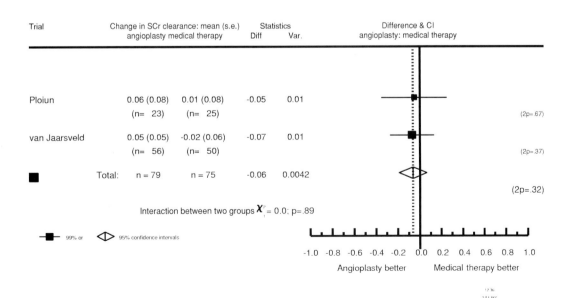

Figure 5. Change in SCr Clearance (between baseline and 6 months): angioplasty vs medical therapy.

The recent clinical trial comparing stenting with PTA[6] although small showed the technical success rate with stenting (88%) to be superior to PTA (57%), difference 31% (confidence interval (CI) 12–50). Again 6-month primary patency was superior with stenting (75%) compared with PTA (29%), difference 46% (CI11-58). The authors advocated a policy of primary stenting. There were no differences, however, between the two groups in the clinical results (blood pressure control or renal function) but clearly the trial was not set up or adequately powered to detect differences in these parameters. Although only a small study this is the only level 1 evidence for primary stenting. It seems unlikely that the trial will be repeated as most operators now feel it is inappropriate to simply perform PTA on ostial atherosclerotic renal artery stenosis.

The remaining three trials[4,5,7] all looked at the effects on blood pressure of revascularization compared with medical treatment alone. Although renal function was monitored, none of the studies were powered to examine renal function and some excluded patients with significantly impaired renal function. The three trials differed in the way blood pressure was measured and reported and likewise the effect on renal function. A recent meta-analysis conducted by the Clinical Trials Unit at Birmingham University[8] conveniently summarizes the combined results (210 patients) of these three trials (Figs 2–5). There were no clear improvements in renal function or blood pressure following revascularization. The confidence intervals (CIs) were compatible with either no benefit or with a moderate but clinically worthwhile, benefit. The different methodology and reporting standards of the trials added further uncertainty. In addition stents were only used in two of the 210 patients. A much larger trial was recommended to answer the question.

ASTRAL (Angioplasty and Stenting for the Treatment of Renal Artery Lesions) and STAR (Stent Trial for Atherosclerotic Renal artery stenosis) have recently been funded and recruitment commenced. They will compare renal stenting plus best medical treatment with medical treatment alone and use renal function as the primary outcome measure. ASTRAL aims to randomize 1000 patients and STAR 250. It is hoped these trials will clarify the role of renal stenting in patients with renal impairment due to atherosclerotic renal artery stenosis. Neither trial aims to examine blood pressure control in any depth.

Conclusion

Atherosclerotic renal artery stenosis is a focal stenotic disease that lends itself to an endovascular approach. Solitary focal lesions in other territories with perhaps the exception of the carotid artery are normally treated by PTA/stent. Although surgical reconstruction can produce excellent results in carefully selected patients it incurs an unavoidable mortality and morbidity. In addition the target population is becoming increasingly elderly with a high incidence of other co-morbid vascular disease which makes an endovascular approach avoiding a general anaesthetic the logical choice. Surgery should be reserved for endovascular failures or complications.

Further research is needed to determine the precise role of renal revascularization and particularly whether it can prevent progressive renal failure. The results of the ASTRAL and STAR trials are awaited with great interest.

Summary

- Primary patency following surgery is superior to PTA. Secondary patency is equal.

- The majority of atherosclerotic renal artery stenosis lesions are treated by PTA/stents in the UK.

- Technical success following stenting is superior to PTA.

- Primary patency following stenting is superior to PTA.

- Meta-analysis of three recent clinical trials shows no clear improvements in renal function or BP following revascularization, but CIs are wide.

- A large clinical trial (several hundred) is required to determine reliably whether renal revascularization improves renal function and blood pressure.

References

1. Mailloux LU, Napolitano B, Belluci AG *et al*. Renal vascular disease causing end-stage renal disease, incidence, clinical correlates and outcomes: a 20 year clinical experience. *Am J Kidney Dis* 1994; 24: 622–629.

2. Zierler RE, Bergelin RO, Isaacson JA *et al*. Natural history of atherosclerotic renal artery stenosis: a prospective study with duplex ultrasonography. *J Vasc Surg* 1994; 19: 250–258.

3. Weibull H, Bergqvist D, Bergentz S-E *et al*. Percutaneous transluminal renal angioplasty versus surgical reconstruction of atherosclerotic renal artery stenosis: a prospective randomised study. *J Vasc Surg* 1993; 18: 841–852.

4. Webster J, Marshall F, Abdalla M *et al*. Randomised comparison of percutaneous angioplasty vs continued medical therapy for hypertensive patients with atheromatous renal artery stenosis. *J Hum Hypertens* 1998; 12: 329–335.

5. Plouin P-F, Chatellier G, Darne B *et al*. Blood pressure outcome of angioplasty in atherosclerotic renal artery stenosis. *Hypertension* 1998; 31: 823–829.

6. Van de ven PJG, Kaatee R, Beutler JJ *et al*. Arterial stenting and balloon angioplasty in ostial atherosclerotic renovascular disease : a randomised trial. *Lancet* 1999; 353: 282–286.

7. Van Jaarsveld BC, Krijnen P, Pieterman H *et al*. The effects of balloon angioplasty on hypertension in atherosclerotic renal artery stenosis. *N Engl J Med* 2000; 342: 1007–1014.

8. Ives N, Wheatley K, Gray R. Continuing uncertainty about the value of revascularisation in atherosclerotic renovascular disease: a meta-analysis of previous trials. 5th UK Renovascular Forum, Glasgow 2001 abst.

Renal artery lesions should be treated by angioplasty and stent

Against the motion
George Hamilton

Introduction

Chronic atherosclerotic renovascular disease is a common and frequently recognized cause of hypertension and renal failure.[1] Up to 40% of elderly hypertensive patients with atherosclerotic risk factors will have renal artery stenosis but many of these lesions will not affect renal function throughout the lifetime of the patient. Progression of renal artery stenosis occurs in a minority of these lesions with high grade stenosis, age, hypertension, female gender and advanced renal failure being associated risk factors. A recent clinical study from the Mayo Clinic of patients with moderately severe renal artery stenosis, (i.e. >70%), treated by medical means alone, revealed only 8–10% progression to severe hypertension and <10% progressive renal failure.[2]

It has been known for many years that patients with atherosclerotic renovascular disease do badly on dialysis with a very high morbidity and mortality from co-existent coronary and cerebral vascular disease.[3] Prevention or delay of onset of dialysis by maintaining renal function and treating hypertension has motivated many policies of aggressive medical endovascular and surgical interventions in the hope that this might reduce the development of coronary and cerebral vascular disease. The challenge in management of these patients remains the timely identification and selection of the small cohort who will benefit from revascularization.

Pathophysiology

Renal artery stenosis causes shrinkage of the renal mass by a process of loss of nephrons and renal atrophy. The details of these underlying changes are beyond the scope of this chapter but it is important in the light of the clinical outcomes reported from interventions, to stress that several factors other than simple ischaemia are at work. Parenchymal changes range from cortical infarction due to diseased intrarenal arteries, to extensive interstitial fibrosis and gross structural damage to the tubules and glomerulus. In addition, patients undergoing angiography and in particular undergoing angioplasty, with or without stents, are susceptible to atheroembolism with occlusion of intrarenal arteries by multiple fragments of atheroma. The common presence of these intrarenal changes has been underestimated and their clinical relevance is highlighted by the indifferent results observed in a significant proportion of patients who have undergone restoration of main-stem renal artery blood flow.

Selection

Best possible assessment of likely intrarenal and segmental disease should form an important part of the pre-intervention assessment. However, there are no reliable methods of assessment which will predict those patients who will benefit from intervention.

Duplex ultrasound is highly operator-dependent providing semi-quantitative assessment of renal artery stenosis but good assessment of renal mass. A bipolar renal length of at least 8cm (without cysts) is the minimum required to allow a successful clinical outcome. Accessory renal arteries are not detected with this method, however.

Radioisotope renography has reasonably good specificity and sensitivity (>90%) in predicting response to revascularization but the accuracy declines with severity of renal failure. This investigation is not frequently used nowadays.

Renal angiography remains the gold standard but is invasive, causes morbidity and is of course associated with a 25% risk of atheroembolism. Recent advances in magnetic resonance angiography have brought this investigation into prominence and this may well become the new gold standard for renal arterial imaging. With either modality, imaging of the coeliac axis should be routine in patients being considered for surgical revascularization by extra-anatomic means.

The ideal investigation would differentiate between renal failure secondary to main-stem arterial stenosis and renal failure from intrarenal segmental or microvascular occlusive disease. As yet this test does not exist and current investigation is based on clinical assessment by repeat functional measurement of renal function, bipolar renal length measurement by ultrasound and angiography. Also certain clinical scenarios are associated with a good outcome from revascularization of significant renal artery stenosis. These include patients with a recent deterioration in renal function, those with flash pulmonary oedema, reversible renal failure following angiotensin-converting enzyme inhibitor therapy (ACE inhibitors), progressive chronic renal failure, patients with bilateral renal artery stenosis or a stenosis to a single functioning kidney, and in patients who have failed medical therapy.

Angioplasty and stent angioplasty

Angioplasty of osteal renal artery stenoses (PTRA) has disappointing short- and long-term results. The introduction of stent angioplasty (PTRAS) has allowed treatment of more severe osteal renal artery stenosis with primary and assisted patency rates reported in most reviews to be well over 90%. Consequently a much more liberal attitude to renal revascularization currently prevails as a result of these seductively good technical results. Alas, the medium- and long-term clinical outcomes are less satisfactory. Recent reviews of the clinical outcomes of PTRAS and PTRA reported improved renal function in only 27%, (15–36%), with maintenance of stable function in 52% (29–91%) and the remaining 21% having worse function (0–45%).[4,5] In addition, during the first 2 years after stenting, average re-stenosis rates of 13–17% have been reported.[6] There have been two recent important randomized studies. One compared PTRA with PTRAS[7] and the second PTRAS with medical treatment.[8] These two studies have shown no significant difference between either form of angioplasty and best medical treatment as regards cure or improvement in hypertension or improvement or stabilization of renal function (Fig. 1). These studies raise major concerns regarding the value of stent angioplasty for renal artery stenosis.

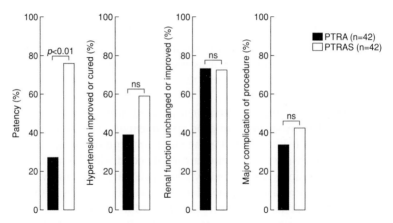

Figure 1. Data from patients randomized to PTRA alone or PTRA with stent (PTRAS) evaluated 6 months after the intervention (mean +/- SEM) for patency, effect on hypertension and renal function. Reproduced from Ref. 7 with permission.

Furthermore, up-to-date analysis of recent stent angioplasty series reveals significant rates of morbidity and mortality, which are similar to those of recent surgical series (Tables 1 and 2). Median morbidity is 8% (range 0–33%) and median mortality is 2% (range 0–14.2%). The risk-benefit ratio of renal artery stenting in these patients is therefore not as favourable as previously believed and the whole rationale of this intervention must now be seriously questioned.

The current randomized comparison of PTRA/PTRAS and medical management, (the ASTRAL study), will provide the level I evidence which is currently lacking.

Table 1. Results of series of renal artery stent angioplasty (PTRAS) for renal failure

First author	Year	No of patients	Technical success (%)	Morbidity (%)	Mortality (%)	Improved (%)	No change (%)	Worse (%)
Rees [9]	1991	28	96	7	3.6	36	36	28
Raynaud [10]	1994	15	100	6.7	0	13	50	37
Iannone [11]	1996	63	99	33	14.2	36	46	18
Rundback [12]	1996	20	96	5	0	25	75	0
Blum [13]	1997	68	100	4.4	0	0	100	0
Boisclair [14]	1997	33	100	21	0	41	35	24
Harden [15]	1997	32	100	0	3	34	34	28
White [16]	1997	100	99	2	1	–	–	–
Gross [17]	1998	30	100	0	3	31	52	17
Dorros [18]	1998	163	99	1	1.8	33	33	34
Tuttle [19]	1998	129	98	4.1	3	13	76	11
Rundback [20]	1998	45				20	52	28
Henry [21]	1999	210	99	1.2	0.5	–	–	–
Xue [22]	1999	39	98	16	0	10	71	8
Bush [23]	2001	73	94	9.1	1.4	30	40	30
Yutan [24]	2001	76	89	5	3.8	10	76	14
Lederman [25]	2001	300	100	12	0	19	54	27
Total		1424	98	5	1.2	25	52	24
Median (range)				(0–33)	(0–14.2)	(0–41)	(0–100)	(0–37)

Table 2. Results of recent series of surgical renal artery revascularization for renal failure.

First author	Year	No of patients	Technical success (%)	Morbidity (%)	Mortality (%)	Improved (%)	No change (%)	Worse (%)
Mercier[26]	1990	43 (24/43 aortic)	–	–	7	41	21	38
Torsello[27]	1990	326 (50 aortic)	94	–	4.3	53	18.6	28.4
Bredenberg[28]	1992	59 (16 aortic)	96	13	3	55	25	20
Libertino[29]	1992	97	83	11	6	63	19	18
Hansen[30]	1992	200 (32 aortic)	98	17.2	2.5	49	36	15
Chaikoff[31]	1994	50 (50 aortic)	98	28	2	42	54	4
Cambria[32]	1994	285 (43 aortic)	95	10.5	5.6	–	–	–
Hallett[33]	1995	304	–	–	10.2	27	51	20
Lamawansa[34]	1995	62	–	–	13	32	26	42
Cambria[35]	1996	139	–	–	8	54	19	27
Darling[36]	1999	568 (77% aortic)	98.7	8	5.5	–	–	–
Hansen[37]	2000	590 (37% aortic)	100	30	7.3	58	35	7
Total		2723	97	13	5.8	51	25.5	20
Median (range)				(8–30)	(2–13)	(27–63)	(18.6–54)	(4–42)

Surgical revascularization

The options for surgical revascularization have evolved in response to the different clinical scenarios in which renal artery stenosis presents as a major problem. Important factors involved in the selection of the intervention include whether one or both kidneys are involved, the condition of the native aorta, the cardiorespiratory status of the patient and whether the stenotic disease is purely osteal, involving the main-stem or the segmental branches of the renal artery. In a small number of patients with difficult to control hypertension, nephrectomy will be required where the bipolar renal length is less than 8cm.

The current population in which revascularization is required is one which is older than before and with many risk factors. Selection is obviously important and based primarily on the patient's cardiac and respiratory status. These patients should be exhaustively assessed prior to surgery and their cardiorespiratory status optimized. Patients with flash pulmonary oedema should have this controlled by medical means with the surgery scheduled to take place in an optimized patient.

The simplest and most direct approach is by aorto-renal bypass grafting. This operation should be reserved for those patients who have a normal or acceptable infrarenal aorta. As in all renal reconstructions, the choice of bypass conduit lies between the use of Dacron, expanded polytetrafluoroethylene (e-PTFE) or saphenous vein; the results for all three conduits are equivalent, (Fig. 2, aorto-renal bypass graft).

Where the aorta requires replacement either for severe aortoiliac occlusive disease or much more commonly for significant aneurysmal disease, simultaneous aortic replacement and renal revascularization may be required. Very careful selection is of paramount importance in this scenario. Renal revascularization should only be added into an aortic intervention if there is a convincing clinical need for renal revascularization as previously outlined, (Fig. 3, simultaneous aortic and renal reconstruction).

Trans-aortic renal endarterectomy performed either as a primary procedure or simultaneously with an aortic reconstruction, is a popular approach to dealing with renal artery stenosis particularly in North America (Fig. 4, trans-aortic renal endarterectomy via longitudinal incision). Endarterectomy of the renal artery stenosis via a transverse incision extending from the aorta into the main stem renal artery with subsequent patch closure is another variation of this operation which is popular in Scandinavia (Fig. 5, trans-aortic renal endarterectomy with patch closure).

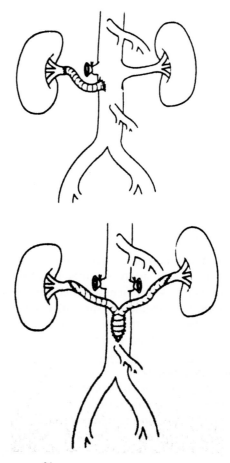

Figure 2. Aorto-renal bypass grafting.

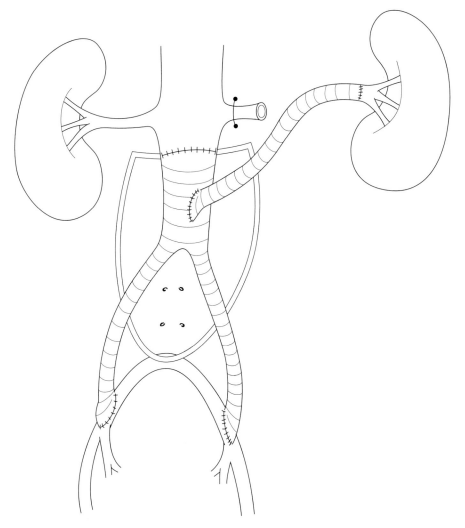

Figure 3. Simultaneous aortic and renal reconstruction where the aorta is significantly aneurismal or occluded.

In those patients where there is branch renal artery disease, extracorporeal reconstruction is required. This is also known as auto-transplantation and requires removal of the kidney from its bed, perfusion with ice cold transplant solutions and maintenance of the kidney in ice cold saline. This allows accurate bench reconstruction of the segmental arteries using either the saphenous vein or the internal iliac artery. The kidney is then re-implanted into the iliac circulation in the classical transplant manner. This operation is very rarely used in treatment of atherosclerotic renal artery stenosis.

Extra-anatomic renal revascularization is the most commonly employed surgical technique in patients with atherosclerotic renal artery stenosis. The aorta rarely needs to be replaced in these patients, the surgical approach is much less traumatic requiring a subcostal or transverse incision, and there is no need for aortic cross-clamping. These factors have obvious advantages for the surgical treatment of these high risk elderly patients. Where there is no significant disease involving the coeliac axis, the kidneys can be revascularized from the hepatic artery on the right or the splenic

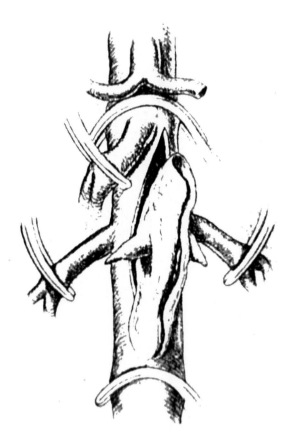

Figure 4. Trans-aortic renal endarterectomy via longitudinal aortic incision.

artery on the left (Fig. 6, extra-anatomical renal revascularization from the hepatic or splenic arteries). Unfortunately, up to 50% of these patients will have significant coeliac artery stenosis and they can be dealt with by aorto-renal bypass grafting or by taking a jump graft from a healthy superior mesenteric artery. A further possible inflow site is the iliac artery but in this class of patients these arteries are so commonly diseased that this approach is rarely used.

Results of renal artery reconstruction

Excellent long-term patency is obtained by surgical revascularization.[38] Perioperative morbidity and mortality, particularly in the earlier series, has been reported to be high with mortality rates of up to 25%. Contemporary clinical series, however, report median perioperative mortality of 5.8%, ranging from 2 to 13% (Table 2). These results reflect improved selection, preoperative optimization of cardiorespiratory status and the advent of extra-anatomical bypass procedures where lower perioperative mortality rates are reported. Analysis of functional outcomes reveal improved renal function in 51%, (range 27–63%), stabilization or no change in 25.5%, (range 18.6–54%), with deterioration in renal function in 20%, (range 4–42%). Comparison of these results with those from renal artery stenting show greater improvement in renal function with surgical intervention, (51% vs 25% respectively), but no difference in those patients undergoing deterioration (Figs 7,8,9). Further analysis of these

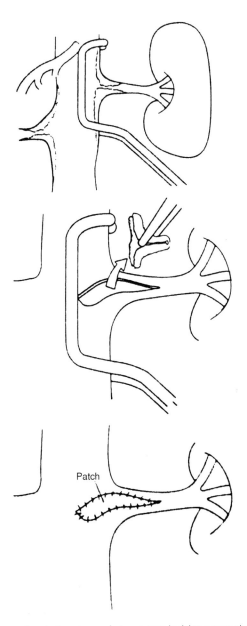

Figure 5. Trans-aortic renal endarterectomy via transverse incision across the renal artery origin with patch closure.

data is required but possible explanations for the improved results with surgery might include differences in patient selection for the two groups (are there more unfit patients treated by stent angioplasty?) with also the very real possibility that surgical reconstruction avoids the effects of atheroembolism.

Surgical revascularization for atherosclerotic renal artery disease provides the best long-term results for any intervention. Contrary to the current bias, peri-procedural mortality in several series of PTRAS is similar to that of surgical revascularization particularly where there is no concomitant aortic procedure. A properly stratified and controlled prospective randomized comparison between renal artery stent angioplasty and renal surgical revascularization is required.

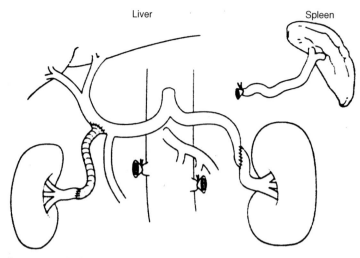

Figure 6. Extra-anatomical renal revascularization from the hepatic or splenic arteries.

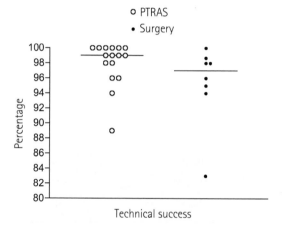

Figure 7. Scattergram comparing median technical success rates between PTRAS and surgical revascularization.

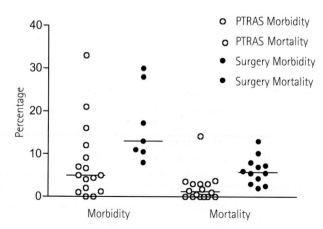

Figure 8. Scattergram comparing morbidity and mortality of PTRAS and surgical revascularization.

230

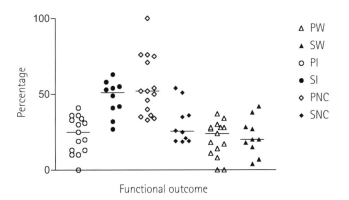

Figure 9. Scattergram comparing median functional outcomes between PTRAS and surgical revascularization.
PI and SI. Improved renal function for PTRAS and surgery respectively.
PNC and SNC: No change in renal function for PTRAS and surgery respectively.
PW and SW. Worse renal function after PTRAS and surgery respectively.

Summary

- Despite superior technical success rates for stent angioplasty, there is no difference in long-term functional outcomes between PTRA and PTRAS.

- There is no long-term difference in renal function between PTRAS and medical treatment.

- Surgical revascularization in current practice can be performed with perioperative mortality rates similar to those reported in several large series of PTRAS.

- Surgical revascularization has superior long-term patency rates and functional outcome, (improved renal function and hypertension, lower restenosis rates).

- There is a need for a prospective randomized comparison between PTRAS and surgical revascularization in patients fit for surgical intervention.

- Medical treatment appears to provide equivalent long-term results to PTRAS; the results of the ASTRAL study are awaited.

References

1. Scoble JE, Hamilton G. Atherosclerotic renovascular disease: A remediable cause of renal failure in the elderly. *BMJ* 1990; **300**: 1670–1671.
2. Chabova V, Schirger A, Stanson AW, McKusick MA, Textor SC. Outcomes of atherosclerotic renal artery stenosis managed without revascularization. *Mayo Clin Proc* 2000; **75**: 437–444.
3. Mailloux LU, Napolitano B, Bellucci AG *et al.* Renal vascular disease causing end-stage renal disease, incidence, clinical correlates, and outcomes: A 20-year clinical experience. *Am J Kidney Dis* 1994; **24**: 622–629.
4. Tuttle KR, Raabe RD. Endovascular stents for renal artery revascularization. *Curr Opin Nephrol Hypertens* 1998; **7**: 695–701.
5. Isles CG, Robertson S, Hill D. Management of renovascular disease: A review of renal artery stenting in 10 studies. *Q J Med* 1999; **92**: 159–167.

6. Leertouwer TC, Gussenhoven EJ, Bosch JL *et al.* Stent placement for renal arterial stenosis: Where to we stand? A meta-analysis. *Radiology* 2000; **216**: 78–85.

7. van de Ven PJ, Kaatee R, Beutler JJ *et al.* Arterial stenting and balloon angioplasty in osteal atherosclerotic renovascular disease: A randomised trial. *Lancet* 1999; **353**: 282–286.

8. van Jaarsveld BC, Krijnen P, Peterman H *et al.* The effect of balloon angioplasty in hypertension in atherosclerotic renal artery stenosis. Dutch Renal Artery Stenosis Intervention Cooperative Group. *N Engl J Med* 2000; **342**: 1007–1014.

9. Rees CR, Palmaz JC, Becker GJ *et al.* Palmaz stent in atherosclerotic stenoses involving the ostia of the renal arteries: Preliminary report on multicentre study. *Radiology* 1991; **181**: 507–514.

10. Raynaud AC, Beyssen BM, Turmel-Rodrigues LE *et al.* Renal artery stent placement: Immediate and mid-term technical and clinical results. *J Vasc Interv Radiol* 1994; **5**: 849–858.

11. Iannone LA, Underwood PL, Nath A *et al.* The effect of primary balloon expandable renal artery stents on long term patency, renal function and blood pressure in hypertensive and renal insufficient patients with renal artery stenosis. *Cathet Cardiovasc Diagn* 1996; **37**: 243–250.

12. Rundback JH, Jacobs JM. Percutaneous renal artery stent placement for hypertension and azotemia: Pilot study. *Am J Kidney Dis* 1996; **28**: 214–219.

13. Blum U, Crumme B, Flugel, P *et al.* Treatment of osteal renal artery stenoses with vascular endo prostheses after unsuccessful balloon angioplasty. *N Engl J Med* 1987; **336**: 459–465.

14. Boisclair C, Therasse E, Oliva VL *et al.* Treatment of renal angioplasty failure by percutaneous renal artery stenting with Palmaz stents: Mid term technical and clinical results. *Am J Roentgenol* 1997; **168**: 245–251.

15. Harden PN, MacLeod MJ, Rodger RS *et al.* The effect of renal artery stenting on progression of renovascular renal failure. *Lancet* 1997; **349**: 1133–1136.

16. White CJ, Ramee SR, Collins TJ *et al.* Renal artery stent placement: Utility and lesions difficult to treat with balloon angioplasty. *J Am Coll Cardiol* 1997; **30**: 1445–1450.

17. Gross CM, Kramer J, Waigan D *et al.* Osteal renal artery stent placement for atherosclerotic renal artery stenosis in patients with coronary artery disease. *Cathet Cardiovasc Diagn* 1998; **45**: 1–8.

18. Dorros G, Jaff M, Mathiak L *et al.* Four-year follow-up of Palmaz-Schatz stent revascularization as treatment for atherosclerotic renal artery stenosis. *Circulation* 1998; **98**: 648–647.

19. Tuttle KR, Choinard RF, Webber JG *et al.* Treatment of atherosclerotic osteal renal artery stenosis with the intravascular stent. *Am J Kidney Dis* 1998; **32**: 611–622.

20. Rundback JH, Gray RJ, Rozenblit G *et al.* Renal artery stent placement for the management of ischemic nephropathy. *J Vasc Interv Radiol* 1998; **9**: 413–420.

21. Henry M, Amor M, Henry I *et al.* Stents in the treatment of renal artery stenosis: Long-term follow-up. *J Endovasc Surg* 1999; **6**: 42–51.

22. Xue F, Bettmann MA, Langdon DR, Wivell WA. Outcome and cost comparison of percutaneous transluminal renal angioplasty, renal arterial stent placement, and renal arterial bypass grafting. *Radiology* 1999; **212**: 378–384.

23. Bush RL, Najibi S, MacDonald MJ *et al.* Endovascular revascularization of renal artery stenosis: Technical and clinical results. *J Vasc Surg* 2001; **33**: 1041–1049.

24. Yutan E, Glickerman DJ, Caps MT *et al.* Percutaneous transluminal revascularization for renal artery stenosis: Veterans Affairs Puget Sound Health Care System experience. *J Vasc Surg* 2001; **34**: 685–693.

25. Laderman RJ, Mendelsohn FO, Santos R *et al.* Primary renal artery stenting: Characteristics and outcomes after 363 procedures. *Am Heart J* 2001; **142**: 314–323.

26. Mercier C, Piquet P, Alimi Y, Turnigand P, Albrand JJ. Occlusive disease of the renal arteries and chronic renal failure: The limits of reconstructive surgery. *Ann Vasc Surg* 1990; **4**: 166–170.

27. Torsello G, Sachs M, Kniemeyer H *et al.* Results of surgical treatment for atherosclerotic renal vascular occlusive disease. *Eur J Vasc Surg* 1990; **4**: 477–482.

28. Bredenberg CE, Sampson LN, Ray FS *et al.* Changing patterns in surgery for chronic renal artery occlusive diseases. *J Vasc Surg* 1992; **15**: 1018–1023.

29. Libertino JA, Bosco PJ, Ying CY *et al.* Renal revascularization to preserve and restore renal function. *J Euro* 1992; **147**: 1485–1487.

30. Hansen KJ, Starr SM, Sands RE *et al.* Contemporary surgical management of renovascular disease. *J Vasc Surg* 1992; **16**: 319–330.

31. Chaikof EL, Smith RB, Salam AA *et al.* Ischemic nephropathy and concomitant aortic disease: A 10-year experience. *J Vasc Surg* 1994; **19**: 135–146.

32. Cambria RP, Brewster DC, L'Italien GJ *et al.* The durability of different reconstructive techniques for atherosclerotic renal artery disease. *J Vasc Surg* 1994; **20**: 76–85.

33. Hallett JW, Textor SC, Kos PB *et al.* Advanced renovascular hypertension and renal insufficiency: Trends in medical co-morbidity and surgical approach from 1970–1993. *J Vasc Surg* 1995; **21**: 750–759.

34. Lamawansa ND, Bell R, Kumar A, House AK. Radiological predictors of response to renovascular reconstructive surgery. *Ann R Coll Surg Engl* 1995; **77**: 337–341.
35. Cambria RP, Brewster DC, L'Italien GJ *et al*. Renal artery reconstruction for the preservation of renal function. *J Vasc Surg* 1996; **24**: 371–380.
36. Darling RC III, Kreienberg PB, Chang BB *et al*. Outcome of renal artery reconstruction: Analysis of 687 procedures. *Ann Surg* 1997; **230**: 524–530.
37. Hansen KJ, Cherr GS, Craven TE *et al*. Management of ischemic nephropathy: Dialysis free survival after surgical repair. *J Vasc Surg* 2000; **32**: 472–482.
38. Steinbach F, Novick AC, Campbell S, Dykstra D. Long-term survival after surgical revascularization for atherosclerotic renal artery disease. *J Urol* 1997; **158**: 38–41.

Renal artery lesions should be treated by angioplasty and stent

Charing Cross Editorial Comments towards Consensus

Who could disagree with this? George Hamilton tries very hard. The enthusiasm for operating upon renal artery stenosis has varied over the decades. It has never been too controversial when considered as an adjunct to aortic surgery when the abdomen is open anyway. But to do an open procedure to the renal artery when there is no other reason for entering the retro-peroneal space has been controversial. Compared with many operations it is technically more demanding and one of the main indications historically has been an attempt to correct hypertension. I think it will be fair to say the results of correcting renal artery stenosis in terms of hypertension have been disappointing but nowadays the hope is to improve renal function more than anything else. If increased blood flow to the renal artery improves renal function and even improves the management of hypertension in some cases, should this be done surgically? Certainly it is a whole lot easier to do by balloon angioplasty with or without stent! The answer is elusive and one of the main reasons is that there have been few data comparing the two for like patients and very few random controlled trials. At the moment angioplasty and stent are simply having the first bite and renal artery surgery is being reserved for complications and instances where angioplasty and stent cannot be arranged. Under these circumstances shall we ever know the answer? These authors have certainly given us the evidence and there are no experts better than the two who have guided us through the difficult thought processes.

Roger M Greenhalgh
Editor

Infected grafts require excision and extra-anatomic reconstruction

For the motion

MA Cairols, JM Simeon, F Guerrero, E Barjau, E Iborra

Introduction

Prosthetic graft infection is one of the most feared complications in vascular surgery, and its management one of the most difficult challenges faced by a vascular surgeon. Whatever the therapeutic approach this complication is associated with a high morbidity and mortality, which makes its management controversial in search of a better outcome. Furthermore, the infected vascular graft is almost always in the most favourable anatomical location for revascularization, making maintenance of adequate lower limb perfusion after graft removal difficult.

Fortunately prosthetic graft infection is relatively uncommon with an incidence average around 0.5 to 2.6% of all vascular reconstructions although the true incidence is unknown.[1-4] Most probably underestimated, in part due to the fact of the long period that elapses from the primary operation to the onset of the infectious clinical syndrome. Because of all these factors, elimination of the infection, limb preservation and survival cannot be achieved in all patients in whom a graft infection is detected.

In this review we will discuss diagnosis and treatment of patients with prosthetic graft infection, placing special emphasis on the basic principles necessary for successful management. Before the best therapeutic option is selected, basic information about all possible factors leading to an individual treatment is necessary. We will discuss our experience and the different therapeutical approaches carried out. Unfortunately there is no level I evidence to stand for a unique option in all patients, therefore individual exceptions must be made for particular patients when treating a prosthetic graft infection. Nevertheless we still think, as most consulted authors, that the standard option is extra-anatomic replacement and graft excision

Pathogenesis

Infection occurs in most cases at the time of the initial surgery and at subsequent early redo procedures involving the graft (e.g. revision in cases of early failure or arteriography through the limb graft) or from involvement of the graft by a nearby infection. Prosthetic graft infection is divided into early and late infection, considering 'early' as before the 4th month of the initial procedure and 'late' infection as beyond this period of time.[5] Most vascular graft infections occur in the early postoperative period, in which the most commonly identified pathogens include coagulase-negative *Staphylococcus aureus* and Gram-negative bacteria, *Escherichia coli*, *Proteus* and *Pseudomonas aeruginosa*.

Micro-organisms can infect the prosthesis at the time of the initial surgery whether by direct implantation, through an infected wound and posterior contamination of the prosthesis or via the blood stream or lymphatic circulation from a remote site. Both, early and late infection are thought to occur at the time of the primary intervention.[1,6]

Infection is defined as the colonization and growth of micro-organisms within the prosthesis and is related to their virulence and concentration. Other predisposing factors are the individual defences and the immunological reaction, as well as the prosthetic material used. Initially, after a graft is implanted an acute inflammatory reaction occurs, followed by a chronic inflammatory response that is associated with fibroblast infiltration of the perigraft space and graft interstices.[7] This is important for the initial healing and subsequent graft incorporation. Some authors use the term 'the race of the surface' to describe the events that arise at the interface after implantation of a prosthesis, a contest between tissue cell integration and bacterial adhesion to the surface.[8,9] If human cells are the first to attach to the graft ahead of micro-organisms, it is likely that no prosthesis-related infection will occur; on the contrary if bacteria adhere and form a nidus, a biofilm may develop which protects the bacteria from the host defences and antibiotics.

It is not uncommon to find multiple organisms particularly in association with systemic sepsis, infected false aneurysms and viscus erosion. *Pseudomonas aeruginosa* is a rare organism infecting prosthesis but quite virulent causing anastomosis suture disruption and an acute haemorrhage.[10] The methicillin-resistant *Staphylococcus aureus* has recently been a main protagonist as one of the relevant aetiological agents in intercurrent infections.

Late graft infections are commonly due to a less virulent bacterium such as coagulase-negative staphylococci and in particular *Staphylococcus epidermidis*. Their diagnoses are difficult, as the clinical syndrome is less evident or absent, although tenderness and erythema not properly evaluated could be present. These bacteria can be inactive at low concentrations for years after the initial operation before the clinical manifestations are apparent. Only after this long period of time may a cutaneous erythema overlying the graft, a perigraft mass or a discharging sinus herald a prosthetic infection.[11]

The pathogenesis of the bacteria coagulase-negative in late infections is well established, as *S. epidermidis* has been the micro-organism more frequently cultured in the explanted prosthesis. This pathogen has a role in the production of aortoenteric fistulae, although in the site of the viscus erosion *E. coli* was the most common, *S. epidermidis* was isolated in prosthetic segments far away from the intestinal lesion.[12]

The clinical manifestation of graft infection is the result of the balance between the pathogenicity of the micro-organism and the host immunological defences. It is reasonable then to think that only a small proportion of grafts contaminated by the micro-organism will develop overt signs of infection.[13] The physiological status of bacterial cells living in biofilms is heterogeneous and determined by the location of each individual cell within the multiple layers of cells forming the biofilm.[14] Cells located in the external layer are metabolically active and frequently reproducing, but they are highly susceptible to antibacterial agents and host defences. Cells located in the deeper layer of the biofilm have scarce access to nutrients and oxygen and show reduced or no reproductive activity. Their metabolism is differentiated towards the synthesis of glicocalyx and, because they are almost dormant are resistant to antibacterial agents and host defences. When the biofilm approaches to the critical mass, the cells in the outer layer may be released to cause acute episodes in the course of otherwise silent infection.[15] The degree of this cellular differentiation is proportional to the age of the film and is an additional factor responsible for the complexity of the clinical syndrome of graft infection.

The causative organism may be difficult to identify. During acute episodes of systemic infection, blood cultures can be useful and should be repeated at short intervals. Samples may also be obtained from wounds, perigraft fluid aspirated under ultrasound or computed tomographic (CT) control or directly from the explanted graft. They must be transported to the laboratory in an adequate liquid medium to be processed immediately. Although culture techniques have improved they still cannot be considered ideal as often an accurate microbiological diagnosis before graft removal is not possible. For those surgeons who decide the surgical option based on the bacteria cultured, identification of the micro-organism is usually not helpful.

Predisposing factors

Graft infection is associated with operative events leading to bacterial contamination or with patients' risk factors that predispose to infection due to impaired host defences. The important association of graft infection with groin incisions has been well documented and the development of complications in a groin wound is frequently the precursor of an infected prosthesis. The inguinal area tends to be relatively dirty as it is close to the perineum and the redundant skin folds increase the chances for contamination. The presence of a groin haematoma following preoperative femoral arteriography may contribute to a vascular graft infection, and a benefit may be observed from increasing the interval between intervention and the surgery in the groin.[3,16]

The incidence of graft infection is increased with emergency surgery, early re-operation, long interventions associated with substantial blood loss and simultaneous gastrointestinal, biliary or urological procedures. Patients who are at increased risk of graft infection are those with malnutrition, diabetes mellitus, chronic renal failure, autoimmune disease, and obesity. Immunodeficiency for malignancy, corticosteroid therapy and leucopenia are also predisposing factors. Infected or gangrenous lesions on the feet are associated with a high rate of wound and graft infections.

The severity of the arterial ischaemia is an important risk factor. The risk of wound infection in patients undergoing lower limb revascularization is augmented in patients with rest pain and skin necrosis compared with claudication or aneurysms.[17] *S. aureus* and *E. coli* were most common and over half of the patients with wound infection had a similar organism isolated from the skin previous to their operation. At least one-third of the patients with late prosthetic infection caused by *S. epidermidis* had evidence of some kind of sepsis or a ruptured aneurysm at the initial surgery.[18]

Finally, the type of prosthesis is also important; in fact graft infection is a problem of prosthetic grafts. Autogenous vein has inherent resistance to infection and it is known that bacterial adherence to Dacron is 10 to 100 times greater than to polytetrafluoroethylene (PTFE), varying according to bacterial pathogen. Unfortunately no clinical differences have been observed in graft infection rates in the two types of prosthesis.[1,3,19]

Diagnosis

Although not proven, an early diagnosis is thought to reduce the incidence of complication after a wound or graft infection. Clinical manifestation depends on different factors – in particular the anatomical location and it is frequently the first sign of alert for diagnosing a graft infection. According to Sharp, in 15% of patients the diagnosis will have confirmation after surgery only, based on the absence of incorporation of the prosthesis into the surrounding tissue.[20] Clinical manifestations such as infected fluid collection, drainage, and exteriorization of prosthetic material, pulsatile inflammatory mass or a haemorrhage confirm the diagnosis. The presence of pseudoaneurysms, even with no inflammatory signs, may be associated with a prosthetic infection.[21] In some patients with retroperitoneal prosthesis and unspecific signs of infection the diagnosis may be more difficult, in cases with general malaise not clearly explained, weight loss and lumbar pain associated with fever might be helpful. Occasionally there is an erythematous rush in the lower extremities caused by microembolization or mycotic aneurysms.

At present, research is directed towards early diagnosis in order to reduce complications linked to redo surgery. If an early diagnosis can be made there may be a significant reduction of mortality rate, therefore germane identification is of relevance. However, isolating the causative organisms of vascular graft infection may be difficult. Culture media even from liquid drained from the inguinal fistulae, from the explanted prosthesis and blood culture may be negative in 25% of prosthetic infections. Aspiration of the perigraft fluid yields leukocytes, but frequently no organisms.[22,23] One explanation for this low rate of positive cultures may be the fact of the fibrous polysaccharide matrix (glycolyx/slime) formation. The negativity of routine sampling culture methods can be reduced by the disruption of the bacterial laden using low energy sound waves. Other specific methods for specific biofilm culture may increase the rate of positive culture.[15]

The main advantage of ultrasound ecographic imaging is its capacity for detecting false anastomotic aneurysms and perigraft fluid. Eco-guided needle aspiration of the detected collection is a valuable tool for improving culture sensitivity.[24]

The widespread availability of the CT scan makes this method almost a mandatory step for diagnosing prosthetic graft infection, since Haaga in 1978 suspected the presence of graft infection by the presence of perigraft gas bubbles.[25] Nowadays, CT scan diagnosis of graft infection includes the presence of perigraft collection, the presence of gas bubbles and altered density of the soft tissue (Fig. 1). However, the absence of these signs does not exclude infection.

Moreover in the immediate postoperative period the CT scan has difficulty in differentiating retroperitoneal haematoma from perigraft infected collection, although haematoma should be gone at 3 months after the operation, and perigraft gas at 3–4 weeks.[26] Therefore after this period of time CT scan images should have a similar density as the normal soft tissue, making the diagnosis be more reliable at 6 months onwards, as proved by some series which have obtained as much as 94% of sensitivity and 85% of specificity.[27,28] As in echography, a CT scan can improve the diagnosis by the use of guided needle aspiration of the perigraft collection. Therefore computed tomography seems a reliable method for confirming the diagnosis when signs are present, although its main disadvantage is that the absence of signs does not exclude infection.[29]

Magnetic resonance imaging (MRI), thanks to its intrinsic characteristics of more accurate differentiation and characterization of tissues, has been accepted as a highly reliable method for prosthetic graft diagnosis. With MRI the main diagnostic cut-off is 6 months from the operation, a period during which modifications take place and

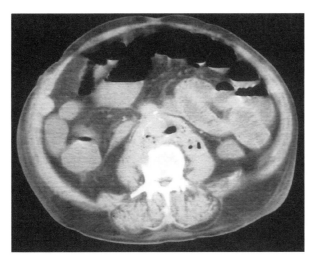

Figure 1. CT scan of an infected prosthetic graft in which a perigraft collection with gas bubbles is seen.

a CT scan is less accurate in differentiating normal from altered prosthetic incorporation. The possibility of accurately evaluating the involvement of the perigraft tissues and the use of paramagnetic contrast which are selectively picked up by infected tissues, makes this method particularly sensitive.[30] Nevertheless MRI is not capable of distinguishing gas from calcified plaques and it is unable to diagnose aortoenteric fistulae and useless for emergency operations.

Fistulography is an easy and simple test that may allow us to assess the extension of the graft involvement. Of particular interest is the involvement of the main prosthetic body, the contralateral limb and any possible ureteral fistulization. Before carrying out a fistulography an appropriate antibiotic systemic therapy is recommended to prevent episodes of bacteraemia (Fig. 2).

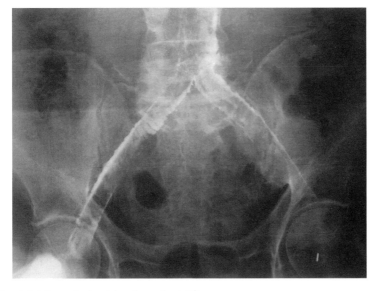

Figure 2. A fistulography involving the entire graft.

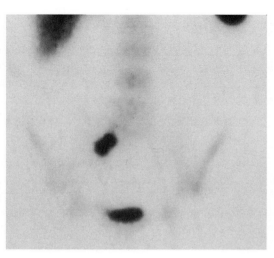

Figure 3. A Technetium 99m-hexametizene scintigraphy showing a localized infection in the left limb with an aorto-bifemoral prosthetic graft.

In comparison with morphological tests, scintigraphic techniques play a role in low-key infections, as it may be capable of making an early diagnosis. Of all the different available techniques, the gallium-67 scan introduced in 1980, is today considered an outdated method due to its unspecific accumulation in the liver, spleen and the gastroenteric tract which makes interpretation difficult. The indium 111-labelled leukocyte scan is more commonly used, although false positive may be linked to the incorporation of platelets. More recently technetium 99m-hexametazine has been introduced as it combines a short time of picture taking with high sensitivity, albeit with an increased number of false negatives, although its main limitation is the false positive cases[31] (Fig. 3).

Evidence for management by graft excision

We have been able to foresee an array of pathogenic doubts, diagnostic difficulties and a variety of clinical manifestation that make treatment of prosthetic graft infection far from settled. A cornerstone of prosthetic graft infection is preoperative prevention, namely the use of prophylactic antibiotics. From 1993 onwards, in our hospital a strict prophylactic antibiotic policy was implemented, and we were able to observe a significant decrease in the number of infections compared with a similar previous period of time. Some reports had striking experience in reducing the rate of graft infection. Kaiser reported on 462 patients undergoing elective vascular procedure; from 6.8% in a placebo group the rate of infection went down to 0.9% in patients under antibiotic prophylaxis.[32]

Although there is no consensus as to its optimal duration, antibiotic prophylaxis reduces wound infection in vascular surgery, and therefore it is recommended. Nevertheless, to date there is no hard data from prospective randomized clinical trials that antibiotic prophylaxis prevents significant graft infection, most probably due to the small incidence of infection and therefore a large study would be needed.[33]

Although prophylaxis should commence before surgery, it is common practice to give the first dose at the induction of anaesthesia, followed by two postoperative doses to cover the first 24 hours. There is no evidence of significant benefit from more prolonged courses of antibiotics, a practice that may be associated with a proliferation of resistant organisms.[34] In situations where the risk is increased, such as lower limb infection or tissue loss, emergency surgery or reoperation, there are no recommendations for prophylaxis, although in these patients it may be justified to give a 5-day course of antibiotics.

The decreased incidence of infection was probably related to a proper antibiotic prophylaxis regime, but improvement in operative technique may have also contributed. All patients, in particular those at high risk, had their underlying medical problem stabilized prior to surgery. The problem arises when the operation must be carried out as an emergency as on some of our patients. Different methods of skin preparation have been suggested to reduce skin contamination (antiseptic baths with chlorhexidine, skin preparation with povidone-iodine, sterile draping) although none of them have proved to be superior. Although their use has not shown a reduction in the incidence of wound infection, even in the groin, we are scrupulously strict in adopting all preventing sterile measures.[35]

The two main therapeutical approaches, total graft excision and extra-anatomic or *in situ* replacements, should be complementary rather than competitive. The authors of these lines are aware that evidence for each of these approaches is needed. Classical total radical excision and extra-anatomic replacement is apparently less attractive, but for most consulted authors, even those defending an *in situ* approach, this still remains the standard procedure.

The surgical management of graft infection depends on the site and the extent of the infection, the virulence of the infecting organism, the need for distal revascularization or the involvement of the anastomoses. The time-honoured radical treatment of total graft excision and extra-anatomic replacement, debridement of the surrounding tissues was first reported by Blaisdell in 1970.[36] However, the Blaisdell procedure has complications in itself such as aortic stump blow out and is associated with mortality of 24–70% and 15–40% of amputation according to the different reported series.[2,4,37] These poor initial results produced new initiatives in the prevention of graft infection based on the use of antibiotic-bonded grafts and *in situ* replacement of the aortoiliac infected graft with autogenous deep lower extremity veins and arterial allografts. However, most published reports are difficult to evaluate as too many different therapies are applied to heterogeneous subjects so that many of the series are biased.

Samuel Johnson in his Dictionary of the English Language of 1746, says, 'knowledge is of two kinds. We know the subject ourselves, or we know where we can find information for it'.

From 1993 to 2000, we have retrospectively reviewed the surgical files in our Department for all patients in whom an infrarenal aortic prosthesis was implanted. During this period of time 627 primary procedures using prosthetic material were performed; of these 13 patients (2.1%, 13/627) had a prosthetic graft infection. All those patients with superficial wounds not involving the prosthetic graft were excluded.

Revascularization is usually done with an extra-anatomic graft through uninfected tissue planes. This is accomplished with a transobturator bypass to the mid-superficial femoral artery or a lateral approach from the pelvis to the profunda or superficial femoral artery usually with PTFE. After completing the extra-anatomic revascularization and closing and bandaging all incisions, the vascular surgeon excises all infected graft through a new groin incision, which is left open to heal secondarily once all infected collection fluid is drained. Ideally the profunda femoris should be maintained patent, then the common femoral artery is ligated before its bifurcation. In the presence of a severe infection a vein patch is frequently used to keep the profunda femoris patent, but since the vein patch may disrupt, this procedure needs to be considered.

Summary of cases of prosthetic graft infection (1993–2000)

The original surgery was performed on 13 males – mean age 69 years (range 47–77 years). There were six cases of abdominal aortic aneurysm and seven cases of atherosclerotic occlusive arterial disease.

We had six early prosthetic infections and four deaths (mortality rate of 66%). One patient died after 2 weeks of an initial surgery for a ruptured abdominal aortic aneurysm and the micro-organism infecting the prosthesis was *Enterobacter cloacae* and multiple flora of coagulase-negative staphylococci. Another patient at 3 weeks from the primary surgery had periprosthetic pus in which *S. aureus*, *E. faecium* had grown and the blood culture showed *B. fragilis*; the patient had fever and a faecaloid fistula. The third early infection was at 1 week from an aortobifemoral bypass after critical limb ischaemia in a patient in whom the prosthetic limb occluding thrombus had grown *Pseudomonas aeruginosa* and multiple flora of coagulase-negative staphylococci. There was a fourth patient with infected graft at 22 weeks (the sample sent to the laboratory did not grow any causative micro-organism), with an onset of massive blood loss from an aortoenteric fistula, who died before we could perform an extra-anatomic replacement.

We had seven patients with late infections and two deaths (mortality of 28%). In one patient infection was seen 54 weeks after surgery, the clinical manifestation was an aortic pseudoaneurysm infected by *Klebsiella oxytoca* and *Streptococcus anginosus*. Death occurred after an unexpected aortic lesion and an intraoperative haemorrhage. Another patient at 217 weeks after surgery, had an aortoenteric fistula and a haemorrhage; he died in the operating theatre. Therefore there is a significant difference between patients with an early infection, most of whom undergo an emergency procedure, and patients with late infection mostly elective.

In only three cases the replacement procedure consisted of an axillofemoral bypass with one limb loss, one death and one alive and well. In three patients a prosthetic limb resection and drainage was the only option available with one patient dead and one limb loss. Drainage and partial graft resection only was the procedure in three cases with one death, one limb loss and one alive and well. *In situ* replacement was attempted in four patients: two iliofemoral PTFE (one death and one alive), and two criopreserved arterial homografts (both alive and needing of reoperation for recurrent infection). The other three patients had conservative treatment such as drainage. Finally in one last case the patient died before surgery was possible. Therefore surgical radical resection and simultaneous extra-anatomic bypass was performed in only three cases, with a mortality of 33%, whereas the different *in situ* methods were attempted in four with a 22% mortality rate; however the recurrent rate of infection needing early reoperation was 50% (Fig. 4).

Seven patients were discharged from hospital and followed up between 12 and 72 months. Of these patients, five had recurrent local wound infection, although no further deaths were registered.

This rather heterogeneous experience reflects the day-to-day clinical reality in a busy vascular department, where in many cases the initial surgical aim was to control haemorrhage. Once haemorrhage was under control and in the presence of an infection the most frequent option was debridement and closure of the area, followed by excision of the infected graft. When possible we prefer to perform the extra-anatomic revascularization first and then later remove the graft and drainage. This limits lower

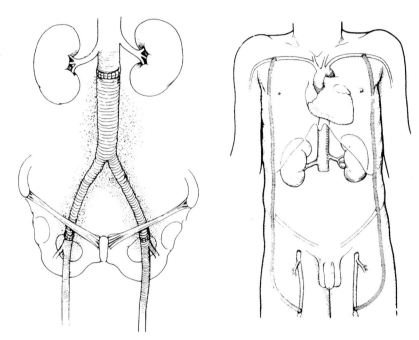

Figure 4a. Schematic drawings of a total excision and simultaneous extra-anatomic replacement with an axillo-superficial femoral.

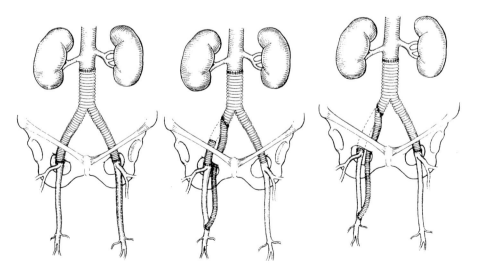

Figure 4b. Partial excision and modalities of replacement *in situ* with an 8-mm thin-wall ringed Gore-Tex graft sutured end-to-end to the proximal limb of the bifurcated graft. Figures 4a,b reproduced with permission from Ref. 57.

limb ischaemia, reduces the cardiovascular changes associated with aortic ligation and lowers the mortality and amputation rates.[38]

Some patients with localized graft infection, partially incorporated and patent prosthesis, were treated by segmental removal of the infected graft followed by a local debridement with an *in situ* placement of a PTFE or criopreserved arterial homograft. In those cases the treatment was infusion of an intravenous antibiotic followed by the coverage of the exposed graft with a muscle flap or a skin graft after adequate granulation. When there was local graft infection involving a thrombosed limb, poor incorporation or evidence of anastomotic breakdown, the procedure followed was resection of that limb, and wide debridement and limb revascularization by an extra-anatomic approach (lateral, obturator, and cross-femoral) (Fig. 5).

Unfortunately from our own experience we cannot advocate any of the therapeutical approaches. Moreover a third conservative option attempted in selected cases (prosthetic limb ligature and drainage without revascularization) has a high rate of mortality and limb loss and recurrent infection. The Mayo Clinic experience is quite similar. Menawat *et al.*[39] reviewed 52 patients from 1980 to 1994, with a peroperative mortality rate of 27% (14/52). However, after emergency procedure the mortality rate was 42% (8/19), whereas elective surgery carried a lower mortality of 18% (6/33). One of their patients died after attempted repair. Additionally, early mortality tended to be higher in patients with bleeding alone (47%, 9/19) compared with patients with

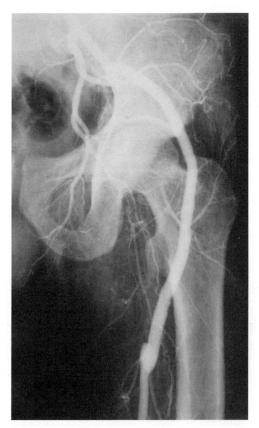

Figure 5.   Groin drainage and localized infection.

infection alone. As in our series the results reflect the difficulties in following a pre-determined algorithm and the need to use different techniques. Graft removal plus staged initial extra-anatomic bypass was feasible in 17% and graft removal plus simultaneous bypass in 33% of patients. Graft removal plus simultaneous *in situ* bypass was carried out in 25% of patients and in 20% an *in situ* replacement plus complete or partial graft removal.

As it is evident that the results are poor, new initiatives in the management of graft infection have been developed. Those new initiatives are based on the following points.

In situ replacement of the aortoiliac infected graft by autogenous deep and superficial lower extremity vein grafts

Nevelsteen *et al.*[40] has reviewed the use of autogenous grafts constructed from deep femoral veins to treat 14 infected graft patients. Postoperative mortality and early amputation rates were 7%. Only three patients had an aortoenteric fistula (21%), and one had an acute haemorrhage, while 11 (79%) presented with isolated graft infection. Most of the presenting symptoms were located at the level of the groin, and only three presented with retroperitoneal abscess. The follow-up period was short with a mean of 16 months and most of the infections were secondary to *S. epidermidis* and *S. aureus* (8/14). Limb swelling was common in the early postoperative period, needing pneumatic compression and elastic stocking in all patients, except in one who developed popliteal vein thrombosis and was treated with prolonged bed rest and anticoagulation.

Clagett *et al.*,[41] reviewed his results in 20 patients with 17 infected aorto-bifemoral prostheses and three other complex aortic problems. Treatment consisted of resection of the infected prosthesis and *in situ* reconstruction with the deep vein the greater saphenous veins or both. The reported mortality and limb loss was 10% each. Infection was cured in all cases and no recurrences were observed. Later in 1997[42]

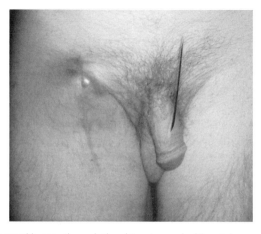

Figure 6. An ilio-femoral bypass through the obturata canal with autologous vein was the treatment carried out (same patient as in Fig. 5).

they reported 15 patients in whom primary and secondary patency rates at 5 years were 83% and 100%, 5 years limb salvage was 86% and significant lower limb oedema was uncommon. However, the mean operative time for *in situ* aortic graft replacement with a graft constructed of superficial femoral vein was 7.9 hours and major postoperative morbidity occurred in 49%, including compartment syndrome in 12% and limb paralysis in 7.5%. Finally in 1999[43] they reviewed 17 patients in whom extra-anatomic bypass was impossible. They conclude: 'extra-anatomic bypass with staged removal of infected vascular prostheses would be the preferred approach, offering the prospect of less physiological stress and improved morbidity and mortality'.

In situ replacement of the aortoiliac infected graft for fresh arterial homograft

Kieffer *et al.*,[44] used allografts to replace infected prosthetic aortic grafts in 43 patients, including 36 with aortic graft infection with a postoperative mortality of 12% and no early amputation. However, allograft-complication occurred in 11 patients (26%) including allograft graft rupture, graft thrombosis and enteric fistula and one late death possibly due to persistent or recurrent infection. Later in 1997[45] they published a review of 100 consecutive patients. In 27, there was an aortoenteric fistula, 26 needed emergency procedures some for lower limb ischaemia, while 74 had planned operations. The reported mortality was 24%, but 38% in patients with aortoenteric fistula. Even more striking was the mortality rate in patients undergoing emergency operations compared with patients on elective surgery (46% vs 16% respectively). There were 13 late deaths of which two were secondary to aortic rupture. Moreover, 20 occlusive lesions were observed in the follow-up with 15 of these requiring re-operation.

Our experience in criopreserved arterial homograft is short and unsatisfactory as the graft is subjected to reinfection and deterioration often with disastrous consequences. Unfortunately, we see an increasing number of extensive infections and emergency cases rather than an increasing number of patients who appear to have isolated film infections appropriate for treatment with *in situ* prosthetic graft replacement. As a matter of fact many consider allografts as a bridge procedure between the initial infection, until a more definitive reconstruction can be undertaken.

In situ replacement of the aortoiliac infected graft for antibiotic bonded grafts

Hayes *et al.*,[46] used rifampicin-bonded polyester graft to replace infected prosthetic aortic grafts in 11 patients with a postoperative mortality of 18.2% and a late mortality of 36%. Their results suggest a poorer long-term outcome (75% mortality rate) in the group of patients who had originally undergone emergency procedures. Besides, the postoperative mortality rate was also significantly higher in those cases involving aortoenteric fistula (three of five presentations, 60%). The authors state 'these figure are comparable with of a number of other series, which used either extra-anatomic bypass grafting procedures or *in situ* replacement'. The conclusion reduces the initial optimism about the use of total graft excision plus *in situ* replacement with rifampicin-bonded Dacron grafts in the management of major aortic infections has been tempered by additional experience.

Twone *et al.*,[47] treated 14 patients who had prosthetic aortic graft infection due to *Staphylococcus* species biofilms with graft excision and *in situ* replacement with a new prosthetic graft. Although there was no mortality or limb loss the patients included in this study had limited infection, and only a portion of the aortic graft was replaced. Speziale *et al.*,[48] retrospectively reviewed 20 patients with infected synthetic abdominal aortic grafts and 18 underwent i*n situ* replacement with standard PTFE. Two patients were excluded from the management protocol because they had more severe clinical disease (positive blood culture, septic lower limb emboli with retroperitoneal collection). All diagnoses were made beyond the 6 months from the original aortic surgery, therefore there were no early infections. In all cases an arteriogram, a 99m-TC scintigraphy and a CT scan was performed. They conclude 'infections caused by coagulase-negative *S. epidermidis* and other bacteria can be successfully treated by *in situ* graft replacement. However, graft infections due to aggressive or mixed bacterial strains still portend an exceedingly poor prognosis'.

It seems that despite the apparent good results with the use of autologous superficial and deep vein, the comments made by these experts emphasizes the selective indication of this procedure.

With regard to limb loss rate, it appears to be similar in all varieties of *in situ* bypass procedures, and significantly lower than the rates between 19% and 27% attributed to extra-anatomic bypass grafting.[4,49] The Mayo Clinic series (39) *in situ* repair showed a better outcome with a 10% limb loss compared with 24% obtained with the extra-anatomic bypass graft procedure and it could be accepted that limb salvage is perhaps the only main advantage.

But if this may be the case some worrying questions remain unanswered. What happens to patients with biofilm graft infections treated with *in situ* prosthetic? Is the infection eradicated or do they live in symbiosis with their infection? If the infection is indolent but still present what is the value of removing the old graft to be replaced by another? What would be the outcome if this type of infection were treated with local measures? If the recurrent infection rate is high at short follow-up, will this rate of clinically evident infections continue to grow as time goes by? There is no doubt, however, that when a significant percentage of patients come back with recurrent infection we will have to manage them when they are older and less able to tolerate a more definitive procedure.

Improved results with radical excision and extra-anatomic bypass replacement

Table 1 lists the most relevant series published in which total excision and extra-anatomic bypass graft have been performed as the procedure of choice after a prosthetic graft infection. Table 2 relates to papers in which the procedure advocated is *in situ* replacement. Comparison between these groups is most probably influenced by the criteria to include a particular patient and by the treatment algorithm. It is clear that different approaches are used in patients with very different potential outcomes to be of value in choosing the best therapeutic management. Outcome after treatment of aortic graft infection with extra-anatomic bypass grafting and graft excision and *in situ* graft replacement appears to be comparable, because the technique is probably not so important as the virulence of infection and the clinical syndrome, in particular acute haemorrhage. Additionally, the catastrophic events associated with allografts and antibiotic-bonded graft *in situ* replacement appear to have a limited indication for those patients in whom no other options are possible.

Table 1. Results of different series in which radical excision and extra-anatomic bypass graft was carried out as replacement

Reference	n (%)	Mortality (%)	Early amputation (%)	Aortic stump blowout (%)	Survival >1year (%)	Extra-anatomic graft infection (%)
Bandyk 1984[50]	18	11	11	0	66	17
O'Hara 1986[4]	84	18	27	22	58	25
Reilly 1987[51]	92	14	25	13	73	20
Yeager 1990[52]	38	14	21	4	76	22
Quinones-Baldrich 1991[49]	45	24	11	0	63	20
Kuestner 1995[53]	33	18	6	6	70 (3 years)	
Yeager 1999[54]	60	13	6.6	1.6	67 (2 years)	10
Seeger 2000[55]	36	11 (19%)	0	2.7	73 (3 years)	2.7
Bandyk 2001[56]	31	21	9	0		3

Table 2. Results of different series in which radical excision and *in situ* bypass graft was carried out as replacement

Reference	n (%)	Mortality (%)	Early amputation (%)	Survival >1 year (%)	Bypass graft infection (%)
Bandyk 1991[18]	28				3.5
Speziale 1997[48]	18	6	0		0
Hayes 1999[46]	11	18.2		63.6	
Clagett 1997[42]	41	7.3	5		0
Bandyk 2001[56]	Prosthesis	25			10
	veins	10			3

In situ replacement using superficial femoral vein is a demanding procedure not appropriate for emergency operations. Furthermore, although operative mortality associated with *in situ* replacement of the infected graft and extra-anatomic bypass grafting are equivalent, postoperative complications associated with autogenous vein graft replacement, in particular limb paralysis and compartment syndrome, are more serious.

A crucial point for comparing series of patients is stratification according to their prognoses. In the reported series on this topic, the heterogeneity of patients, as well as the wide variance of mortality and morbidity is of relevance. It looks as if we were comparing apples and oranges. We have reporting standards in other areas in vascular surgery and we must also develop reporting standard for this problem. Both tables have common authors giving evidence for different therapeutic approaches, which confirms the lack of standardization for prosthetic graft reporting.

Conclusions

Our data suggest that success depends primarily on patient selection determined by clinical presentation and cultured organism. *In situ* graft replacement is a reasonable option in properly selected patients (i.e. indolent coagulase-negative staphylococcus prosthetic infection or when no organism is cultured), where apparently there is a low mortality rate and higher rate of limb salvage. In contrast, this therapy failed in 100% of the patients with either mixed organism or Gram-negative infection.

Graft removal with extra-anatomic bypass is durable although associated with mortality. Graft preservation may be successful with low-grade early staphylococcal infection.

Sepsis and its complications were the most common cause of death and systemic sepsis as the presenting symptom of aortic graft infection predicted an almost 60% mortality associated with treatment. Treatment using staged extra-anatomic bypass and aortic graft excision was associated with the lowest mortality but when patients presented with evidence of systemic sepsis, mortality was high regardless of how they were treated. At present, staged axillofemoral bypass prior to aortic graft removal is used preferentially for treatment of aortic graft infection. In addition, significant effort is made to control retroperitoneal sepsis, as this seems to be a major determinant of mortality after treatment of this complex problem.

The introduction of multiple new techniques for managing patients with this complex problem appears to have improved the outcome for individual patients with this feared complication, but also has made the selection of the 'best' treatment for an individual patient more critical and more difficult.

Thus until all questions are answered, and gradation of infected grafts comes into the methodology for stratifying prognoses, the sound knowledge but not evidence that we have for prevention and treatment of graft infection can be summarized as follows:

1. Antibiotic prophylaxis reduces wound (but not graft) infections.
2. With sepsis, extensive retroperitoneal infection and secondary aortoenteric fistula (in particular with active bleeding) are associated with a poor result whatever the repair technique used.
3. Total graft excision and extra-anatomic bypass remains the standard treatment for aortic graft infection as results have improved recently.
4. *In situ* graft replacement is an acceptable alternative in selected patients with minimal contamination.

Summary

- 100% failure of *in situ* graft replacement in the presence of mixed organisms or Gram-negative infection.

- Ongoing sepsis is the most common cause of death.

References

1. Calligaro KD, Veith FJ. Diagnosis and management of infected prosthetic aortic grafts. *Surgery* 1991; 110: 805–813.
2. Yeager RA, Porter JM, Arterial and prosthetic graft infection. *Ann Vasc Surg* 1992; 6: 485–491.
3. Lorentzen Nielsen OM, Arendrup H *et al.* Vascular graft infection: an analysis of sixty-two graft infection in 2411 consecutively implanted synthetic vascular grafts. *Surgery* 1985; 98: 81–86.
4. O'Hara PJ, Hertzer NR, Beven EG, Krajewsky LP. Surgical management of infected abdominal aortic grafts: review of 25-year experience. *J Vasc Surg* 1986; 3: 725–731.
5. Hicks RCJ, Greenhalgh RM. Pathogenesis of vascular grafts infection. *Eur J Vasc Endovasc Surg* 1997; 14 (Suppl A): 5–9.

6. Moore WS, Cole CW. Infection in prosthetic vascular grafts. In *Vascular Surgery: A Comprehensive Review*. Moore WS (ed). Philadelphia: WB Saunders. 1991: 471–485.

7. Olofsson P, Rabahie GN, Matsumoto K *et al*. Histopathological characteristics of explanted human prosthetic grafts: implications for the prevention and management of graft infection. *Eur J Vasc Endovasc Surg* 1995; 9: 143–151.

8. Ratliff DA. New initiatives in the prevention and treatment of graft infection. In *The Evidence for Vascular Surgery*. Earnshaw JJ, Murie JA (eds). TFM Publishing 1999: 173–181.

9. Gristina AG. Biomaterial-centred infection: microbial adhesion versus tissue integration. *Science* 1987; 237: 1588–1595.

10. Calligaro KD, Veith FJ, Schwartz ML, Savarese RP, DeLaurentis DA. Are Gram-negative bacteria a contra-indication to selective preservation of infected prosthetic arterial graft. *J Vasc Surg* 1992; 16: 337–346.

11. Bunt TJ. Synthetic vascular graft infections. I. Graft infections. *Surgery* 1983; 93: 733–746.

12. Vinard E, Eloy R, Descotes JR *et al*. Human vascular grafts failure and frequency of infection. *J Biomed Mat Res* 1991; 25: 499–513.

13. Wooster DL, Louch RE, Kradjen S. Intraoperative bacterial contamination of vascular grafts: a prospective study. *Can J Surg* 1985; 28: 407–419.

14. Selan L, Pasarriello C. Microbiological diagnosis of aortofemoral grafts infection. *Eur J Vasc Endovasc Surg* 1997; 14 (Supp A): 10–12.

15. Tollefson DF, Bandyk DF, Kaebuch HW, Seabrook GR, Towne JB. Surface biofilm disruption: enhanced recovery of micro-organisms from vascular prostheses. *Arch Surg* 1987; 122: 38–43.

16. Landrenau MD, Raju S. Infections after elective bypass surgery for lower limb ischaemia: the influence of perioperative transcutaneous arteriography. *Surgery* 1981; 90: 956–961.

17. Earnshaw JJ, Slack RCB, Hopkinson BR, Makin GS. Risk factors in vascular surgical sepsis. *Ann Roy Coll Surg Engl* 1988; 70: 139–143.

18. Bandyk DF, Bergamini TM, Kinney EV *et al*. *In situ* replacement of vascular prostheses infected by bacterila biofilm. *J Vasc Surg* 1991; 13: 575–583.

19. Schmidt DD, Bandyk DF, Pequet AJ, Towne JB. Bacterial adherence to vascular prosthesis. *J Vasc Surg* 1986; 3: 732–740.

20. Sharp W, Hoballah JJ, Mohan CR *et al*. The management of the infected aortic prosthesis: a current decade of experience. *J Vasc Surg* 1994; 19: 844–850.

21. Relly LM, Altman H, Lusby RJ *et al*. Late results following surgical management of vascular graft infection. *J Vasc Surg* 1984; 1: 36–44.

22. Padberg FT Jr, Smith SM, Eng RH. Accuracy of disincorporation for identification of graft infection. *Arch Surg* 1995; 130: 183–187.

23. Bandyk DF, Esses GE. Prosthetic graft infection. *Surg Clin North Am* 1994; 74: 571–590.

24. Gooding GA, Effeney DJ, Goldstone J. The aortofemoral graft: detection and identification of healing complications by ultrasonography. *Surgery* 1981; 89: 94–101.

25. Haaga JR, Baldwin GN, Reich NC. CT detection of infected synthetic grafts: preliminary reports of a new sign. *Am J Roentgenol* 1978; 131: 317–320.

26. Brown OW, Stanson AW, Pairolero PC *et al*. Computerised tomography following abdominal aortic surgery. *Surgery* 1982; 91: 716–722.

27. Qvafordt PG, Reilly LM, Mark AS *et al*. Computerised tomographic assessment of graft incorporation after reconstruction. *Am J Surg* 1985; 150: 227–231.

28. Low RN, Wall SD, Jeffrey RB, Sollito R, Reilly L. Aortoenteric fistula and perigraft infection: evaluation with CT. *Radiology* 1990, 175: 157–162.

29. Aufferman W, Olofsson PA, Rabahie GN. Incorporation versus infection of retroperitoneal aortic grafts. MR imaging features. *Radiology* 1989; 172: 359–362.

30. Spartera C, Morettini G, Petrassi C *et al*. The role of MRI in the evaluation of aortic graft healing, perigraft fluid collection and graft infection. *Eur J Vasc Endovasc Surg* 1990; 4: 69–73.

31. Fiorani P, Speziale F, Rizzo L *et al*. Detection of aortic graft infection with leukocytes technetium 99m-hexametazime. *J Vasc Surg* 1993; 17: 87–96.

32. Kaiser AB, Clayson KR, Mulherin JL *et al*. Antibiotic prophylaxis in vascular surgery. *Ann Surg* 1978; 188: 283–289.

33. Strachchan CJL. Antibacterial prophylaxis in peripheral vascular and orthopaedic prosthetic surgery. *J Antimicrob Chemother* 1993; 31 (Suppl B): 65–78.

34. Santini C, Baiocchi P, Serra P. Perioperative antibiotic prophylaxis in vascular surgery. *Eur J Vasc Endovasc Surg* 1997; 14 (Suppl A): 13–14.

35. Cruse PJE, Foord R. The epidemiology of wound infection. A 10-year prospective study of 62,939 wounds. *Surg Clin North Am* 1980; 60: 27–40.

36. Blaisdell FW, Hall AD, Lim RC Jr, Moore WC. Aortoiliac arterial substitution utilizing subcutaneous grafts. *Ann Surg* 1970; 172: 775–780.

37. Reilly LM, Altman H, Lubsby RH *et al.* Late results following surgical management of vascular graft infection. *J Vasc Surg* 1984; **1**: 36–44.

38. Seeger JM, Pretus HA, Welborn MB *et al.* Long-term outcome after treatment of aortic graft infection with staged extra-anatomic bypass grafting and aortic graft removal. *J Vasc Surg* 2000; **32**: 451–461.

39. Menawat SS, Gloviczki P, Serry RD *et al.* Management of aortic graft enteric fistula. *Eur J Vasc Endovasc Surg* 1997; (Suppl A) **14**: 74–81.

40. Nevelsteen A, Lacroix H, Suy R. Infrarenal ortic graft infection: *in situ* aortoiliofemoral reconstruction with the lower extremity deep veins. *Eur J Vasc Endovasc Surg* 1997; **14** (Suppl A): 88–92.

41. Clagett GP, Bowers BL, Lopez-Veigo MA *et al.* Creation of a neo-aortoiliac system for lower extremity deep and superficial veins. *Ann Surg* 1993; **218**: 239–249.

42. Clagett GP, Valentine RJ, Hagino RT. Autogeneous aortoiliac/femoral reconstruction from superficial femoral-popliteal veins: feasibility and durability. *J Vasc Surg* 1997; **25**: 255–270.

43. Gordon LL, Hagino RT, Jackson MR, Modrall JG, Valentine RJ, Clagett GP. Complex aorto femoral prosthetic infection. The role of autogeneous superficial femoropopliteal vein reconstruction. *Arch Surg* 1999; **134**: 615–621.

44. Kieffer E, Bahnini A, Koskas F *et al. In situ* allograft replacement of infected infrarenal aortic prosthetic grafts: results in forty-three patients. *J Vasc Surg* 1993; **17**: 349–356.

45. Routolo C, Plissonnier D, Bahnini A, Koskas F, Kieffer E. *In situ* arterial allografts: A new treatment for aortic prosthetic infection. *Eur J Vasc Endovasc Surg* 1997; **14** (Suppl A): 102–107.

46. Hayes PD, Nasim A, London NJM *et al. In situ* replacement of infected graft with rifampicin-bonded prostheses: the Leicester experience (1992–1998). *J Vasc Surg* 1999; **30**: 92–98.

47. Twone JB, Seabrook GR, Bandyk D, Freischlag JA, Edmiston CE. *In situ* replacement of arterial prosthesis infected by bacterial biofilms: long-term follow-up. *J Vasc Surg* 1994; **19**: 226–235.

48. Speziale F, Rizzo L, Sbarigia E *et al.* Bacterial and clinical criteria relating to the outcome of patients undergoing in situ repalcement of infected abdominal aortic grafts. *Eur J Vasc Endovasc Surg* 1997; **13**: 127–133.

49. Quinones-Baldrich BW, Hernandez JJ, Moore WS. Long-term results following surgical management of aortic graft infection. *Arch Surg* 1991; **126**: 507–511.

50. Bandyk DF, Berni GA, Thiele BL *et al.* Aortofemoral graft infection due to *Staphylococcus epidermidis*. *Arch Surg* 1984; **119**: 102–108.

51. Reilly LM, Stoney RJ, Goldstone J, Ehrenfeld WK. Improved management of aortic graft infection: the influence of operation sequence and staging. *J Vasc Surg* 1987; **5**: 421–431.

52. Yeager RA, Moneta GL; Taylor LM *et al.* Improving survival and limb salvage in patients with aortic graft infection. *Am J Surg* 1990; **159**: 466–469.

53. Kuestner LM, Reilly LM, Jicha DL *et al.* Secondary aortoenteric fistula: contemporary outcome using extraanatomic bypass and infected graft excisio. *J Vasc Surg* 1995; **21**: 185–196.

54. Yaeger RA, Taylor LM, Moneta GL *et al.* Improved results in conventional management of infrarenal aortic infection. *J Vasc Surg* 1999; **30**: 76–83.

55. Seeger JM, Petrus HA, Welborn MB *et al.* Long-term outcome after treatment of aortic graft infection with staged extra-anatomic bypass grafting and aortic removal. *J Vasc Surg* 2000; **32**: 451–461.

56. Bandyk DF, Novotney ML, Back MR *et al.* Expanded aplication of in situ replacement for prosthetic graft infection. *J Vasc Surg* 2001; **34**: 411–420.

57. Hollier L. Management of aortic graft infection. In *Vascular and Endovascular Surgical Techniques* 4th edn. Greenhalgh RM (ed). London: WB Saunders, 2001: 153–160.

Infected grafts require excision and extra-anatomic reconstruction

Against the motion

Max Zegelman, Gisela Günther

for the Working Group *Graftinfections**

Introduction

Thesis

Infection of vascular prostheses is a rare but serious complication in vascular surgery. The infection has a dramatic effect on the course and can result in loss of the limb, functional disorder or death. Even in successful treatment, the complication 'graft infection' may give rise to a greater deficit than the actual vascular condition which occasioned the first operation.[1] It is therefore important that the effect of surgery applied is as definitive as possible and that it is safe and relatively simple. The risk and inconvenience for the patient and surgeon must be acceptable. This can best be achieved with *in situ* reconstruction after complete removal of all infected prosthesis material.

General

The incidence of vascular prosthesis infection varies from 0.5% to 5%.[1] It depends on the site of implantation, the urgency of the operation, the underlying diseases and the immunological status. Graft infections are more frequent after emergency operations, in anastomosis with the femoral artery or in subcutaneous prosthesis position.[1,2,3] The route of infection can result from direct contamination during the operation or from disorders of wound healing, or spread may be haematogenous. When the formation of pseudointima is not complete, bactaeremia may also cause microbial colonization of a prosthesis even more than 1 year after implantation. Moreover, the prosthesis can also be infected by erosion with the skin or the gastrointestinal tract. Early (up to 4 months after implantation) and late infections are distinguished. Half of all graft infections occur early. Infections of aortic prostheses occur an average of 40 months and infections of peripheral prostheses an average of 7 months after implantation.[1] *Staphylococcus aureus* is the most frequent cause in the group of early infections. Late infections are based in particular on infection with *Staphylococcus epidermidis*, *Candida* and other microbes.[1,4]

---

*For details of the Working Group *Graftinfections* see p. 258.

Surgical therapy is always necessary since antibiotic therapy alone will not clear the infection. There are quite divergent views on the kind of surgical treatment. Complete removal of all infected materials may be combined with extra-anatomical or with *in situ* reconstruction. The rationale for the 'most simple' approach of removing all infected material completely in combination with *in situ* reconstruction will be described. The preliminary results of our data collection for the use of silver-coated Dacron prostheses in treating vascular prosthesis infections will be presented.

Infection-protected grafts

Since 1992, we have gathered experience in treating vascular prosthesis infections with a Dacron prosthesis soaked in triclosane. This was inserted after official approval in individual cases. Triclosane is an antiseptic which has been used for 20 years, mainly in dermatology, wound treatment and dental medicine. It is added to toothpaste, mouth washes and deodorants. In more than 30 patients, all prosthesis material was explanted without exception. Debridement and *in situ* repair were carried out. Antibiotic cover was always given. There were no reinfections in this group of patients with a mean duration of observation of 2 years. However, this prosthesis was not used on a broad scale, since triclosane did not have any approval for this indication nor had the manufacturer applied for a certification.[5]

On the basis of the positive experience with triclosan as an antiseptic, the well-documented experience with silver suggested that this might be used as an alternative. Medical application of silver has been known for a long time. The disinfectant action of silver compounds was already documented in antiquity and the middle ages. Silver compounds are used clinically today in ophthalmology, wound treatment, cardiac surgery and intensive-care medicine. Silver-coated implantable medical products such as heart valves, Foley catheters or net transplants are licensed and CE-certified for European approval.[6,7,8,9] It was shown in several test series[10] that the silver-coated Dacron vascular prosthesis has normal haemocompatibility. The antimicrobial property was also demonstrated in several test series.[10] The silver prosthesis fulfils the licensing criteria for implants and is CE-certified.

Evidence
Patients and methods

In 1999, we commenced a prospective multicentre data survey on the implantation of the silver-impregnated Dacron prosthesis in cases of vascular prosthesis infections. The data were recorded with a questionnaire completed in the event of a replacement operation and reconstruction with the Intervascular InterGard Silver™. Besides demographic data (patient coding, age, date of operation, gender), the date and kind of vascular prosthesis previously implanted, microbes detected, clinical signs of infection, clinical test values for leukocytes and C-reactive protein were obtained.

Information was collected in a questionnaire (with a text box for notes) on the replacement operation, the position of the freshly implanted prosthesis, the extent of prosthesis explantation, organisms detected and antibiotic cover during the operation and in the course of treatment. The clinical finding at the time of discharge was recorded with documentation of possible complications. At 3 months as well as 6 months after the operation, a fresh documentation was made on the clinical findings, patency and signs of infection. Further data were collected 1 and 2 years after operation. Endpoints of the study were reinfection of the replaced graft or death. In the meantime, the first questionnaires have now been supplemented in some instances. In addition, a computed tomography scan of the abdomen should be taken in central intra-abdominal anastomoses in the 1st and 2nd postoperative year, and a duplex ultrasonogram should be taken in anastomoses that are only peripheral. The questionnaire is now available on the internet at the website www.graftinfections.de. Additional telephone calls were made to clarify or to establish the further course when the data given was not unequivocal.

Up to October 2001, data were obtained from 88 patients with *in situ* reconstruction in vascular prosthesis infections. Forty-five hospitals participated, sending us data from one to eight patients. The age and sex distribution is as usual for vascular surgery patients, and the same applies to the concomitant illnesses. The mean duration of follow-up observation is 11 months. Attention must be drawn to immunocompromised patients with diabetes mellitus, malignancy, liver cirrhosis and kidney failure."

The latency period from the first operation up to occurrence of infection shows three peaks. One peak is in the first 8 months after the first implantation. A further peak occurs in the course 1–7 years after the first implantation. The third peak is a consequence of very late infections up to 10 years after the first implantation. There was increased incidence of infections after interventions a short time previously or second operations such as embolectomies.

We encountered 47 instances of *Staphylococcus aureus*, 11 *Pseudomonas* and six *Staphylococcus epidermidis*. Infections were mainly in the aortoiliac region as well as peripheral reconstructions involving the groin.

The location of the re-implants meets the requirements, i.e. a location corresponding to that of the infected grafts. Altogether, 73 showed an anatomical course and 24 showed an extra-anatomical course with at least one anastomosis *in situ*.

Results

In 26 patients with vascular prosthesis infection, only part of the prosthesis was explanted. Reinfections occurred in 13 of these patients. Of the remaining 13 patients, one patient showed a perigraft reaction in the course without clinical signs of reinfection. Six of the patients from the group with reinfections died (30-day mortality 15.4%, four of 26). One death was independent of infection and attributable to cardiomyopathy. The other five patients died of the consequences of reinfection: multi-organ failure from persistent infection, aortic rupture with the proximal part of the prosthesis left in, pneumonia and sepsis in recurrence of infection. In 62 patients, the prosthesis was removed in its entirety. Fifty-eight patients remained free of infection. In four patients, there was a fresh prosthesis infection (6.5%). Of the 58 patients, eight died in consequence of sepsis, cerebral infarction, intestinal necrosis or myocardial infarction without a fresh infection of the prosthesis (Fig. 1) with a 30-day lethality of 6.5% (four of 62). The recurrences of infection occurred in patients in whom several bacterial strains were detected. In the case of aortic stent removal, a silver tube prosthesis had been implanted. Coils to control endoleaks had been left in. A young drug addict with fixer groin was given an iliacofemoral bypass which became infected. The *in situ* reconstruction with silver-coated prosthesis became infected after several bypass thromboses and thrombectomies. One patient with iliacoprofunda *in situ* reconstruction and net plug as a biological safeguarding operation

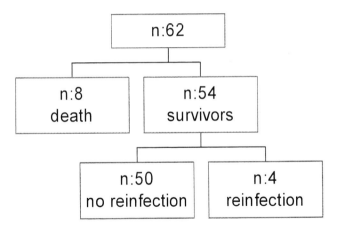

Figure 1. Complete removal of the infected prosthesis: mean follow-up 11 months.

developed an infected fistula to the prosthesis that emanated from a disorder of wound healing in the groin. A further iliacofemoral bypass developed a reinfection without perceptible cause.

Discussion

In the literature, very diverse approaches to treatment of vascular prosthesis infection have been suggested. Up to now there have been no ideal means of treatment that reliably ensure optimal results. There is little controversy on the need to remove all infected prosthesis material (as a rule, the entire implant, especially in late infection).[4,12,13] This is impressively underscored by our results with the silver prosthesis. The incomplete removal of the infected graft results in a hardly tolerable rate of reinfection of 50%. A partial explantation of the prosthesis has been suggested when the remainder of the prosthesis left behind is securely incorporated and has no connection to the infected prosthesis segment.[1] However, the surgeon concerned may also have made the same assumption in our series and infected prostheses were nevertheless left in place. An attempt to salvage the prosthesis by extensive local measures may only be possible in an early and circumscribed disorder of wound healing/infection.[12] Antibiotic cover on its own is ineffective and the infection may persist even if local measures are applied.[1]

Still, what should the revascularization look like? Bandyk makes the following apposite observation: '*In situ* replacement avoids the failure-prone, extra-anatomic reconstruction, aortic stump blowout, and increased physiologic stress associated with multiple or staged procedures.'[12]

Moreover, depending on the area affected, the extra-anatomical reconstruction with an allograft may entail disadvantages in consequence of the lower flow, poorer patency rate, gluteal ischaemia, higher mortality and increased reinfection.[14,15,16]

Numerous working groups were able to present favourable results with *in situ* reconstruction. The biological materials used were mainly deep leg veins[12,17] and homografts.[11,16,18] The Dacron prosthesis soaked in rifampicin was also used successfully.[15,19] Whereas very much more dissection and corresponding trauma is required for the deep leg veins,[17,18] attention must be drawn to the problem of availability and the possible later degeneration in the case of homografts.[11,14,16,18] A raised rate of reinfection in methicillin-resistant *Staphylococcus aureus*,[12,15] a relatively short residence time of the antibiotic in the prosthesis[19,20] and its limited activity spectrum must be mentioned as drawbacks of the rifampicin prosthesis.[15] On the other hand, silver acts as an antiseptic with all advantages: lack of development of resistance, wide activity profile including methicillin-resistant *Staphylococcus aureus*, sustained availability at an effective dose (2–4 weeks) on the prosthesis.[10]

The low 30-day lethality of 6.5% and the rate of reinfection of only 6.5% in complete removal of an infected prosthesis in our survey can be rated as very favourable compared with other methods of treatment. This is especially the case since the patient population investigated comprised 50% infected aortic or iliac reconstructions including prosthetoenteral fistulae (n = 5, without reinfection). It must be pointed out that these silver prostheses can only be regarded as (readily available) part of the treatment concept. Extensive wound debridement and systemic antibiotic treatment are indispensable. Biological safeguarding with vital tissue is always advisable. Additional local measures such as application of antibiotics (after taking an antibiogram) may be appropriate. Intraoperative lavage with disinfectant solutions should be performed, but only before implantation of the silver-coated prosthesis, since the silver may otherwise be washed out. For this reason, the area of surgery should hence be kept as dry of blood as possible. The objective of the systemic antibiotic administration is to control the infection whereas the silver is simultaneously intended to prevent adherence of the bacteria to the implant. Since the protective action of silver is greatly reduced after approximately 4 weeks, the graft must be evaluated like any other fabric. The justification for a protracted or indeed long-term antibiotic therapy might be inferred from this, especially when possible foci of infection are present or when there is prolonged lymph secretion. This also explains why it may make sense to replace once more the silver-coated prosthesis that was prophylactically implanted and then became infected.

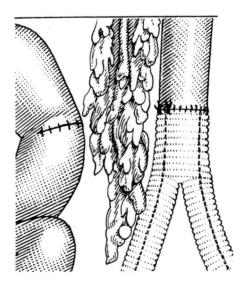

Figure 2. Local repair either by 2–3 prolene sutures to close the defect or by inserting a short Dacron tube to link the prosthesis to a more proximal aortic suture line without tension. Reproduced with permission from Ref. 22.

In establishing the indication for *in situ* replacement of infected allografts, iliac or aortic reconstructions are more important than peripheral reconstructions. If possible, veins should be used as *in situ* reconstruction for peripheral vessels because of the better patency rate. Although a period of follow-up observation of 11 months is the basis for the data presented, longer follow-up is necessary. A period of follow-up observation of at least 2 years was stipulated initially in a study comprising 100 patients, and results will only be available after this period has elapsed.

Conclusion

Treatment of vascular prosthesis infections must be established individually in each single case. Our survey indicates that *in situ* reconstruction with the infection-protected silver Dacron prosthesis in conjunction with thorough wound debridement and possible biological safeguarding techniques (Sartorius muscle flap, graft covering) and systemic antibiotic administration are a new approach that promises to be successful. However, this procedure is unreliable when explantation of the prosthesis is incomplete. In complete prosthesis explantation, it is a superior alternative to extra-anatomical procedures that has also advantages over other *in situ* reconstruction techniques. The evident drawbacks of extra-anatomical methods and the trauma entailed in removing autologous material (e.g. deep leg vein) can be avoided. It is conceivable that it will perform better than homografts. It can therefore be concluded that all infected foreign material must be removed. According to various working groups, reconstruction can be carried out *in situ*. It is left to the reader to conclude whether the silver-coated prosthesis is already an established (advantageous) component of a therapeutic concept.

Summary

- Various working groups have impressively proved the value of *in situ* reconstruction.

- When a vascular prosthesis is infected, it should be explanted completely.

- This silver-coated Dracon® prosthesis is a promising therapeutic option. The results obtained up to now are favourable.

- Questionnaires and current information under: www.graftinfections.de

References

1. Bandyk DF. Infection in prosthetic vascular grafts. In: *Vascular Surgery*. Rutherford (ed). Philadelphia: WB Saunders 2000; 733–751.
2. Chiesa R, Melissano G, Castellano R *et al.* Postoperative arterial infection: Epidemiology, bacteriology and pathogenesis. In *Complications in Vascular and Endovascular Surgery* Part 1 (EVC). Branchereau A, Jacobs M (eds). Armonk: Futura, 2001; 61–73.
3. Goeau-Brissoniere O, Coggia M. Prevention and treatment of arterial graft infections. In *Complications in Vascular and Endovascular Surgery* Part 1 (EVC). Branchereau A, Jacobs M (eds). Armonk: Futura, 2001; 75–84.
4. Edwards WH, Martin RS, Jenkins JM, Edwards WH, Mulherin JL. Primary graft infections. *J Vasc Surg* 1987; 6: 235–239.

5. Zegelman M, Schmidt A. Klinische Erfahrungen mit einer antimikrobiell beschichteten Dacronprothese. Abstractbook. Karlsruher Gefäßtage, Karlsruhe/Germany 10–11.10.1997.
6. Ahearn DG, Grace DT. Effects of hydrogel/silver coatings on in vitro adhesion to catheters of bacteria associated with urinary tract infections. *Curr Microbiol* 2000; 41: 120–125.
7. Nissen S, Furkert FH. Antimikrobielle Wirksamkeit einer Silberbeschichtung von Hydrogellinsen. *Ophthalmologie* 2000; 97: 640–643.
8. Raad I, Hanna H. Intervasular catheters impregnated with antimicrobial agents: a milestone in the prevention of bloodstream infections. *Support Care Cancer* 1999; 7: 386–390.
9. Tweden KS, Cameron JD. Biocompatibility of silver-modified Polyester for antimicrobial protection of prosthetic valves. *J Heart Valve Dis* 1997; 6: 553–561.
10. Intervascular^R Bensheim/Germany; NamSa^R Inc. USA.
11. Verhelst R, Lacroix V, Vraux H *et al.* Use of cryopreserved arterial homografts for management of infected prosthetic grafts: a multicentric study. *Annls Vasc Surg* 2000; 14: 602–607.
12. Bandyk DF, Novotney ML, Back MR, Johnson BL, Schmacht DC. Expanded application of *in situ* replacement for prosthetic graft infection. *J Vasc Surg* 2001; 34: 411–419.
13. de Virgilio C, Cherry KJ, Gloviczki P *et al.* Infected lower extremity extra-anatomic bypass grafts: management of a serious complication in high-risk patients. *Annls Vasc Surg* 1995; 9: 459–466.
14. Camiade C, Goldschmidt P, Koskas F *et al.* Optimization of the resistance of arterial allografts to infection: Comperative study with synthetic prostheses. *Annls Vasc Surg* 2001; 15: 186–196.
15. Hayes PD, Nasim A, London NJM *et al.* *In situ* replacement of infected aortic grafts with rifampicin-bonded prostheses: The Leicester experience (1992–1998). *J Vasc Surg* 1999; 30: 92–98.
16. Kieffer E, Gomes D, Plissonnier D, Koskas F, Bahnini A. Current use of allografts for infrarenal aortic graft infection: experience with 133 patients. *27th Global Vascular and Endovascular Issues, Techniques and Horizons.* New York, XVI 3.1/3.2. 2000.
17. Nevelsteen A, Lacroix H, Suy R. Autogenous reconstruction with the lower extremity deep veins: An alternative treatment of prosthetic infection after reconstructive surgery for aortoiliac disease. *J Vasc Surg* 1995; 22: 129–134.
18. Leseche G, Castier Y, Petit MD *et al.* Long-term results of cryopreserved arterial allograft reconstruction in infected prosthetic grafts and mycotic aneurysms of the abdominal aorta. *J Vasc Surg* 2001; 34: 1–7.
19. Earnshaw JJ. The current role of rifampicin-impregnated grafts: Pragmatism versus science. *Eur J Vasc Endovasc Surg* 2000; 20: 409–412.
20. Lovering AM, White LO, MacGowan AP, Reeves DS. The elution and binding characteristics of rifampicin for three commercially available protein-sealed vascular grafts. *J Antimicrob Chemother* 1996; 38: 599–604.
21. Eugene M, Gerota J. Cryopreserved aortic allograft replacement of infected prosthetic grafts in man: processing and clinical results. *Transpl Int* 1998; 11: 452–454.
22. Baird RN. Surgical management of secondary aortoenteric fistulae. In *Vascular and Endovascular Surgical Techniques* 4th edn. Greenhalgh RM (ed). London: WB Saunders, 2001; 161–164.

Working Group *Graftinfections*

H-H Eckstein, D Mitsch, *Ludwigsburg*
P Langenscheidt, D Kreisler-Haag, *Homburg*
D Meyer, F Endter, *Würzburg*
V Mickley, M Cazzonelli, *Baden-Baden*
D Raithel, M Klein, *Nürnberg*
T Schmitz–Rixen, R Ritter, *Frankfurt*

Infected grafts require excision and extra-anatomic reconstruction

Charing Cross Editorial Comments towards Consensus

This old chestnut runs on and on. At one stage it was suggested that there was an American solution and a European solution. The implication was that in the USA infected grafts were taken out and extra-anatomic bypass was performed whereas in Europe they were left in, washed and cleaned locally with iodine and other materials in the hope that they would not need to be removed. There is a smattering of truth about this old view but one has heard and seen many surgeons holding extreme views on both sides of the Atlantic. Just when we thought that infected prosthetic grafts would be taken out in the USA, Denton Cooley and his group excised grafts and inlaid new prosthetic grafts. Quite satisfactory results were reported. There are those in the UK who have had a similar approach. It beggars belief but it seemed to work in their hands. Equally there have been those enthusiasts in the UK and the continent of Europe to remove infected prosthetic grafts and to reconstruct by an extra-anatomic bypass in the same way as mentioned above. Personally I have never had good results leaving an infected prosthetic bypass behind. In the end it has always had to be removed but others have had different experience.

Roger M Greenhalgh
Editor

Aortoiliac reconstruction should avoid femorofemoral crossover

For the motion
André Nevelsteen, K Daenens,
I Fourneau, H Lacroix

Introduction

The value of direct aortoiliac reconstruction has already been recognized for 50 years and according to Szilagyi, it is considered the best standardized therapeutic procedure available to the vascular surgeon.[1] It was in fact René Leriche who as early as 1923 stated that resection and substitution of the aortic bifurcation should be the most appropiate treatment for aortoiliac occlusive disease. The first aortofemoral Dacron graft reconstruction was performed by M DeBakey in the late 1950s. By the late 1960s, prosthetic graft reconstruction had become the method of choice in direct reconstruction for aortoiliac occlusive disease. Prosthetic grafts offer indeed the most definitive and durable revascularization in aortoiliac occlusive disease and they are currently used to treat more than 90% of patients by most surgeons (Fig.1).

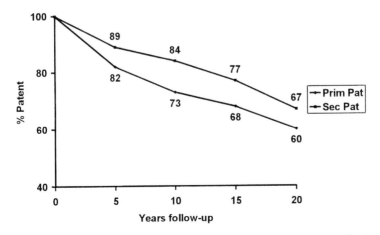

Figure 1. Long-term outcome of prosthetic aortobifemoral grafting in 930 patients (authors' experience) (Prim Pat: primary patency; Sec Pat: secondary patency).

Evidence

The operative technique for direct aortoiliac reconstruction has been well described. Endarterectomy has been abandoned in most centres in favour of prosthetic insertion, and aortobifemoral grafting remains the prototype. The operation is usually performed by midline laparotomy or a left retroperitoneal approach. Although several surgeons prefer a proximal end-to-end anastomosis, the end-to-side technique might be an alternative in many cases (Fig.2) and in each case the reconstruction should be performed taking into account the preservation of blood supply to the pelvic organs.

In addition the proximal anastomosis should be placed immediately below the renal arteries and the body of the graft has to be kept as short as possible in order to prevent kinking of the limbs at the bifurcation. The diameter of the graft should be appropiately matched to the native vessels and, although knitted grafts are generally preferred, equal results might be obtained with woven grafts or the more recent poly-tetrafluoroethylene (PTFE) bifurcation grafts. Concomitant femoropopliteal occlusive disease, most frequently present at the superficial femoral artery, is a significant factor with regard to long-term outcome. Therefore the construction of the distal anastomosis at the level of the femoral bifurcation is probably the most important step of the operation. An anastomosis to the common femoral artery is only acceptable in a minority of patients without femoropopliteal involvement and concomitant profundaplasty produces superior results in the majority of the cases (Figs 3 and 4).

Operative mortality and morbidity rates after direct aortoiliac reconstruction have been cited as a disadvantage with regard to extra-anatomic reconstruction. The mortality rate after direct aortofemoral grafting is around 2–3% but should not exceed 5%. Over the last few years there has been a substantial improvement thanks to the use of epidural catheters and the introduction of perioperative blockade of beta-adrenergic receptors. In the DECREASE study, 112 high-risk patients for major vascular surgery were randomized between standard care (n=53) and bisoprolol treatment (n=59).[2] The operative mortality in the bisoprolol group was 3.4% vs 17% in the standard care group (p=0.02). Non-fatal myocardial infarction occurred in nine

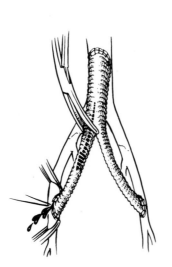 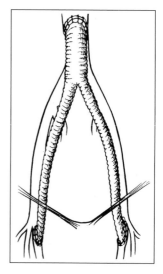

Figure 2. Proximal anastomosis in a case of aortobifemoral grafting.

patients in the standard care group (17%) and in none of the bisoprolol group (p<0.001).

The importance of the surgical approach was demonstrated by Lacroix in 1997.[3] He randomized 200 candidates for infrarenal aortic reconstruction between midline laparotomy (n=62), transverse laparotomy (n=73) and left retroperitoneal approach (n=65). Although there were no differences in operative mortality, the incidence of perioperative complications, especially gastrointestinal problems was significantly lower in the retroperitoneal group. The mean hospital stay for the retroperitoneal group was 8.6 days vs 10.5 days in the midline laparotomy group (p=0.05). Podore reported more recently his experience with a clinical pathway for elective infrarenal aortic surgery that targeted hospital discharge on postoperative day 3.[4] He described

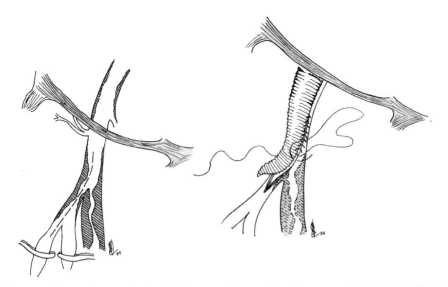

Figure 3.   Concomitant profundaplasty in a case of concomitant femoropopliteal occlusive disease.

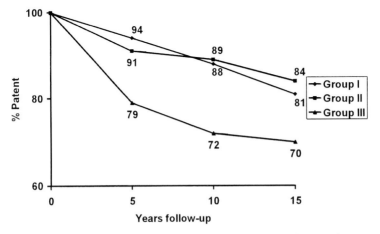

Figure 4.   Long-term outcome in relation to the femoral anastomosis and concomitant femeropopliteal occlusive disease (FPOD) (authors' experience in 930 patients).
Group I: No FPOD (n=498).
Group II: Concomitant FPOD – concomitant profundaplasty (n=718).
Group III: Concomitant FPOD – no profundaplasty (n=340).

a consecutive series of 50 patients of whom 80% were discharged on postoperative day 3. Compliance improved with increasing experience, with 92% of the most recent 25 patients being discharged on postoperative day 3. He concluded that such early discharge, resulting in reduced hospitalization costs, proved to be routinely achievable, safe and well accepted by the patients. This reduced hospital stay has also been reported in association with the recently developed laparoscopic and videoscopic techniques for direct aortoiliac surgery.[5]

Disturbance of sexual function might be seen as another disadvantage of direct aortoiliac reconstruction. It should, however, not be forgotten that over 60% of the patients have already presented with sexual function disturbances in association with aortoiliac occlusive disease. In a prospective study of 62 males, performed in our Department, erectile function after aortofemoral reconstruction remained unchanged in 77% of the patients.[6] Improvement or deterioration was observed in 11.3% and 20.5% of the cases respectively but impotence occurred in only one patient (6%) with normal function preoperatively.

Long-term complications after aortofemoral prosthetic reconstruction are seen in 20–25% of the patients and include thrombosis, anastomotic aneurysm, anastomotic stenosis and infection (both primary infection and graft enteric fistula). They are seen most frequently in the first years postoperatively, but patients remain at risk lifelong. When compared with extra-anatomic grafting, graft enteric fistula is the only complication specifically related to direct aortoiliac reconstruction and the incidence is around 1% (bladder trauma has, however, been documented also in relation with femorofemoral crossover graft). Anastomotic aneurysms may be observed at the proximal anastomosis of an aortofemoral graft but over 90% occur at the femoral anastomosis.

Long-term patency after aortofemoral grafting is primarily dependent on the operative indication (claudication vs ischaemia), the operative technique and concomitant femoropopliteal occlusive disease. The site of the proximal anastomosis (end-to-side vs end-to-end) and the graft material do not seem to be of great importance, but less favourable results have been reported in patients who continue smoking postoperatively. In our own experience with 930 patients the graft limb related patency at 10 and 15 years was 84% and 78% respectively. The respective patient related patency rates were 73% and 68% (Fig.1). When considering secondary patency rates, these increased to 84% and 77% respectively. This compares very well with patency rates as reported in the literature (Table 1). De Vries and Hunink presented in 1997 a well performed meta-analysis of 23 studies.[13] The primary patency rates for patients with claudication were 86% and 79% at 5 and 10 years, respectively, compared with 80% and 72% for patients with ischaemia.

Table 1.   Long-term patency rates after prosthetic aortobifemoral reconstruction

Author	% Patent		
	5 years	10 years	15 years
Brewster and Darling[a7]	88	75	
Martinez *et al.*[a8]	88	78	
Szilagyi *et al.*[b1]	77	76	73
Poulias *et al.*[b9]	82	76	72
van den Akker *et al.*[b10]	86		
Passman *et al.*[b11]	80		
Mingoli *et al.*[b12]	80		

[a]Graft limb related patency.
[b]Patient related patency.

Indications for **femorofemoral crossover bypass graft** are limited. It was originally introduced for high-risk patients who could not safely tolerate an aortic reconstruction. Proponents argue that it is easy to perform, it avoids the haemodynamic stress of aortic clamping and it does not require an abdominal operation. The facts are (1) that these high-risk patients most frequently present with diffuse bilateral disease, (2) that, thanks to the modern techniques and anaesthesiological developments, the number of patients who cannot tolerate a direct reconstruction diminishes from year to year and (3) that the long-term results are inferior to these of direct reconstruction (Table 2).

Table 2. Primary patency rates after reconstruction occlusion for unilateral iliac occlusion

Author	5 years patency (%)
Direct reconstruction	
Cham[14]	86
Cormier[15]	86
Ricco[16]	90
Crossover graft	
Harrington[17]	64
Criado[18]	60
Brener[19]	55
Berce[20]	72
Ricco[16]	65
Mingoli[12]	70

Patients with an occcluded aortofemoral graft limb are frequently considered as such a 'high-risk'. Here also, over 80% of the patients can be successfully managed by simple graft thrombectomy and reconstruction of the distal anastomosis.[21]

In 1997, Ricco et al. presented the results of 143 'low-risk' patients with unilateral iliac occlusion who were randomized between direct bypass (n=69) and femorofemoral crossover bypass (n=74).[16] There were no significant differences in operative mortality and morbidity rates. The primary patency rate at 7 years was 49% for the crossover bypass vs 86% for direct reconstruction (p=0.006); 32% of the patients in the crossover group needed a secondary intervention because of graft failure, compared with 10% in the direct bypass group. Progression of disease at the contralateral side after direct reconstruction was observed in 12 patients (17.4%).

Summary

- Direct prosthetic reconstruction for aortoiliac occlusive disease offers durable results.

- Most patients are in need of bilateral reconstruction.

- Unilateral direct prosthetic reconstruction is justified in selected cases and produces superior results compared with femorofemoral crossover.

- Femorofemoral crossover grafts should be reserved for high-risk patients, who cannot tolerate a direct reconstruction.

References

1. Szilagyi DE, Elliott JP, Smith RF *et al.* A thirty-year survey of the reconstructive surgical treatment of aortoiliac occlusive disease. *J Vasc Surg* 1985; 3: 421–436.

2. Poldermans D, Boersma E, Bax JJ *et al.* The effect of bisoprolol on perioperative mortality and myocardial infarction in high-risk patients undergoing vascular surgery. Dutch Echocardiographic Cardiac Risk Evaluation Applying Stress Echocardiography Study group. *N Engl J Med* 1999; 341:1789–1794.

3. Lacroix H. The optimal approach for elective reconstruction of the infra- and juxta-renal abdominal aorta: A randomised prospective study. Doctoral Thesis. Belgium: Leuven University Press, 1997.

4. Podore PC, Throop EB. Infrarenal aortic surgery with a 3-day hospital stay: A report on success with a clinical pathway. *J Vasc Surg* 1999; 29: 787–792.

5. Alimi YS, Hartung O, Valerio N, Juhan C. Laparoscopic aortoiliac surgery for aneurysm and occlusive disease: when should a minilaparotomy be performed? *J Vasc Surg* 2001; 33: 469–475.

6. Nevelsteen A, Beyens G, Duchateau J *et al.* Aorto-femoral reconstruction and sexual function: a prospective study. *Eur J Vasc Surg* 1990; 4: 247–251.

7. Brewster DC, Darling RC. Optimal methods of aortoiliac reconstruction. *Surgery* 1978; 84: 739–748.

8. Martinez BD, Hertzer NR, Beven NG. Influence of distal arterial occlusive disease on prognosis following aortobifemoral bypass. *Surgery* 1980; 88: 795–805.

9. Poulias GE, Doundoulakis N, Prombenas E *et al.* Aortofemoral bypass and determinants of early success and late favourable outcome: experience with 1000 consecutive cases. *J Cardiovasc Surg* 1992; 33: 669–678.

10. van den Akker PJ, van Schilfgaarde R, Brand R *et al.* Long-term results of prosthetic and non-prosthetic reconstruction for obstructive aortoiliac disease. *Eur J Vasc Surg* 1992; 6: 53–61.

11. Passman MA, Taylor LM, Edwards JM *et al.* Comparison of axillofemoral and aortofemoral bypass for aortoiliac occlusive disease. *J Vasc Surg* 1996; 23: 263–269.

12. Mingoli A, Sapienza P, Feldhaus RJ *et al.* Comparison of femorofemoral and aortofemoral bypass for aortoiliac occlusive disease. *J Cardiovasc Surg* 2001; 42: 381–387.

13. de Vries SO, Hunink MGM. Results of aortic bifurcation grafts for aortoiliac occlusive disease: A meta-analysis. *J Vasc Surg* 1997; 26: 558–569.

14. Cham C, Myers C, Scott DF *et al.* Extra-peritoneal unilateral iliac artery bypass for chronic lower limb ischemia. *Austr NZ J Surg* 1988; 58: 859–863.

15. Cormier JM. Résultats des pontages aorto-fémoraux unilatéraux en PTFE. In *Les lésions occlusives aorto-iliaques chroniques.* Kieffer E (ed). Paris: AERCV, 1991: 233–242.

16. AURC & Ricco JB, Bouin-Pineau MH, Demarque C *et al.* Late results of femorofemoral crossover bypass surgery. In *Long-term Results of Arterial Interventions.* Branchereau A, Jacobs M (eds). New York: Futura Publications 1997: 155–166.

17. Harrington ME, Harrington EB, Haimov M *et al.* Iliofemoral versus femorofemoral bypass: the case for individualized approach. *J Vasc Surg* 1992; 16: 841–854.

18. Criado E, Burnham SJ, Tinsley EA *et al.* Femoro-femoral bypass graft: analysis of patency and factors influencing long-term outcome. *J Vasc Surg* 1993; 18: 495–505.

19. Brener BJ, Brief DK, Alpert J *et al.* Femoro-femoral bypass. A twenty-five year experience. In *Long Term Results in Vascular Surgery.* Yao JST, Pearce WH (eds). Norwalk; NJ: Appleton & Lange, 1993: 385–394.

20. Berce M, Sayers RD, Miller JH. Femorofemoral crossover grafts for claudication: a safe and reliable procedure. *Eur J Vasc Endovasc Surg* 1996; 12: 437–441,

21. Nevelsteen A, Peeters P, Suy R. Late thrombosis of the aortofemoral graft: thrombectomy or graft replacement? *Angéiologie* 1984; 36: 137–144.

Aortoiliac reconstruction should avoid femorofemoral crossover

Against the motion
William Paaske

Introduction

Femorofemoral bypass grafting, a classical, extra-anatomical vascular operation, was first suggested by Vetto in 1962 for treatment of unilateral iliac artery obstruction;[1] an interesting essay on the background and historical development has been given by Eastcott.[2]

Initially, the procedure was reserved for patients considered to have too high a risk to permit open surgical aortoiliac reconstruction, but due to the reported, reasonably high, patency rates in combination with low perioperative mortality and complications, it is now considered more as a choice than as a compromise.[3] With endovascular techniques for establishing inflow to a groin, the technique is considered as an option for a safe, low-risk procedure in cases where ipsilateral procedures to create, or improve, groin run-in are considered technically problematic and/or dangerous.

Consequently, primary femorofemoral bypass can be considered as an isolated procedure to ensure inflow to a leg below an iliac occlusion or one or more haemodynamically significant stenoses where contralateral groin run-in is not compromised.

In clinical practice, it has found a place as an adjunct, or supplementary, procedure to ensure inflow to a leg below an iliac occlusion, or one or more haemodynamically significant stenoses unfit for balloon angioplasty (PTA) +/- stent, where contralateral groin run-in is compromised but where these contralateral lesions can be treated with PTA, thrombendarterectomy, or bypass graft, as appropriate.

The technique is also suitable as part of a two- or multiple level (segment) procedure with contralateral, proximal revascularization, local groin reconstruction, and procedures for establishing or increasing run-off, e.g. profundaplasty, or, as part of sequential grafting, with femoropopliteal or *in situ* saphenous vein bypass, etc.

Femorofemoral bypass is the reconstructive method of choice in a variety of secondary instances as a complete or a partial operation, either as redo or as other site intervention, e.g., in patients with a thrombosed aortofemoral bifurcation graft limb that can be opened neither by thrombolysis nor by surgical manoeuvres.

The femorofemoral bypass constitutes a part of the extra-anatomical axillo-bifemoral procedures, and finally this bypass technique has found a place as an adjunct to endovascular treatment of abdominal aortic or aortoiliac aneurysms.[4,5]

In Denmark, where exact procedural numbers covering the whole country are available through the Danish Vascular Registry (Karbase), 247 primary femoro-femoral reconstructions were made in 1998, and 225 in 1999 as well as in 2000; this corresponds to a frequency of 4.4 procedures per 100 000 inhabitants (all ages) per year and to 3.5% of all primary procedures. The Swedish national registry (Swedvasc) recorded 153 operations in 1999 corresponding to a frequency of 1.7 per 100 000.

Technique

The operation can be performed under local anaesthesia with infiltration of both groins and of the subcutaneous tunnel.

The procedure is simple.[6] The vessels in both groins are exposed, and arteriotomies, in typical situations, are made into the distal, anterior parts of the common femoral arteries (with the incisions going $\frac{1}{2}$ to 1 cm into the superficial femoral arteries to control run-in if these vessels are patent). A synthetic tube graft with calibre 6–8 mm is mounted with an end-to-side anastomosis using parachute technique and mono-filament, continuous polypropylene 5-0 suture. The toe of the graft is placed distally. A plane of cleavage is dissected digitally from both sides in the deepest part of the subcutaneous tissue just above the symphysis. An appropriate instrument (e.g., a large, curved DeBakey aneurysm clamp) is led through this tunnel from the receiving side to the side where the anastomosis has been placed (the donor side), and the distal, free end of the graft is grasped. The graft is then led through the subcutaneous tunnel to the receiving side, and an anastomosis is mounted, as before, with the toe distally. This way of positioning the graft is called 'inverted C' mounting. Care is taken to avoid graft kinking by positioning of the graft in comfortable curvatures just above the anastomoses before it enters the orifices of the subcutaneous channel. The result is monitored by intraoperative ultrasound Doppler examination with papaver-ine tests over the run-off vessels.

Which graft?

The literature does not provide information as to the fact whether Dacron is prefer-able to expanded polytetrafluoroethylene (ePTFE) or *vice versa*.[7] An American Veterans Affairs Cooperative Study with 340 patients did not show any difference between the patencies of externally supported Dacron and PTFE grafts;[8] the assisted primary patency rate at 5 years was 50% for Dacron and 47% for PTFE (72% limb salvage cases); this is the only available prospective and randomized study of this aspect in the literature. I prefer an externally ring-supported ePTFE graft, but this strategy is not evidence based.

In selected cases, e.g., infection, autologous arteries (endarterectomized superficial femoral artery) can be used.[9]

Alternative techniques

Oblique groin incisions have been shown to be associated with a lower incidence of wound infection.[10]

The anastomosis on the inflow side can be placed high on the common femoral artery just below the inguinal ligament (or on the distal external iliac artery) with the receiving side anastomosis placed as above. In this way, a 'lazy S' mounting is achieved.

If only the profunda femoris artery is open on the receiving side, the anastomosis can be placed on the first or second part of this artery.

Oblique incisions on the femoral vessels have been proposed to reduce the risk of neointimal hyperplasia formation, but the evidence for a beneficial effect of this is scarce.

Positioning of the graft in the space of Retzius (behind the rectus muscle) does not provide better results, although, in theory, the graft should be better 'protected' towards external compression.

The steal phenomenon (ischaemia of the donor limb side) rarely occurs, if the iliac inflow to the donor groin is uncompromised,[11,12] but subclinical steal (decline of >0.1 in ankle blood pressure index) is common.[12]

Crossover iliofemoral bypass grafting is beyond the scope of this presentation, but a recent European series was published by Defraigne et al.[13] It should also be noted that there is some controversy whether anatomical iliofemoral bypasses are preferable to extra-anatomical femorofemoral grafting.[14,15]

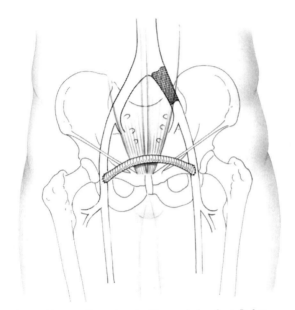

Figure 1. Femorofemoral bypass. Reproduced with permission from Ref. 6.

Evidence

The literature was searched through Medline in October 2001 and shall be interpreted in the systematic terms of *Categories of evidence* & *Strength of recommendation* as defined by Ellis *et al.* (see Table 1).

Table 1. Categories of evidence & Strength of recommendation[a]

Categories of evidence

I a	Evidence from meta-analysis of randomized controlled trials
I b	Evidence from at least one randomized controlled trial
II a	Evidence from at least one controlled study without randomization
II b	Evidence from at least one other type of quasi-experimental study
III	Evidence from descriptive studies, such as comparative studies, correlation studies, and case control studies
IV	Evidence from expert committee reports or opinions or clinical experience of respected authorities, or both

Strength of recommendation

A	Directly based on category I evidence
B	Directly based on category II evidence or extrapolated recommendation from category I evidence
C	Directly based on category III evidence or extrapolated recommendation from category I or II evidence
D	Directly based on category IV evidence or extrapolated recommendation from category I, II, or III evidence

[a] As defined in Ref. 33.

Durability and outcomes

Femorofemoral crossover bypass as a primary, isolated procedure

The Swedvasc data year 1999 yielded a <30 days occlusion rate of 7.8% in the 153 procedures, but a scientific report is not available, and there is no information published as to the frequency of simultaneous PTA (not classifiable).

From Hong Kong, Lau *et al.* recently reported a 5-year patency rate of 71% in operations for limb salvage in 61 poor-risk patients collected over 18 years[16] (Evidence category IV). In Australia, graft patencies in claudicants were 72% (primary) and 89% (secondary) at 5 years[17] (Evidence category IV). A retrospective study was performed in the USA on 91 patients with femorofemoral bypass with a primary graft patency after 5 years of 60%; decision to use this technique was based on an estimate of excessive operative risk for aortobifemoral reconstruction or because of an ideal donor iliac system in a patient in the good risk category[18] (Evidence category IV). Similar results were reported in another American study[19] (Evidence category IV). In Europe, Ricco found a primary patency of direct revascularizations of 89.8% at 4 years, and 52% for crossover bypass,[20] a statistically significant difference (Evidence category Ib). In Vienna, Kretschmer *et al.* analysed 57 consecutive patients with PTFE grafts; the cumulative primary patency rate was 52% at 5 years, the secondary 63%[21] (Evidence category IV).

An overview with a table of the primary patency rates (55–86%) in older materials of varying scientific quality (1972–1993) can be found in the works by Criado *et al.*[22,23]

Femorofemoral crossover bypass for atherosclerosis in connection with contralateral inflow procedures as documented in the literature since 1990

Shah and coworkers collected 99 patients who had 111 femorofemoral bypass grafts placed over a 10-year period; bypass alone was made in 89 cases, and preoperative donor iliac PTA was used in 22.[24] The overall graft failure did not differ between these two groups with failures of 21/89 and 2/22, respectively, at a mean follow-up of 36 ± 28 months (Evidence category IV).

Criado *et al.* found a 1-year primary patency rate of 78% in patients who had pre-operative PTA of the donor iliac artery; the patency was 93% in those patients where PTA was not performed, but this difference was not statistically significant;[22] grafts placed for limb-threatening ischaemia or in patients with occlusion of the superficial femoral artery had a similar patency rate compared with those placed for claudication or in patients with patent superficial femoral artery (Evidence category IV).

A 5-year primary patency rate of 79% was recorded by Perler and Williams in 26 patients who had femorofemoral bypass grafting and PTA, but the corresponding primary patency rate in 44 patients who did not have PTA was 59%[25] (Evidence category IV).

In a study on ten patients with critical ischaemia and severe co-morbidities, Chalmers *et al.* found a median duration of primary graft patency of 50 months in a mixed material comprising 10 patients[26] (Evidence category IV). A similar American study had a 5-year patency of 82%[15] (Evidence category IV).

On an intention to treat basis, patency at 6 months was 100% in the complex material of Whatling and coworkers.[27] It was suggested that the stenting of occluded iliac arteries should be reserved for patients with limited life expectancy, but younger and fitter patients should be offered femorofemoral crossover grafting as a primary procedure (Evidence category IV).

The retrospective work by Mingoli and coworkers comprised 228 patients where 67.5% were judged as having high risk for surgery, and 82.5% of the procedures were made for limb-threatening ischaemia.[28] The material is mixed, with 150 patients having femorofemoral bypass as the primary procedure, and 78 patients having previous graft failure or infection. PTA was made in 25% of the material, and 55.7% had a supplementary procedure to improve outflow. Overall, the long-term results of femorofemoral bypass grafting were similar to those obtained with reconstructions originating from the aorta when performed as a primary operation. An interesting finding was that the 5 and 10 years primary and secondary patency rates were significantly higher when externally supported grafts were used (Evidence category IV). Another study by the same author[29] indicates that primary ePTFE externally supported femorofemoral grafts in high-risk patients is a safe procedure which produces long-term results similar to those of aortofemoral reconstruction (Evidence category IV).

Aburahma and coworkers recently studied 41 patients with long iliac occlusion and significant contralateral iliac stenosis treated with combined femorofemoral bypass grafting and PTA and stenting.[30] The primary patency rates at 1, 2 and 3 years were 96%, 85% and 85% for patients with an iliac stenosis <5 cm. The secondary patency rates for this group were 100%, 96% and 87%. The patients with >5 cm stenosis had primary patency rates of 46%, 46% and 31%, secondary 62%, 54% and 27%. The overall limb salvage rates were 96% in the group with the short iliac lesions, and 85% for the long. Thus it appeared that combined use of PTA and stenting plus femorofemoral crossover bypass was effective and durable if the iliac stenoses were <5 cm, but stenoses of >5 cm failed to support the femorofemoral procedure (Evidence category IV).

The question of femorofemoral bypass and occlusion of one aortofemoral bifurcation graft limb was addressed by Testini et al. who collected retrospective material on 40 patients.[31] The median follow-up time was 51 months [range 1–14 years], and all had non-externally supported Dacron grafts. There was no operative mortality, two grafts occluded in the postoperative course, and a total of nine occlusions were seen (Evidence category IV). The material of van Andrichem et al. included 19 patients with bifurcation limb occlusion.[32] The overall primary patency rate was 80% after 3 years (Evidence category IV).

Femorofemoral crossover bypass in connection with contralateral inflow procedures for aortic and aortoiliac aneurysmal disease

Rehring et al. studied 51 consecutive patients in whom 28 custom-made and 22 commercially available endovascular devices were implanted.[4] The endograft was extended to the external iliac artery in 42% of the cases, and the contralateral iliac artery was occluded either by a closed covered stent or by intraluminal coils. The result, in terms of primary and secondary patencies, was 98% and 100% (mean follow-up 15.8 months). The incidence rate of femorofemoral bypass occlusion after aorto-uni-iliac endovascular repair was 0.7% (Evidence category IV). Further, femorofemoral bypass in conjunction with an unilateral endovascular device has been shown to have results similar to those with bifurcated types[5] (Evidence category IV).

Mortality data

In Sweden, the <30 day mortality for femorofemoral crossover bypass was 4.7% (Swedvasc) for the entire material.

As usual, the mortality rates are dependent on case mix, but from the aggregated literature, including that dealing with endovascular repair, it appears that the <30 day mortality for these often high-risk patients lies around 0–6%, also in cases including PTA, with myocardial infarction, cardiac arrhythmias, pulmonary and renal complications, and an occasional deep vein thrombosis as causes of death.[5,17,22,23,25,27,28,30]

Complications

From the Swedvasc data it is seen that 76% of all procedures were not followed by any surgical complication, and 91.3% did not have any general complication, but detailed analysis is not yet available. Some series report no major complications,[27] but from the published data, an infection rate of 0–6% must be expected.[5,22,25,26] The Veterans Administration study[23] had a similar rate of infected grafts (3.5%) in both the Dacron and the PTFE group. Seroma and lymph leaks occur in around 2% of the cases,[5,22,26] and in addition to this, the occasional groin or scrotal haematoma can be encountered.[5,26]

Quality of life

The literature does not provide information as to the quality of life after these reconstructive procedures. The reported survival rates are about 71% at 3 years, with limb salvage rates at the same point in time of around 88%.[18]

Cost benefit

Whatling *et al.*[27] demonstrated that stenting of the iliac arteries is not as cost-effective as femorofemoral crossover bypass grafting in unilateral iliac artery disease. The hospital stay time for femorofemoral crossover bypass was 4 days with a cost of UKP 3072 +/– 201 (SEM) per case in the UK. In the USA, the total hospital and professional charges, adjusted to 1991 US$, were in median US$ 22061 ± 1773 (SEM) (no PTA).[18] Formal cost benefit analyses are not available.

Conclusion

Femorofemoral crossover bypass grafting, whether performed as an isolated, primary procedure or as a component of aortoiliac balloon dilatation with or without stent, as a secondary reconstruction, or as a supplement to endovascular prosthesis deployment for aneurysmal disease, is a simple and safe procedure but the scientific documentation is rudimentary and based on Evidence category IV information and, consequently, the recommendation for its use can be classified as a type D recommendation (Table 1).

It can be performed in even high-risk patients with low perioperative mortality caused by general complications and with primary and secondary patency rates of the same order of magnitude as that found in other, often more complex, traditional vascular surgical procedures but, again, this statement is based on Evidence category IV information and the recommendation remains a type D. The local, surgical complications are few, and the rates of groin infection is similar to those reported on other vascular operations where the groin vessels are exposed.

Quality of life and cost benefit analyses are not available.

Summary

The clinical usefulness of femorofemoral crossover bypass grafting is based on Evidence category IV information. In purely clinical terms, it:

* is simple,

* is safe,

* is associated with low perioperative mortality, almost exclusively from general causes,

* has few local, surgical complications,

* has good 5 years primary and secondary patency rates,

* is a pertinent alternative to aortoiliac-femoral reconstruction,

* is well suited as a supplementary procedure to iliac PTA,

* is the treatment of choice in high-risk patients.

But: Evidence category Ia information from meta-analysis of randomized clinical trials is not available in the literature.

References

1. Vetto RM. The treatment of unilateral iliac artery obstruction with a transabdominal subcutaneous femorofemoral graft. *Surgery* 1962; **52**: 542–545.
2. Eastcott HHG. Femoro-femoral crossover grafting. In *Indications in Vascular Surgery*. Greenhalgh RM (ed.) London: W.B.Saunders, 1988: 429–438.
3. Sethi GK, Crawford FA, Scott SM, Takaro T. Femorofemoral bypass graft: choice or compromise? *Am Surg* 1975; **41**: 61–66.
4. Rehring TF, Brewster DC, Cambria RP *et al.* Utility and reliability of endovascular aortouniiliac with femorofemoral crossover graft for aortoiliac aneurysmal disease. *J Vasc Surg* 2000; **31**: 1135–1141.
5. Walker SR, Braithwaite B, Tennant WG, MacSweeney ST, Wenham PW, Hopkinson BR. Early complications of femorofemoral crossover bypass grafts after aorta uni-iliac endovascular repair of abdominal aortic aneurysms. *J Vasc Surg* 1998; **28**: 647–650.
6. Fiorani P, Faraglia V, Taurino M, Speziale F, Colonna M. Femorofemoral bypass. In *Vascular and Endovascular Surgical Techniques*. Greenhalgh RM (ed). London: W.B.Saunders, 2001: 177–180.
7. Lau H, Cheng SW. Is the preferential use of ePTFE grafts in femorofemoral bypass justified? *Ann Vasc Surg* 2001; **15**: 383–387.
8. Johnson WC, Lee KK. Comparative evaluation of externally supported Dacron and polytetrafluoroethylene prosthetic bypasses for femorofemoral and axillofemoral arterial reconstructions. Veterans Affairs Cooperative Study #141. *J Vasc Surg* 1999; **30**: 1077–1083.
9. Blaisdell FW, Hall AD, Lim RC Jr, Moore WC. Aorto-iliac arterial substitution utilizing subcutaneous grafts. *Ann Surg* 1970; **172**: 775–780.
10. Chester JF, Butler CM, Taylor RS. Vascular reconstruction at the groin: oblique or vertical incisions? *Ann R Coll Surg Engl* 1992; **74**: 112–114.
11. Lee RE, Baird RN. A haemodynamic evaluation of the femoro-femoral cross-over bypass. *Eur J Vasc Surg* 1990; **4**: 167–172.
12. Vogt KC, Rasmussen JG, Schroeder TV. The clinical importance and prediction of steal following femoro-femoral cross-over bypass: study of the donor iliac artery by intravascular ultrasound, arteriography, duplex scanning and pressure measurements. *Eur J Vasc Endovasc Surg* 2000; **19**: 178–183.
13. Defraigne JO, Vazquez C, Limet R. Crossover iliofemoral bypass grafting for treatment of unilateral iliac atherosclerotic disease. *J Vasc Surg* 1999; **30**: 693–700.
14. Ng RL, Gillies TE, Davies AH, Baird RN, Horrocks M. Iliofemoral versus femorofemoral bypass: a 6-year audit. *Br J Surg* 1992; **79**: 1011–1013.
15. Nazzal MM, Hoballah JJ, Jacobovicz C *et al.* A comparative evaluation of femorofemoral crossover bypass and iliofemoral bypass for unilateral iliac artery occlusive disease. *Angiology* 1998; **49**: 259–265.
16. Lau H, Cheng SW, Hui J. Eighteen-year experience with femoro-femoral bypass. *Aust N Z J Surg* 2000; **70**: 275–278.
17. Berce M, Sayers RD, Miller JH. Femorofemoral crossover grafts for claudication: a safe and reliable procedure. *Eur J Vasc Endovasc Surg* 1996; **12**: 437–441.
18. Schneider JR, Besso SR, Walsh DB, Zwolak RM, Cronenwett JL. Femorofemoral versus aortobifemoral bypass: outcome and hemodynamic results. *J Vasc Surg* 1994; **19**: 43–55.
19. Harrington ME, Harrington EB, Haimov M, Schanzer H, Jacobson JH. Iliofemoral versus femorofemoral bypass: the case for an individualized approach. *J Vasc Surg* 1992; **16**: 841–852.
20. Ricco JB. Unilateral iliac artery occlusive disease: a randomized multicenter trial examining direct revascularization versus crossover bypass. Association Universitaire de Recherche en Chirurgie. *Ann Vasc Surg* 1992; **6**: 209–219.
21. Kretschmer G, Niederle B, Schemper M, Polterauer P. Extra-anatomic femoro-femoral crossover bypass (FF) vs. unilateral orthotopic ilio-femoral bypass (IF): an attempt to compare results based on data matching. *Eur J Vasc Surg* 1991; **5**: 75–82.
22. Criado E, Burnham SJ, Tinsley EA Jr, Johnson G,Jr., Keagy BA. Femorofemoral bypass graft: analysis of patency and factors influencing long-term outcome. *J Vasc Surg* 1993; **18**: 495–504.
23. Criado E, Farber MA. Femorofemoral bypass: appropriate application based on factors affecting outcome. *Semin Vasc Surg* 1997; **10**: 34–41.
24. Shah RM, Peer RM, Upson JF, Ricotta JJ. Donor iliac angioplasty and crossover femorofemoral bypass. *Am J Surg* 1992; **164**: 295–298.
25. Perler BA, Williams GM. Does donor iliac artery percutaneous transluminal angioplasty or stent placement influence the results of femorofemoral bypass? Analysis of 70 consecutive cases with long-term follow-up. *J Vasc Surg* 1996; **24**: 363–369.
26. Chalmers RT, Kerr J, Gillies T, Brittenden J. The crossover femoropopliteal bypass: a useful option for unilateral iliofemoral occlusive disease. *Eur J Vasc Endovasc Surg* 1996; **11**: 330–334.

27. Whatling PJ, Gibson M, Torrie EP, Magee TR, Galland RB. Iliac occlusions: stenting or crossover grafting? An examination of patency and cost. *Eur J Vasc Endovasc Surg* 2000; **20**: 36–40.

28. Mingoli A, Sapienza P, Feldhaus RJ, Di Marzo L, Burchi C, Cavallaro A. Femorofemoral bypass grafts: Factors influencing long-term patency rate and outcome. *Surgery* 2001; **129**: 451–458.

29. Mingoli A, Sapienza P, Feldhaus RJ, Di Marzo L, Burchi C, Cavallaro A. Comparison of femoro-femoral and aortofemoral bypass for aortoiliac occlusive disease. *J Cardiovasc Surg (Torino)* 2001; **42**: 381–387.

30. Aburahma AF, Robinson PA, Cook CC, Hopkins ES. Selecting patients for combined femorofemoral bypass grafting and iliac balloon angioplasty and stenting for bilateral iliac disease. *J Vasc Surg* 2001; **33**(Suppl): S93–S99.

31. Testini M, Todisco C, Greco L, Impedovo G, Fullone M, Regina G. Femoro-femoral graft after unilateral obstruction of aorto-bifemoral bypass. *Minerva Cardioangiol* 1998; **46**: 15–19.

32. van Adrichem LN, van Berge Henegouwen DP, Lobach HJ, van der Werken C. The femoro-femoral cross-over bypass. *Neth J Surg* 1991; **43**: 67–70.

33. Ellis M, Freemantle N, Mason J. North of England evidence based guidelines development project: methods of developing guidelines for efficient drug use in primary care. *BMJ* 1998; **316**: 1232–1235.

Internet websites

The Danish Vascular Registry, Karbase:
http://www.karbase.dk/English/english.htm
The Swedish Vascular Registry, Swedvasc:
http://www.sos.se/mars/kva013/kva013.htm

Aortoiliac reconstruction should avoid femorofemoral crossover

Charing Cross Editorial Comments towards Consensus

The authors have argued this issue extremely well. When Dr Michael DeBakey and colleagues first considered aortoiliac reconstruction they drew attention to the bilateral nature of disease in most instances. The DeBakey solution was to prescribe an aortic bifurcation graft to jump the whole segment on both sides. The operation was the gold standard for many decades, had an approximate 90% 5-year patency but of course with some mortality risk of major aortic surgery. The argument for the bifurcation graft was that it would avoid the so-called 'extra-anatomic' femorofemoral crossover which was regarded by some pioneers with great suspicion. The aorto-uni-iliac Dacron tube was criticised because it often lead to the need for a second operation on the contralateral side in due course. Few surgeons in the early days performed endarterectomy of the whole segment but those who did including Edwin J Wylie of San Francisco reported 95% 5-year patency for endarterectomy. However, Jack Wylie and his colleagues preferred the endarterectomy technique for lesser disease just down to the termination of the common iliac artery and regarded the external iliac artery with great suspicion and when it was diseased preferred bypass rather than endarterectomy.

The advent of endovascular techniques and balloon angioplasty has revolutionized the whole of the approach to aortoiliac reconstruction. Arteriograms and aortoiliac images are looked at afresh with new techniques in mind. Almost always it is possible to overcome at least one side with aortoiliac reconstruction using either plain balloon or balloon and stent. With one femoral pulse normally restored the second side is considered and either this is corrected by endovascular techniques or there now emerges the possibility of a femorofemoral bypass with two small incisions at the groin level to reconstruct the second side. Clearly the femorofemoral crossover has gained a new lease of life because of the endovascular revolution.

Nor is that the end of the endovascular story as far as femorofemoral crossover is concerned. Currently aortic bifurcation endovascular repair is preferred for abdominal aortic aneurysm repair but there are emerging techniques for emergency aneurysm repair and the first-line treatment could easily be an aorto-uni-iliac procedure with femorofemoral crossover performed as a second stage with occlusion of the contralateral iliac by a basket technique. The waxing and waning of enthusiasm for the femorofemoral crossover over the last 30 years has been one of the fascinations of vascular surgery.

Roger M Greenhalgh
Editor

Pull-through pressures improve outcome quality for aortoiliac angioplasty

For the motion

Tony Nicholson

Introduction

The haemodynamic significance of an arterial stenosis can be judged by both morphological and haemodynamic means. Morphological information can be obtained from a number of imaging tests. Duplex ultrasound combined with B-mode imaging can provide a combination of physiological and anatomical information. Unfortunately the iliac artery is deep, while bowel gas, body habitus, tortuosity and the difficulty of judging the exact gate angle in the iliac arteries hinder the resolution, localization and accuracy of measurements. Though computed tomographic and magnetic resonance angiography are evolving rapidly, contrast angiography is still the gold standard providing excellent spatial and contrast resolution. Because stenoses are often eccentric, and because arteries overlap each other, angiography needs to be performed in more than one plane in order to accurately assess the pelvic arteries. There are several features on an angiogram that allow an assessment of the haemodynamic significance of an area of narrowing. These include slow flow of contrast on one side compared with the other, the development of collateral arteries around a lesion and the presence of post-stenotic dilatation. However, there is intra-observer and inter-observer variability in the estimation of the degree of a stenosis diagnosed at angiography (Fig. 1a–e).[1-3] In addition eccentric stenoses can be under-assessed even with two views. Therefore the information provided about the functional significance of an arterial stenosis is limited. Sensitivities as low as 45%, and specificities as low as 63% have been reported for the angiographic estimation of area reduction.[3]

Angiographic visual estimation and unreliability is most pronounced for intermediate grades of stenosis and in judging the results of angioplasty (Fig. 2a–d). Intravenous ultrasound has been shown to be superior to angiography in these two areas.[4] However, in most centres intravenous ultrasound is still a research tool in peripheral arteries or preserved for problem solving. It is expensive, requires the use of a much larger sheath than is necessary for angiography and is not without its own complications. In addition it cannot be used for judging the haemodynamic significance of an arterial occlusion; 90% of the peer reviewed literature on intravenous ultrasound concerns the coronary arteries. It has been conclusively shown in comparisons of intravenous ultrasound and coronary pressure measurements that both are of similar value with respect to the assessment of arterial stenoses and the result

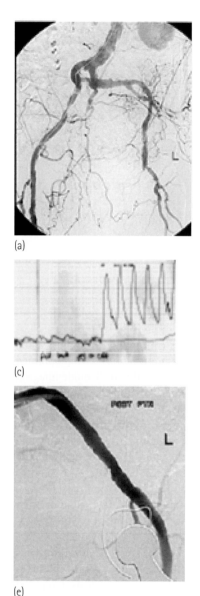

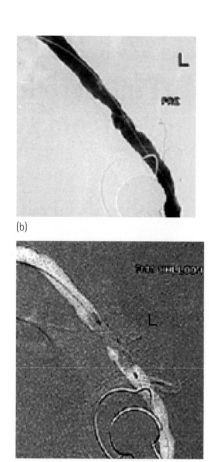

Figure 1a–e. A 68-year-old man with rest pain and ulceration of his left foot. (a) Iliac angiography reveals an occluded left superficial femoral artery. However, his left common femoral pulse was poor but apart from slight irregularity (b) in the distal external iliac artery no reason for this was seen. A pull-back pressure measurement (c) revealed a systolic gradient of 90 mmHg without a vasodilator. Confirmation of the stenosis and its degree can be seen by the wasting of the 7 mm balloon used to angioplasty the lesion (d). A good angiographic result was obtained (e) with abolition of the gradient.

of endovascular intervention.[5] Intra-arterial pressure measurements are cheap, relatively non-invasive if performed at the same time as angiography or intervention and there are no reported complications.

Intra-arterial pressure measurements for assessing the haemodynamic significance of iliac disease

The pressure decrease across a stenosis (the gradient) is a direct indicator of the haemodynamic effect of that stenosis. It is a more accurate measure of the significance of a stenosis or occlusion than morphologic criteria, especially where a stenosis

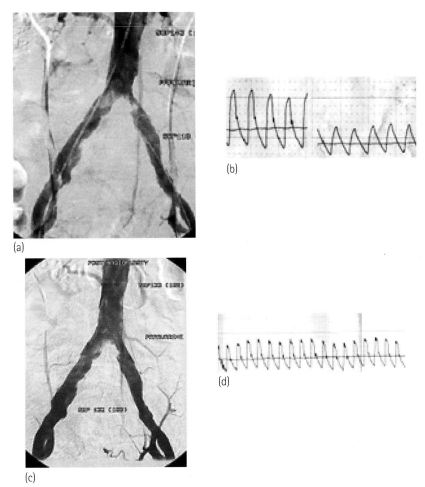

Figure 2 a-d. A 55-year-old man with significant claudication and an absent left femoral pulse was shown to have a 70% stenosis of his left common iliac origin at angiography (a). A mean pressure gradient of 20 mmHg without vasodilatation was demonstrated on simultaneous pressure measurement (b). Following 10 mm balloon angioplasty there was still a 20–30% stenosis (c) but the gradient was abolished (d) and no further intervention was undertaken. He remains well with no claudication 4 years after PTA.

appears to be of moderate severity or the results of an endovascular intervention are being judged.[3,6–8] The recent Dutch randomized control trial[9] randomized patients to angioplasty (PTA) alone or secondary stenting for a poor angioplasty result. The post-PTA result was judged by the presence or absence of a pressure gradient. The mean pressure gradient chosen was 10mmHg mean gradient at rest or after vasodilatation. A later study by Kamphuis *et al.*[10] demonstrated that patients with residual stenoses, where the pressure gradient was between 5–10, fared as well as patients with gradients of less than 5 mm of mercury. In the Dutch study no significant difference was found between primary stent placement in iliac stenosis or selective stent insertion for poor angiographic result. Using the same haemodynamic criteria the latter study[10] showed that 41% of patients became eligible for stent placement following PTA. If more liberal criteria are used and stents are only placed when the mean systolic pressure is greater than 20mm of mercury without a vasodilator, only 4% of patients would be eligible for a stent but the Dutch study does not support this approach.

Mean pressure gradients are probably a better measure of haemodynamic significance than peak systolic gradients. Clearly a 10 mmHg systolic gradient in a patient with a blood pressure of 200/90 mmHg is far less significant than a similar gradient in a patient with a blood pressure of 100/70 mmHg. Mean pressure gradient also provides a good balance between systolic flow rates and peripheral resistance. Finally, mean gradients negate respiratory variations in systolic peaks. Where mean pressure gradients are equivocal (i.e. between 5 and 10 mmHg) it is vital to decrease peripheral resistance in order to mimic limb exercise. Such manoeuvres are physiologically sound especially in patients complaining of claudication. The easiest way of simulating this exercise is to employ an intra-arterial vasodilator such as nitroglycerine (100–200 µg), tolazoline (25–40 mg) or papavarine (15–30 mg).

Pitfalls of intra-arterial pressure measurements and how to overcome them

Air bubbles in either the catheter or the transducer apparatus in fluid-fill systems can dampen pressure waveforms considerably.[11] This is easily prevented by simple attention to detail and careful and thorough flushing of all equipment before pressure is measured.

It has been reported that the diameter of a catheter across a stenosis can exaggerate a pressure gradient downstream.[12] Whilst this may be overcome in very small arteries by using pressure wires rather than catheters, in the aortoiliac system it is not a significant problem because morphologically highly significant stenoses do not necessarily need a pressure gradient to measure their significance. Diameters of 1.3 mm are highly unlikely to reproduce this effect in the aortoiliac segment.

There is really no difference in the use of endhole or sidehole catheters for measuring pressure providing that sideholes do not bridge the stenosis or any adjacent lesions. Patterns of flow disruption adjacent to a stenosis may induce variations in the pressures recorded by sidehole catheters. However, this effect is negligible beyond 2 cm of a stenosis where there are high flow rates.[12] In addition the direction of a hole relative to the direction of blood flow has little practical relevance when measuring pressures upstream or downstream of a stenosis.[12]

Clearly very low systemic blood pressure could eliminate an otherwise significant pressure gradient across a stenosis. However, this is not a practical problem: patients as hypotensive as this would have more severe problems requiring attention in other systems.

Pressures can either be measured simultaneously above and below a stenosis or can be measured by pull-back of a catheter across the stenosis. Simultaneous pressures have the temporal advantage of negating variations in blood pressure and the transient action of vasodilators. They also allow the maintenance of position above and below a stenosis that is lost by pull-back pressure.

Summary

- It is clear from the peer reviewed literature that careful measurement of pressure gradient offers significant advantages over the use of morphological criteria alone for assessing the haemodynamic significance of iliac stenoses and occlusions and for assessing the adequacy of endovascular intervention.

- A number of studies exist that provide data in favour of a significant threshold of a post-vasodilator mean gradient of 10 mmHg.

- The literature suggests that intra-arterial pressure gradients are as good as intravenous ultrasound when evaluating stenotic disease.

- Intra-arterial pressure measurements are cheap, relatively non-invasive, easy to perform and able to assess the significance of occlusive disease with no complications.

- The assessment of aorto-iliac disease and evaluation of the results of endovascular treatment is incomplete without intra-arterial pressure measurements.

References

1. Kinney TB, Rose SC. Intra-arterial pressure measurements during angiographic evaluation of peripheral vascular disease: Techniques, interpretation, applications and limitations. *AJR* 1996; **166**: 277–284.
2. Brewster DC, Waltman AC, O'Hara PJ *et al*. Femoral artery pressure measurement during aortography. *Cardiovasc Surg* 1978; **60**: 1120–1124.
3. Tettaroo E, van Englen AD, Spithoven JH *et al*. Stent placement after iliac angioplasty: comparison of haemodynamic and angiographic criteria. *Radiology* 1996; **201**: 155–159.
4. Vogt KG, Schroeder TV. Intra vascular ultrasound for iliac artery imaging. Clinical review. *J Cardiovasc Surg* 2001; **42**: 69–75.
5. Hanekamp CE, Koolen JJ, Pijls NH *et al*. Comparison of quantitative coronary angiography intravascular ultrasound and coronary pressure measurement to assess optimum stent deployment. *Circulation* 1999; **99**: 1015–1021.
6. Kaufman SL, Barth KH, Kadir S *et al*. Haemodynamic measurements in the evaluation of follow-up of transluminal angioplasty of the iliac and femoral arteries. *Radiology* 1982; **142**: 329–336.
7. Gunn IG, Cowie TN, Forest H *et al*. Haemodynamic assessment following iliac artery dilatation. *Br J Surg* 1981; **68**: 858–860.
8. Udoff EJ, Barth KH, Harrington DP *et al*. Haemodynamic significance of iliac artery stenosis: pressure measurements during aortography. *Radiology* 1979; **132**: 289–293.
9. Tetteroo E Van der Graf Y Bosch JL. Randomised comparison of primary stent insertion vs. primary angioplasty and selective stent insertion in iliac artery occlusive disease *Lancet* 1998; **351**: 1153–1159.
10. Kamphius AG, van Englen AD, Tettaroo E *et al*. Impact of different haemodynamic criteria for stent placement after sub-optimal iliac angioplasty. Dutch Iliac Stent Trial Study Group. *JVIR* 1999; **10**: 741–746.
11. Ganz P, Harrington DP, Gasper J, *et al*. Phasic pressure gradients across coronary and renal artery stenoses in humans. *Am Heart J* 1983; **106**: 1399–1406.
12. McWilliams RG, Robertson I, Smye SW *et al*. Sources of error in intra-arterial pressure measurements across a stenosis. *Eur J Vasc Endovasc Surg* 1998; **15**: 535–540.

Pull-through pressures improve outcome quality for aortoiliac angioplasty

Against the motion
Trevor Cleveland

Introduction

Balloon angioplasty, with or without the addition of metallic stenting, has become a widely used tool in the treatment of patients with symptomatic aortoiliac atheromatous disease. Balloon angioplasty became possible with non-compliant balloons following Gruntzig's description in 1974[1]. In common with all medical operations and procedures, it is necessary to assess whether balloon angioplasty has been successful, and this translates into assessment of the patients symptoms and if they improve. Assuming that it has been possible to correctly identify the symptoms as being attributable to a stenosis or occlusion of an iliac artery segment, then the outcome will often correlate with the long-term patency of that segment following balloon angioplasty. This is not always the case as a result of multiple factors including concurrent disease locally or remotely, incorrect selection of lesions for balloon angioplasty and patient-related factors. However, having made the clinical decision to treat an aortoiliac lesion the intention is to perform this in the best way possible to achieve short- and long-term patency of that segment.

At the time of the procedure, there are a number of methods which may be used to assess whether the balloon angioplasty has been successful or if a different size balloon (length and/or diameter), a different type of inflation technique (e.g. prolonged low-pressure inflation) or a stent may be needed. These techniques include:

1. angiography,
2. iliac pressure measurements,
3. pulse palpation,
4. iliac duplex,
5. flow wires,
6. pressure wires.

The later four are not commonly used. This is because palpation of the femoral pulse is difficult when the vessel already has an arterial sheath in position, and even if it were easy this is a very crude method of assessing residual proximal arterial disease. Iliac duplex has the potential to give information regarding the haemodynamic situation during balloon angioplasty; however, few interventional vascular suites have easy access to the necessary machinery. Should ultrasound be available, the transcutaneous site would be very close to the sterile field with the risk of contamination, and anxious patients tend to swallow air obscuring the acoustic window. Even in optimal circumstances a significant proportion of iliac arteries may not be possible to visualize, although some authors indicate high success rates.[2]

Flow wires and pressure wires have been extensively investigated in the coronary circulation, but have made little impact in the peripheral circulation and almost no peripheral vascular laboratories have access to this technology. The cost of such devices is high for both the static machine and also for the disposable catheters.

In practical terms this leaves angiography and iliac pressure measurements as the mainstay of assessment at the time of balloon angioplasty to attempt to predict the outcome of the procedure.

The arterial response to balloon angioplasty

In 1980 Casteneda-Zuniga *et al.*[3] proposed a mechanism for balloon angioplasty, which has subsequently been supported by others.[4-13] It seems likely that atherosclerotic plaque compresses little at the time of balloon angioplasty, rather the high balloon pressure causes the plaque to crack and be sheared away from the arterial media, which explains the 'subintimal' tracking of contrast which is seen angiographically after balloon angioplasty. Fortunately the separation of the plaque from the media is only partial otherwise there would be significant embolization following balloon angioplasty. The dilatation causes the media to be stretched, but its integrity is maintained, thus avoiding rupture. There is histological evidence that there is irreversible stretching of the media[4] as evidenced by a 'corkscrew' appearance of the smooth muscle nuclei. It is then thought that the media is freed from the rigid constraints of the atheromatous lining and able to respond to the local circulatory needs by further dilating – positive remodelling. This has indeed been documented angiographically following balloon angioplasty,[4,14] adding credence to Gruntzig's description that balloon angioplasty is 'controlled injury' following which there is healing. It appears that if the media is stretched then the muscle fibres remain permanently overstretched, which is an essential part of positive remodelling; however, if the media is over stretched and ruptures, then healing is by scar formation which may result in negative remodelling and restenosis.

In addition, neointimal hyperplasia may be formed, which seems to be related to platelet adhesion and release of platelet-derived growth factors,[15] stimulating smooth muscle cells to migrate to the inner lining of the artery with deposition of ground substance. This fills space and causes loss of the gain achieved by balloon angioplasty. However, this process is not completely understood, as for example intimal hyperplasia may occur in the presence of profound thrombocytopenia.[16] That smooth muscle cells migrate and are seen to deposit ground substance[17] seems clear and the process of neointimal formation appears to accentuated by stent placement. In the coronary circulation the insertion of a stent is associated with a greater late loss in lumen diameter than non-stent balloon angioplasty. The increased intimal proliferation after stenting is thought to be a result of a biological reaction to foreign material. Indeed this may be further accentuated by the continued stimulus to smooth muscle cells provided by self-expanding stents.[18-22] There is, therefore, histological and clinical evidence that following appropriately sized balloon angioplasty, positive remodelling of the artery can be expected and that by placing a stent this positive remodelling may be inhibited by the stent causing neointimal formation, which may result in a loss of luminal gain.

How are iliac pressures measured?

The conventional method for assessment of the aortoiliac segment is to cannulate the common femoral artery along with the brachial artery and to compare the two pressures. Papavarine (20 mg) is injected into the femoral artery and a fall in the index of >20% is deemed significant.[23] In the context of endovascular interventional procedures the intra-arterial blood pressure may be measured using the following methods:

1. Pull-back measurements from the ipsilateral femoral artery.
2. Pull-back measurements from the contralateral femoral artery.
3. Simultaneous measurements from the aorta and the ipsilateral femoral artery using a catheter in the aorta placed from the contralateral side.
4. Simultaneous measurements of aortic and femoral artery pressures from the ipsilateral groin.

All of the above have potential drawbacks. Pull-back pressures from the ipsilateral groin following balloon angioplasty require that wire access is maintained across the angioplasty segment, otherwise further damage may occur when the lesion is recrossed. This wire must be sufficiently small so as not to alter the pressure measured and the seal around this wire sufficiently secure to ensure an accurate recording. The major problem with this technique is that a patients blood pressure may change from beat to beat, particularly if the patient has a dysrhythmia. This variation may be accentuated by the addition of vasodilators especially if they are short acting, such as papavarine. If the pull-back is performed from the contralateral side the catheter used to measure the pressure distal to the treated side is placed across the angioplasty site and may accentuate any pressure drop. To compound this a downstream facing catheter hole may give falsely reduced pressure readings.[24]

If the measurements are taken simultaneously then this removes the problems with beat-to-beat variation of blood pressure and allows for more accurate usage of vasodilators. However, if this is all performed from the ipsilateral side then the catheter across the balloon angioplasty site may falsely accentuate any residual gradient, particularly in the presence of the high flows following vasodilatation.[24] In addition the sheath from which the distal pressure is measured must be of sufficient size to ensure that the measurement from this site is not impeded by the presence of the catheter within it.

It is therefore most accurate and reproducible to perform iliac pressure measurements by placement of a sheath in the downstream ipsilateral femoral artery with a separate catheter placed in the aorta from either the contralateral femoral artery, or the brachial artery.[25] Unfortunately many authors do not use this method, do not specify their technique or use a mixture depending on changing circumstances. This makes comparison difficult and the shortcomings may be overlooked. However, despite these problems the measurements taken are considered accurate and the 'gold standard'.

Is a pressure gradient significant?

The following have all been used as levels of haemodynamic assessment of iliac balloon angioplasty, above which the balloon angioplasty is considered to have been insufficient:

1. >or equal to 5 mmHg mean arterial gradient,[26-28]
2. >or equal to 5 mmHg, mean or systolic not mentioned,[29,30]

3. >or equal to 5 mmHg systolic,[31]
4. >or equal to 10 mmHg mean,[32–34]
5. >or equal to 20 mmHg.[35]

Along with the various gradients noted above, a range of vasodilators have been used to simulate exercise, including:

1. papavarine,
2. glycerol trinitrate,
3. tolazoline.

Not only have different vasodilator substances been used, but also differing doses. This results from a lack of basic data indicating what dose of which substance produces maximal vasodilatation.

In the only prospective study in which stents have not been placed when there is a residual pressure gradient, Kamphuis *et al.*[35] found that if a mean pressure gradient of up to 5 mmHg was left following balloon angioplasty, the outcome of these patients was the same as those who had no pressure gradient following balloon angioplasty. This supports the histological data detailed above indicating that remodelling occurs after balloon angioplasty which may be positive as well as negative.

Do iliac pressure measurements avoid acute thromboses?

There are no data to support the view that angiographic or haemodynamic measurements are able to predict when a lesion treated by balloon angioplasty is likely to thrombose in the immediate period following the procedure. Some practitioners are concerned that if a 'significant' pressure gradient is allowed to remain then the vessel may acutely occlude. There is no scientific basis to this assumption, indeed the placement of a metallic stent may promote thrombosis despite a seemingly good result. Furthermore, intravenous ultrasound and post-mortem studies show clearly that dissection flaps occur following balloon angioplasty, even when there is no residual pressure gradient. Similarly there is no evidence that this situation is more or less likely to promote thrombosis than when the flap causes a gradient. There is anecdotal data to suggest that large (up to 70 mmHg systolic) gradients may be allowed to remain, with modern antiplatelet medications, and the remodelling process allowed to work. Angiographically and haemodynamically these may result in satisfactory outcomes as well as being symptomatically satisfactory.

Do pull–back pressures predict outcome?

Whilst it may be true that measurement of iliac pressures can be better than angiography at defining the haemodynamic result following balloon angioplasty,[36,37] patients with haemodynamic gradients have not been allowed to proceed without stent placement. As a result there are no data on the outcome of patients with residual iliac pressure gradients, to compare either with those who have been stented or those who have no gradient following balloon angioplasty. It is only possible to look at the patency of successful balloon angioplasty, as assessed haemodynamically, with those who have gone on to secondary stenting. This provides no information as to whether pull-back pressures predict outcome. There are no prospective trials of the iliac pressures measured at balloon angioplasty comparing these with the outcome, be that patency, effectiveness or cost-effectiveness.

Conclusion

The method by which the pressure in the aortoiliac segment is measured is variable and frequently suboptimal. The definition of a significant pressure gradient is not resolved with different authors using different definitions. There are no dose-response curves constructed for the vasodilators in common use, with various doses of various vasodilators used in the different studies. There is no standard way to measure aortoiliac pressures.

Taking an arbitrary gradient as being significant, patients are immediately subjected to stent placement. Thus:

1. The remodelling process so essential to balloon angioplasty is inhibited by stenting.
2. The stent itself may be promoting restenosis.
3. Patients with these gradients have not been followed up to scientifically test if these gradients do or do not predict outcome.

The data does not support the suggestion that iliac pressure measurements improve the outcome of balloon angioplasty.

Summary

- Arteries are known to remodel following balloon angioplasty.

- Stents inhibit remodelling and promote neointimal formation.

- If pull-through pressures are measured, residual gradients are treated with stents.

- Iliac pressures are measured using differing catheter arrangements and different vasodilatation regimes.

- It has not been decided what constitutes a 'significant pressure gradient'.

- Patients with residual gradients have not been followed without the results being confounded by stents.

- There is no evidence that pull-through pressure measurements improve outcome quality for aortoiliac balloon angioplasty.

References

1. Gruntzig A, Hopff H. Perkutane Rekanalisation chronischer arterieller Verschlusse mit einem neuen Dilatations-Katheter. *Dtsch Med Woechenschr* 1974; **99**: 2502.
2. De Smet AAEA, Kitslaar PJEHM. A duplex criterion for aorto-iliac stenosis. *Eur J Vasc Surg* 1990; **4**: 275–278.
3. Casteneda-Zuniga WR, Formanek A, Tradavarthy M *et al*. The mechanism of balloon angioplasty. *Radiology* 1980; **135**: 565.
4. Zollikofer C, Cragg A, Hunter D *et al*. Mechanism of transluminal angioplasty. In *Interventional Radiology* 2nd edn, Vol. 1. Casteneda-Zuniga WR, Tadavarthy SM (eds). Baltimore: Williams & Wilkins, 1992; 249–297.
5. Laerum F, Vlodaver Z, Casteneda-Zuniga WR *et al*. The mechanism of angioplasty: Dilatation of iliac cadaver arteries with intravascular pressure control. *ROFO* 1982; **136**: 573.
6. Zollikofer CL, Chain J, Salomonowitz E *et al*. Percutaneous transluminal angioplasty of the aorta. *Radiology* 1984; **151**: 355.

7. Faxon DP, Sanborn TA, Haudenschild CC, Ryan TJ: Effect of antiplatelet therapy on restenosis after experimental angioplasty. *Am J Cardiol* 1984; **53**: 72C.

8. Sanborn TA, Faxon DP, Haudenschild C *et al*. The mechanism of intraluminal angioplasty: Evidence for formation of aneurysms in experimental atherosclerosis. *Circulation* 1983; **68**: 1136.

9. Faxon DP, Weber VJ, Haudenschild C *et al*. Acute effects of transluminal angioplasty in three experimental modules of atherosclerosis. *Arteriosclerosis* 1982; **2**: 125.

10. Block PC, Myler RK, Sertzer S, Fallon JT. Morphology after transluminal angioplasty in human beings. *N Engl J Med* 1981; **305**: 382.

11. Hoffman MA, Fallon JT, Greenfield AJ *et al*. Arterial pathology after percutaneous transluminal angioplasty. *AJR* 1981; **137**: 147.

12. Clouse ME, Tomashefski JF Jr, Reinhold RE *et al*. Mechanical effect of balloon angioplasty: Case report with histology. *AJR* 1981; **137**: 869.

13. Saffitz JE, Totty WG, McLennan BL *et al*. Percutaneous transluminal angioplasty: Radiological-pathological correlation. *Radiology* 1981; **141**: 651.

14. Crawley F, Clifton A, Markus H, Brown MM. Delayed improvement in carotid artery diameter after carotid angioplasty. *Stroke* 1997; **28**: 574–579.

15. Ferns GA, Raines EW, Sprugel KH *et al*. Inhibition of neointimal smooth muscle accumulation after angioplasty by an antibody to PGDF. *Science* 1991; **253**: 1129.

16. Guyton JR, Karnovsky MJ: Smooth muscle cell proliferation in the occluded rat carotid artery: Lack of requirement for luminal platelets. *Am J Pathol* 1979; **94**: 585.

17. Liu MW, Roudin GS, King SB: Restenosis after coronary angioplasty. Potential biologic determinants and role of intima hyperplasia. Point of view. *Circulation* 1989; **79**: 1374.

18. Mintz GS, Popma JJ, Pichard AD *et al*. Arterial remodeling after coronary angioplasty. A serial intravascular ultrasound study. *Circulation* 1996; **94**: 35–43.

19. Hoffman R, Mintz GS, Mehran R *et al*. Late tissue proliferation both within and surrounding Palmaz-Schatz stents is associated with procedural vessel wall injury (abstract). *J Am Col Cardiol* 1997; **29** (Suppl): 397A–3970.

20. Mintz GS, Pichard AD, Kent KM *et al*. Endovascular stents reduce restenosis by eliminating geometric arterial remodeling: a serial intravascular ultrasound study (abstract). *J Am Coll Cardiol* 1995; **25** (Suppl): 36A–360.

21. Karas SP, Gravanis MB, Santoian EC *et al*. Coronary intimal proliferation after balloon injury and stenting in swine: an animal model of restenosis. *J Am Coll Cardiol* 1992; **20**: 467–474.

22. Chronos N, Dieineman ME, Cipolla GD *et al*. Stent implantation induces late arterial wall cellular proliferation compared to angioplasty in normal rabbits (abstract). *Eur Heart J* 1997; **18** (Suppl): 451.

23. London N. JM. Vascular laboratory investigation. *Essential Vasc Surg* 1999; **4**: 47–61.

24. McWilliams RG, Robertson I, Smye SW, Wijesinge L, Kessel D. Sources of error in intra-arterial pressure measurements across a stenosis. *Eur J Vasc Endovasc Surg* 1998; **15**: 535–540.

25. Tomlinson M *et al*. Intra-arterial Pressure Measurements. *Eur J Endovasc Surg* 1999; **17**: 458–459. Article No. ejvs 1998.0765.

26. Palmaz JC, Garcia OJ, Schatz RA *et al*. Placement of balloon-expandable intraluminal stents in iliac arteries: first 171 procedures. *Radiology* 1990; **174**: 969–975.

27. Palmaz JC, Laborde JC, Rivera FJ, Encarnacion CE, Lutz JD, Moss JG. Stenting of the iliac arterias with the Palmaz stent: experience from a multicenter trial. *Cardiovasc Intervent Radiol* 1992; **15**: 291–297.

28. Murphy KD, Encarnacion CE, Le VA, Palmaz JC. Iliac artery stent placement with the Palmaz stent: follow-up study. *JVIR* 1995; **6**: 321–329.

29. Martin EC Katzen BT, Benenati JF *et al*. Multicentre trial of the Wallstent in the iliac and femoral arteries. *JVIR* 1995; **6**: 843–849.

30. Long AL, Sapoval MR, Beyssen BM *et al*. Strecker stent implantation in iliac arteries: patency and predictive factors for long-term success. *Radiology* 1995; **194**: 739–744.

31. Henry M, Amor M, Ethevenot G *et al*. Palmaz stent placement in iliac and femoropopliteal arteries: primary and secondary patency in 310 patients with 2-4 year follow-up. *Radiology* 1995; **197**: 167–174.

32. Hausegger KA, Lammer J, Hagen B *et al*. Iliac artery stenting: clinical experience with the Palmaz stent, Wallstent and Strecker stent. *Acta Radiologica* 1992; **33**: 292–296.

33. Cikrit DF, Gustafson PA, Dalsing MC *et al*. Long-term follow-up of the Palmaz stent for iliac occlusive disease. *Surgery* 1995; **118**: 608–614.

34. Tetteroo E, van Engelen AD, Spithoven JH, Tielbeek AV, van der Graaf Y, Mali WPTM. Stent placement after iliac angioplasty: comparison of hemodynamic and angiographic criteria. *Radiology* 1996; **201**: 155-159.

35. Kamphius Zollikofer CL, Antonucci F, Pfyffer M, *et al*. Arterial stent placement with the use of the Wallstent: mid-term results of clinical experience. *Radiology* 1991; **179**: 449–456.

36. Kaufman SL, Barth LH, Kadir S *et al*. Hemodynamic measurements in the evaluation and follow-up of transluminal angioplasty of the iliac and femoral arteries. *Radiology* 1982; **142**: 329-336.

37. Tetteroo E, Haaring C, van Engelen AD, van der Graaf Y, Mali WPTM. Therapeutic consequences of variation in intraarterial pressure measurements after iliac angioplasty. *Cardiovasc Intervent Radiol* 1997; **20**: 426–430.

Pull-through pressures improve outcome quality for aortoiliac angioplasty

Charing Cross Editorial Comments towards Consensus

Here are two leading vascular radiologists from the same part of the same country taking an absolutely diametrically opposite position. Dr Tony Nicholson, current President of the British Society of Interventional Radiology, has summarized his certainty that pull-through pressures are valuable and that they should be performed at the time of angioplasty. Dr Trevor Cleveland argues that such is the uncertainty of the methodology they are not worth recommending. Perhaps the evidence in favour of the value of pull-through pressures at the time of angioplasty is firmer for the larger aortoiliac segment than for the smaller femoral popliteal segment. As the arteries become smaller, relative to the stenoses and available lumen through the stenoses, the catheters are effectively larger and it can be argued that this could distort the pressure difference measurements in the femoral-popliteal segment particularly in the distal vessels of smaller arteries of smaller patients. There are simply inadequate studies to be certain about the point and from the evidence presented I conclude that we need much more information to be certain about this important issue but both authors are likely to acknowledge that on-table proof of excellence of procedure needs to be achieved if at all possible. Any radiologist 'worth his or her salt' does not need to measure pull-through pressure to know if an angioplasty is done properly. It would seem that it would be necessary to image any lesion in a number of planes to be about to take this view. At the very best, pull-through pressures are here depicted as an additional assessment supported by Tony Nicholson but not by Trevor Cleveland.

Roger M Greenhalgh
Editor

Vascular brachytherapy is preferable to drug–eluting stents to reduce peripheral artery restenosis

For the motion

Erich Minar, Boris Pokrajac,
Roswitha Wolfram, Richard Poetter

Introduction

Peripheral vascular disease from the aortic bifurcation to the run-off vessels is common, and the efficacy of percutaneous transluminal angioplasty (PTA) has been well documented in numerous trials. The advantages of PTA include low morbidity and mortality and the necessity of shorter hospital stay. However, restenosis has remained until now a major limitation of the clinical usefulness of PTA, especially in the femoropopliteal and crural region. A poor long-term patency rate after PTA of longer femoropopliteal lesions was repeatedly reported, and complex and longer areas of stenosis may have a 6-month patency rate as low as 23%.[1] Therefore, angioplasty is not generally accepted for treatment of longer (> 10 cm) femoropopliteal lesions by many interventional radiologists and especially by vascular surgeons, despite the increasing primary success rates due to experience and technical improvements. Angioplasty for recurrence after previous PTA has a further reduced long-term success rate.[2] A 1-year patency rate of 41% and a 3-year patency rate of only 11% was reported after PTA of recurrent femoropopliteal lesions with lesion lengths between 1 and 5 cm.

The use of newer interventional devices such as stents has not improved these long-term results. While stents can reduce the constricting effect of vascular remodelling, the major drawback of stent implantation is the enhanced occurrence of neointimal proliferation within the stent (Fig. 1). Results of three randomized trials[3–5] in patients with femoropopliteal lesions revealed no improvement of long-term success rate after primary stent placement, compared with PTA alone. Vroegindeweij *et al.*[3] reported a 12-month patency rate of 62% in the group with stents vs 74% in the PTA group, and Cejna *et al.*[4] reported a cumulative 1-year angiographic primary patency rate of 63% in both groups. Grimm *et al.*[5] recently reported the results of a randomized study comparing PTA alone vs PTA with Palmaz stent placement for femoropopliteal lesions. No significant differences in primary or secondary patency rates could be observed at 12 or 39 months. Therefore, the recent recommendations by the TransAtlantic InterSociety

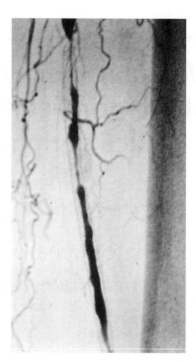

Figure 1. Angiogram obtained 6 months after stent implantation in the femoropopliteal region demonstrates severe long-distance recurrence caused by neointimal hyperplasia.

Consensus Working Group[6] stated that femoropopliteal placement of stents as a primary approach is not indicated.

Since pharmacological adjuncts have been tried without success after peripheral angioplasty with/without stent implantation, there is urgent need for new approaches to deal with the problem of restenosis. Increasing knowledge about the pathophysiology of the process leading to restenosis has given the rationale to investigate the potential role of radiation in the prevention of restenosis. Compared with the rapidly increasing experience in the coronary circulation, there is until now only a very limited number of studies with clinical data concerning the use of brachytherapy in the peripheral circulation. Most of the studies in the peripheral system have been done in the femoropopliteal region.

Evidence supporting the use of endovascular brachytherapy

Frankfurt Trial

The first clinical trial using endovascular brachytherapy after femoropopliteal angioplasty was initiated in the early 1990s by the Frankfurt group. Böttcher *et al.*[7] were the first to present data showing that endovascular irradiation is both feasible and safe in humans. Between 1990 and 1997, 30 patients were treated with PTA followed by endovascular brachytherapy for in-stent restenosis in the superficial femoral artery. The length of the stented vascular segments ranged from 4.5 cm to 14 cm with a mean of 6.7 cm. This group used a dose of 12 Gy because of the long experience and positive results with this dose in the prevention of keloids and hypertrophic scars. The optimistic primary results have been confirmed recently by long-term results, with a range of follow-up of 7-84 months (median 33 months). In the 28 patients available for follow-up, the 5-year patency rate (determined clinically and by ultrasound) was 82%. Three patients developed restenosis within the treated segment, while two patients presented with acute thrombotic occlusion after 16 and 37 months, respectively.[8]

PARIS Trial

PARIS (Peripheral Artery Radiation Investigational Study) is a US multicentre, randomized, double-blind control study in 300 patients following PTA of femoropopliteal lesions. Eligible for inclusion are patients between 40 and 80 years of age with claudication (Rutherford category 2 or 3) or critical leg ischaemia. Target lesions should be stenosis between 5 and 15 cm in length or combined stenosis and occlusions of 5-15 cm with the length of the totally occluded segment not exceeding 5 cm. Furthermore, at least one patent crural vessel providing straight run-off to the foot is mandatory. The gamma-radiation 192-Ir source is delivered via a centred segmented end-lumen balloon catheter. The treatment dose of 14 Gy is prescribed to the adventitia of the artery, which is defined as the radius of the centring balloon catheter plus 2 mm to compensate for the arterial wall thickness. The target length is the total length of the dilated segment plus a 1.0 cm margin on each end.

The results of the PARIS feasibility clinical trial have been reported recently.[9] Forty patients with claudication and superficial femoral artery lesions with a mean lesion length of 9.8 cm were enrolled. The angiographic binary restenosis rate at 6 months was 17% and the clinical restenosis rate at 12 months was 13%. There were no angiographic or clinical adverse events related to the radiation therapy. The authors concluded that intra-arterial radiation after PTA of superficial femoral artery lesions with use of high-dose rate gamma radiation represents a potent anti-restenotic therapy for peripheral arteries.

The randomized phase of PARIS was initiated in 15 centres in 1998 and enrolment of the patients was completed in the meantime.

The Vienna experience

In May 1996, our group in Vienna began to investigate the feasibility and efficacy of endovascular brachytherapy after femoropopliteal angioplasty.

In all trials, an Iridium-192 source with a diameter of 1.1 mm was delivered by using a high-dose-rate remote afterloader (micro-Selectron; Nucletron).

Vienna 01 Trial[10]

In this pilot study, ten patients with long-segment (mean length: 16 cm; range: 9-22 cm) restenosis after former PTA underwent angioplasty followed by endovascular irradiation. A dose of 12 Gy was targeted to the inner intimal layer of the vessel. Endovascular BT was technically feasible in all patients without complications. In six patients, the dilated and irradiated segment remained widely patent on colour duplex sonography, with corresponding excellent haemodynamic and clinical results after 12 months. In four patients, arteriography demonstrated 60-90% diameter restenosis.

Considering the negative selection of patients with a high risk of restenosis, the results of this pilot study were promising concerning the possibility of reduction of restenosis by means of endovascular brachytherapy after long-segment femoro-popliteal PTA without stent implantation.

Vienna 02 Trial[11]

From November 1996 to August 1998, 113 patients (63 male, 50 female; mean age 71 years) with de-novo ($\geq$ 5 cm) or recurrent (any length) femoropopliteal lesions were included in this randomized trial comparing the angiographically verified restenosis rate after PTA plus brachytherapy (n=57) vs PTA (n=56) without stent implantation. The mean treated length of the artery was 16.7 cm (PTA + brachytherapy) vs 14.8 cm (PTA), respectively. In patients randomized to PTA + brachytherapy, a reference dose of 12 Gy was prescribed in 3 mm distance from the source axis.

The primary endpoint of the study was patency of the recanalized segment after 6 months. Restenosis was defined as an angiographically verified stenosis of greater than 50% narrowing of the luminal diameter within the recanalized segment compared with the diameters of normal segments of the vessel on the follow-up angiograms. Clinical success of the procedure was defined by immediate improvement by at least one clinical category according to the criteria defined by Rutherford. Patients with tissue damage had to move up at least 2 categories and reach the level of claudication to be considered improved. Clinical patency was defined by sustained improvement without further intervention.

In 107 patients information concerning patency could be obtained after 6 months (Fig. 2). The overall angiographically verified recurrence rate was 15/53 (28.3%) in the PTA + brachytherapy-group vs 29/54 (53.7%) in the PTA-group (chi-square test; p < 0.05). The cumulative patency rates at 12 months of follow-up were 63.6% in the PTA + brachytherapy-group and 35.3% in the PTA-group (log rank test, p < 0.005). The significant improvement in patency was also maintained after 2 years (see Fig. 3).

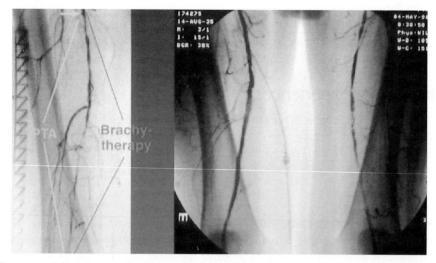

Figure 2. *Left:* angiogram of a 63-year old male with long-distance recurrent femoropopliteal lesion after former angioplasty. The lesion was treated by further angioplasty followed by brachytherapy. *Right:* control angiogram 6 months later demonstrating excellent follow-up result without restenosis on the right leg (restenosis developed in the contralateral artery after PTA without brachytherapy).

The cumulative clinical patency rates at 12 months of follow-up were 51.9% in the PTA-group and 73.6% in the PTA + brachytherapy-group, respectively (log rank test, $p < 0.05$).

The angiographic appearance of restenosis after brachytherapy was quite different compared with the well known kind of restenosis after long-segment angioplasty without brachytherapy. While in these patients the typical pattern of long-segment recurrence with a high degree of stenosis covering mostly the total length of the former dilated segment was observed, the morphologic pattern in case of restenosis after brachytherapy was characterized by only circumscript stenosis with segments of normal lumen width between. These findings suggest a detectable radiation effect also in patients classified as recurrence.

Despite the significant reduction of recurrence in this randomized trial, we could not prevent restenosis in about one-third of the patients. The nominal dose employed in this trial was lower than the dose given in most intracoronary trials using γ-sources. This may not be adequate for complete inhibition of neointimal hyperplasia. Another important factor that can account for the observed restenoses in this study may be the dose inhomogeneity due to an eccentric catheter position. With long treatment lengths, a non-centred catheter can often be eccentrically located at various points along the vessel length. An eccentric plaque can further accentuate this non-centring, resulting in significant dose inhomogeneity to the target volume. In our experience, decentring of the source with the technique applied was not uncommon although some centring may be achieved by the 5-F radiation delivery catheter and the 6-F sheath. Otherwise, source centring for γ-emitters such as Ir-192 is not as critical as it is for β-emitters. New catheters with centring capabilities have been designed and are being used in ongoing clinical trials. The reduction in 'hot spots' along the intimal surface by a source centring system may also improve the overall therapeutic ratio, by reducing restenosis rates without a corresponding increase in toxicity.

In summary, this was the first randomized study to demonstrate the efficacy of endovascular brachytherapy for prophylaxis of restenosis after femoropopliteal PTA.

Vascular brachytherapy is preferable to drug-eluting stents • For the motion • E Minar et al.

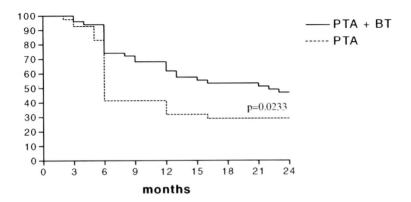

Figure 3. Vienna-2 trial. Plot of cumulative patency rate after 24 months (Kaplan-Meier) after femoropopliteal PTA according to assigned treatment (BT = brachytherapy).

Vienna 03 Trial

In November 1998, enrolment began in an Austrian multicentre trial employing a new catheter with source-centring capabilities similar to the one used in the PARIS trial. This study was also designed as a randomized double-blinded study comparing the restenosis rate after PTA + brachytherapy vs the rate after PTA alone.

However, in contrast to the PARIS protocol, patients with longer lesions (total occlusions > 5 cm) were eligible and the prescribed dose was 18 Gy delivered to the adventitia of the artery. The primary endpoint is angiographically demonstrable restenosis after 12 months. The results will be available at the end of 2002.

Vienna 04 Trial[12]

To evaluate the interaction of endovascular brachytherapy and peripheral arterial stenting, a pilot study was completed in patients with long-segment femoropopliteal angioplasty + stent implantation. Thirty-three patients with femoropopliteal lesions (mean treated length, 17 cm; range, 4-30 cm) underwent PTA and stent implantation followed by brachytherapy with a centring catheter. A dose of 14 Gy was delivered to the adventitia. Long-term pharmacotherapy with acetylsalicylic acid was combined with clopidogrel for 1 month.

The overall 6-month recurrence rate was 30% (10 of 33 arteries). Seven patients developed sudden late thrombotic occlusion of the segment with the stent 3.5-6 months after stent implantation. Considering the overall results after successful local thrombolysis in six of these seven patients, only four (12%) of 33 arteries with a stent had in-stent restenosis caused by neointimal hyperplasia.

The study results are promising concerning the possibility of reducing in-stent restenosis by means of brachytherapy after long-segment femoropopliteal placement of stents. However, the high incidence of late thrombotic occlusion requires optimization of the antithrombotic regimen. Such late thrombotic events have also been reported in patients receiving intracoronary brachytherapy in conjunction with stenting, and are believed to be due to delayed re-endothelialization of the newly implanted stents in the irradiated vessels. Therefore, we have changed our antithrombotic regimen and all patients now continue on clopidogrel for at least 12 months.

Based on the results from the Vienna 04 study, we have initiated a double-blind randomized trial comparing the angiographically verified recurrence rate after femoropopliteal stenting and brachytherapy vs stenting alone (an angiographic example is given in Fig. 4). The results will be available at the end of 2002.

Are there any data supporting the use of drug-eluting stents in the peripheral vessels?

No clinical trials have been published studying the effect of drug-eluting stents on the restenosis rate after peripheral angioplasty.

The results of randomized trials in patients with femoropopliteal lesions revealed no improvement of long-term patency after primary stent placement.[3-5] This is in contrast to the coronary trials, where patients who received a coronary stent compared with balloon angioplasty alone had a reduction in angiographic restenosis and in clinical revascularization events (e.g. STRESS; BENESTENT I; REST). This means

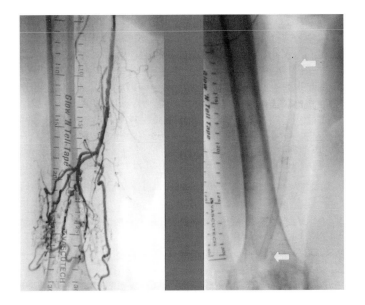

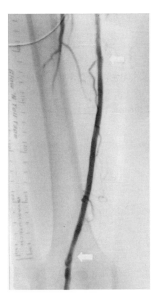

Figure 4. *Top left:* angiogram of a 75-year-old female with long-distance femoropopliteal stenosis/occlusion before PTA. *Top right:* the stented segment is marked by the arrows. *Bottom centre:* control angiogram obtained 14 months after stent implantation followed by brachytherapy with excellent follow-up result (the stented segment is between the arrows).

that the data from coronary trials cannot be extrapolated to the peripheral circulation. Therefore also the data from coronary trials with drug-coated stents – e.g. antithrombotic coating with heparin as in BENESTENT II or antiproliferative coating with sirolimus (as in the recently reported RAVEL trial) and paclitaxel (ASPECT) do not allow to draw conclusions for the peripheral vessels.

The results of these recently reported trials seem striking, and they rise the hope that the combination of a stent with optimal mechanical scaffolding properties and the dynamic bioactive effect of a site-specific antiproliferative drug might have the potential to virtually eliminate restenosis after coronary interventions. Many cardiologists are already convinced that such drug-coated stents will certainly represent the most important advance in the history of interventional vascular therapy. However, caution is recommended for the cardiologist with such prognosis in light of the relatively short follow-up period. Even more scepticism is recommended for the vascular specialist dealing with peripheral interventions. This is due to the former differences in results of coronary and peripheral trials and to the complete lack of trials with drug-eluting stents in the non-coronary vessels.

Therefore the correct answer to the question cited in the heading of this paragraph is: No !

Summary

- The feasibility and safety of endovascular brachytherapy after femoropopliteal angioplasty has been demonstrated in pilot studies.

- The efficacy of endovascular brachytherapy for prophylaxis of restenosis after femoropopliteal PTA has been demonstrated in a randomized study.

- Further improvements of the results of this approach can be expected by modification of the brachytherapy procedure – e.g. use of a centring device; optimization of dose – and by combination with stent implantation with optimized antithrombotic regimen.

- In contrast to coronary trials, stent placement did not improve long-term patency in the femoropopliteal region compared with balloon angioplasty alone.

- No clinical trials have been published studying the effect of pharmacocoated stents on the restenosis rate after peripheral angioplasty.

- The data from coronary trials cannot be extrapolated to the peripheral vessels.

References

1. Murray RR Jr, Hewes RC, White RI Jr *et al.* Long-segment femoropopliteal stenoses: is angioplasty a boon or a bust? *Radiology* 1987; 162: 473–476.
2. Treiman GS, Ichikawa L, Treiman RL *et al.* Treatment of recurrent femoral and popliteal artery stenosis after percutaneous transluminal angioplasty. *J Vasc Surg* 1994; 20: 577-587.
3. Vroegindeweij D, Vos LD, Tielbeek AV, Buth J, Bosch HC. Balloon angioplasty combined with primary stenting versus balloon angioplasty alone in femoropopliteal obstructions: A comparative randomized study. *Cardiovasc Intervent Radiol* 1997; 20: 420-425.
4. Cejna M, Thurnher S, Illiasch H *et al.* PTA versus Palmaz stent placement in femoropopliteal artery obstructions: a multicenter prospective randomized study. *J Vasc Interv Radiol* 2001; 12: 23-31.
5. Grimm J, Müller-Hülsbeck S, Jahnke T *et al.* Randomized study to compare PTA alone versus PTA with Palmaz stent placement for femoropopliteal lesions. *J Vasc Interv Radiol* 2001; 12: 935-941.
6. Dormandy JA, Rutherford RB. Management of peripheral arterial disease (PAD): TASC Working Group – TransAtlantic Inter-Society Consensus (TASC). *J Vasc Surg* 2000; 31: S1-S296.
7. Böttcher HD, Schopohl B, Liermann D, Kollath J, Adamietz IA. Endovascular irradiation – a new method to avoid recurrent stenosis after stent implantation in peripheral arteries: technique and preliminary results. *Int J Radiat Oncol Biol Phys* 1994; 29: 183-186.

8. Liermann DD, Bauernsachs R, Schopohl B. Intravascular irradiation therapy. In *Vascular Brachytherapy* 2nd edn. R Waksman (ed). Armonk, NY: Futura Publishing, 1999: 395-405.

9. Waksman R, Laird JR, Jurkovitz CT *et al.* for the PARIS Investigators. Intravascular radiation therapy after balloon angioplasty of narrowed femoropopliteal arteries to prevent restenosis: results of the PARIS feasibility clinical trial. *J Vasc Interv Radiol* 2001; 12: 915-921.

10. Minar E, Pokrajac B, Ahmadi R *et al.* Brachytherapy for prophylaxis of restenosis after long-segment femoropopliteal angioplasty: pilot study. *Radiology* 1998; 208: 173-179.

11. Minar E, Pokrajac B, Maca T *et al.* Endovascular brachytherapy for prophylaxis of restenosis after femoropopliteal angioplasty: results of a prospective, randomized study. *Circulation* 2000; 102: 2694-2699.

12. Wolfram RM, Pokrajac B, Ahmadi R *et al.* Endovascular brachytherapy for prophylaxis against restenosis after long-segment femoropopliteal placement of stents: initial results. *Radiology* 2001; 220: 724-729.

Vascular brachytherapy is preferable to drug-eluting stents to reduce peripheral artery restenosis

Against the motion
Takao Ohki, Frank J Veith

Introduction

Restenosis remains the chief limitation of percutaneous transluminal angioplasty (PTA) for the treatment of most peripheral vascular lesions as well as those in the coronary artery system. This is especially true when PTA is applied to the femoropopliteal region.[1-3] The application of metallic stents to the coronary artery system has improved the results of percutaneous transluminal coronary angioplasty (PTCA) in a dramatic fashion. This has been substantiated in well designed, prospective randomized trials.[4,5] For example, in the Stent Restenosis Study and the Benestent Study, the restenosis rate at 6 months following PTCA decreased from 42% to 32% and 32% to 22%, respectively, with the use of stents.[4,5] These landmark studies have revolutionized the treatment of coronary artery disease and the utilization of stents. Currently, over 500 000 coronary stenting procedures are performed annually in the USA. However, the same benefit of stenting was not found when applied to the femoropopliteal region as shown by two randomized trials comparing the efficacy of PTA vs PTA+stenting in lower extremities.[6,7] The application of stenting in the femoropopliteal artery appeared to hamper the already dismal patency rate as suggested by the primary patency at 1 year of 62% for the PTA+stent arm and 74% for the PTA–alone arm.[7]

Moreover, although stenting improved the outcome following PTCA, restenosis was not completely prevented, and 20-35% of stented patients still developed restenosis, usually within 6-9 months after their procedure.[4,5,8] Stents provide a metal scaffolding that reduces the risk of restenosis by providing a greater initial gain in vessel luminal diameter and eliminating vascular contraction (negative vascular remodelling). Stents, however, do not inhibit intimal hyperplasia but, rather, induce greater intimal hyperplasia than PTA alone. Thus, prevention of intimal hyperplasia has been a major theme in the field of vascular intervention.

Intimal hyperplasia is primarily a function of intimal thickening due to excessive cellular growth and production of extracellular matrix. To understand how to minimize restenosis it is necessary to examine the process of intimal hyperplasia. Intimal hyperplasia occurs as a response to injury.[9] It is caused by vascular smooth muscle cells that migrate from the media into the intima where they proliferate and secrete extracellular matrix. This phenomenon is regulated by a number of factors released by various cells. These 'bad actor' cells include inflammatory cells (which secrete TNF, IL1b), smooth muscle cells, and adventitial fibroblasts (which secrete TGFb, basic FGF, etc), and platelets (which produce thrombin, PDGF). The endothelial cell is a 'good actor' cell that secretes a number of anti-thrombotic factors as well as anti-proliferative factors.

A number of drugs have been evaluated in an attempt to prevent restenosis or intimal hyperplasia. Angiotensin-converting enzyme inhibitors, cytotoxic agents, anti-thrombotic agents and anticoagulants have all been unsuccessful in preventing intimal hyperplasia. These drugs were administered systemically and probably an inadequate dose of the drug reached the target site. The current focus is to administer agents to the lesion in a more targeted manner and to inhibit only the 'bad actor' cells while trying to preserve the 'good actors'.

In the early 1990s, vascular brachytherapy and more recently pharmacologically coated stents have emerged as promising technologies to prevent intimal hyperplasia and these therapies are the topic of this debate.

We believe that drug-eluting stents are superior to brachytherapy for a number of reasons. In fact, we believe that drug-eluting stents will make brachytherapy obsolete. This article will summarize the pros and cons of both approaches and will provide a basis for our position. Since there is no clinical experience with the use of drug-eluting stents in the peripheral vasculature at this time, comparison will mainly be made from data derived from PTCA. In addition, the data available from PTCA are very quantitative and the reporting of these data is more standardized than those available in the peripheral literature. By analysing the existing data from PTCA, it will be easy to extrapolate how these two technologies will perform when applied to peripheral vascular lesions.

Basic mechanism of drug-eluting stents

The basic idea of drug-eluting stents is to bind drugs to a stent so that it will not only act as a metal scaffolding that will maintain a larger lumen but also function as a means to deliver drugs to the site of the injury where intimal hyperplasia takes place. Preserving the beneficial mechanical properties of a stent while synergistically delivering an active therapeutic agent to the target site is the goal of drug-eluting stents.[10,11] The critical components of drug-eluting stents include the stent, the drug and the carrier matrix.

Stent

Ongoing clinical trials dealing with drug-eluting stents currently utilize pre-existing balloon-expandable coronary stents.[12,13] However, to maximize the capacity of drug a stent can carry and to accomplish more complex drug-release kinetics, several dedicated stents have been designed. Such stents have multiple small wells in the struts of the stents to accommodate various drugs that can be programmed to be released at various doses at various timing depending on the carrier used (see below).[12–14] An equally important advancement includes the use of self-expanding stents that can be used as drug-eluting stents. Self-expanding stent technology will be an important step toward the application of drug-eluting stents for some peripheral applications such as the femoropopliteal artery and the carotid artery. Cordis (Warren, NJ) is conducting a randomized trial comparing PTA alone vs rapamycin-eluting SMART stent (SIROCCO trial) to treat femoropopliteal lesions.

Drug

The drug or drugs of choice are ones that work on many parts of the processes that lead to intimal hyperplasia. For example, a drug that inhibits restenosis might be one that acts on inflammation, migration, proliferation and/or secretion of extracellular matrix. It is not clear whether or not inhibiting only one of these factors will reduce intimal hyperplasia. However different compounds are being investigated to target these different factors with the goal of attenuating the overall response.[15]

Additional physical properties are important in determining the efficacy of a drug for stent-based local delivery. These drug properties include the ability to undergo sterilization without degrading functionality of drug, stability for reasonable shelf-life, lipophilic qualities to facilitate tissue uptake of the drug, and effectiveness in very small doses so that the stent will maintain a low profile.

The Boston Scientific Corporation's (Natick, MA) TAXUS programme utilizes paclitaxel, which is the active ingredient of Taxol®.[12] Paclitaxel is a widely used compound which has been well-studied for its anti-inflammatory and anti-proliferative effects. It possesses a unique mechanism of action to polymerize microtubules rendering them non-functional. Microtubules are involved with cellular migration, proliferation, signal transduction and secretion, all of which contribute to the formation of intimal hyperplasia. Proper dosimetry of paclitaxel can selectively inhibit pathological smooth muscle cells ('bad actors') while minimizing collateral damage to endothelial cells ('good actors').[15,16] Cook, Inc. (Indianapolis, IL) is also investigating paclitaxel for their drug-eluting stents programme (ELUTE trial).

Another promising drug is rapamycin (Sirolimus), which is a macrolide antibiotic that possesses immunosuppressant activity. It is a potent inhibitor of DNA synthesis and inhibits cell proliferation. It inhibits cell-dependent kinases (CDK) via CDK inhibitor p27 and inhibits phophorylation of the retinoblastoma protein. Selective inhibition of smooth muscle cells may be difficult with rapamycin.[15] Rapamycin is currently utilized in Cordis's (Warren, NJ) RAVEL programme.[13]

Actinomycin D is being investigated by Guidant (Minneapolis, IL). By creating carrier wells on the stent struts, larger compounds such as proteins and oligonucleotides as well as nitric oxide can be used.

Carrier

There are three basic mechanisms by which drugs are attached to and released by the stent:

1. Inert coatings (protein polymers, diamond-like coatings, phosphorylchloine coatings). The idea is to 'hide' the implant from the body; however, no data suggest any long-term benefit.
2. Active surfaces. Covalently attached drugs such as heparin to help prevent a negative effect on the stent, such as thrombus deposition. No data are available to suggest any benefit of intimal hyperplasia inhibition.

3. Controlled release of drug from stents to impact the various pathways leading to restenosis These can be released from a polymer in a controlled manner depending on the target and can last as long as necessary as polymers can be tailored to influence release.[10,11] For example, with the Boston Scientific Corporation TAXUS stent paclitaxel elutes over a 30-40 day period. Designing a carrier that effectively adheres to the struts of the stent without altering the mechanical properties of the stent is an important feature. Future drug-eluting stents will be able to deliver multiple drugs at varying release rates and doses.[10,11]

Evidence

Drug–eluting stents will make brachytherapy obsolete

Clinical evidence: data will speak for itself

Preliminary results of a prospective randomized trial evaluating the feasibility, safety and efficacy of two different types of drug-eluting stents compared with standard stenting have recently been presented. The TAXUS-1 trial randomized 61 patients with de novo coronary artery disease to paclitaxel-coated NIR stents and standard NIR stents[12] (Tables 1 and 2). The results of the RAVEL trial have also been presented. This trial compared rapamycin-coated BX Velocity stents with standard BX Velocity stents.[13] Results of these trials have yet to be published. Both trials showed an impressive zero restenosis at 6 months based on follow-up angiograms. The restenosis rates for the control arm were 11% for the NIR stents and 25% for the BX Velocity stents. More impressive was the near zero late loss in luminal diameter. Most of the brachytherapy studies have dealt with in-stent restenosis and only a few studies have evaluated it in de novo coronary lesions. Four studies have mainly dealt with de novo lesions and we have selected these studies to make a fair comparison with the two drug-eluting stents trials.[17-21] As shown in Table 2, the efficacy of drug-eluting stents dwarfs that of brachytherapy. Although brachytherapy decreased the rate of restenosis and target vessel revascularization, it is not as dramatic as that following drug-eluting stents (Fig. 1). Of note is the fact that brachytherapy increased death, and thrombosis of the target site by 64–160% compared with the control.[18,21]

Logistics and practicality

Administration of both gamma– and beta-emitting brachytherapy represents a difficult logistical problem. The guideline published by the American Board of Brachytherapy mandates the involvement of multiple specialties and personnel.[22] This includes a therapeutic radiologist, a qualified medical and health physicist and a radiation safety officer. When a gamma-emitting source is used, the angiosuite needs to be structurally shielded. In most cases, the patients have been transferred to the radiation oncology department after PTA and after the radiation delivery catheter has been placed. This step itself has been responsible for an additional 30-45 minutes of procedure time.[23,24] A beta-emitting source is more user-friendly in this regard, but because of the limited tissue penetration capability and because it can only be applied to a short lesions (5-10 mm per pass), its use in peripheral vascular lesions is not practical.[22] For these reasons, all the studies applying brachytherapy for femoropopliteal lesions have utilized gamma sources.[23-26] The need to use intravenous ultrasound for accurate dosimetry poses an additional burden on the operator.[25]

Table 1. Comparison between drug-eluting stent trials and brachytherapy trials for the treatment of coronary lesions

Trial	TAXUS-1[12]	RAVEL[13]	Verin V[17]	PREVENT[18]	Colonado JA[19]	BERT[20]	GAMMA-1[21]
Type of trial	Randomized against stent	Randomized against stent	Feasibility	Randomized against stent	Feasibility	Feasibility	Randomized against stent
Number treated (number control)	61 (31)	238 (118)	45	105 (25)	21	23	252 (121)
De novo (%) lesion	100%	100%	100%	70% (30% ISR)	100%	100%	0%
Drug/source	Paclitaxel	Rapamycin	Beta(Yttrium90)	Beta (P 32)	Gamma (Ir192)	Beta (Sr90/Y)	Gamma (Ir192)
Stenting (%)	100%	100%	28%	61%	9%	0%	100%
F/U mos	6	6	6	6 (12 for MACE)	6	6	6 (9 for MACE)

ISR: in-stent restenosis, MACE: major adverse cardiac events.

Table 2. Comparison in outcome between drug-eluting stent trials and brachytherapy trials

Trial/Author	TAXUS-1[12]	RAVEL[13]	Verin V[17]	PREVENT[18]	Colonado JA[19]	BERT[20]	GAMMA-1[21]
Restenosis at 6 months (treatment)	0%	0%	15%	8%	27%	15%	32%
Restenosis rate at 6 months (control)	7%	26%	NA	31%	NA	NA	55%
RRR for restenosis	100%	100%	NA	79%	NA	NA	42%
Late loss (mm)	0.02	−0.01	0.18	0.2	0.2	0.05	0.73
TVR % (treatment)	0%	0.8%	11%	21%	9%	9%	31%
TVR % (control)	0%	23%	NA	32%	NA	NA	46%
RRR for TVR %	100%	96%	NA	34%	NA	NA	33%
SAT %	0%	0%	10%	10%	9%	5%	5.3%
MACE %	0%	3.3%	18%	26%	?	9%	35%
RRR for MACE	100%	88%	NA	19%	NA	NA	27%
MI or death	0%	2.6%	7%	11%	0%	0%	13%
MI or death in control arm	0%	4.2%	NA	4%	NA	NA	5%
RRR for MI or death	100%	38%	NA	−64%	NA	NA	−160%

NA: not applicable, RRR: relative reduction rate compared with control arm, TVR: target vessel revascularization within 6 months, subacute thrombosis: subacute thrombosis of treated vessel during 1–6 months, major adverse cardiac events: major adverse cardiac events, MI: myocardial infarction.

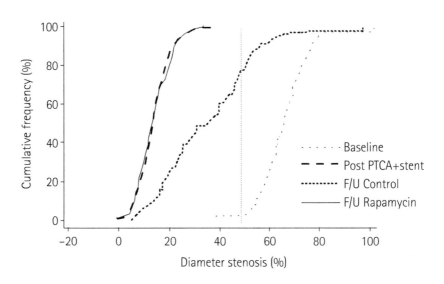

Figure 1. Cumulative % stenosis analysis. Diameter stenosis at baseline (control stent and rapamycin-coated stent), immediate post-stenting, and at 6 months follow-up (F/U). Note the complete overlap between immediate post-stenting and F/U rapamycin coated stent curve. Modified from Ref 13.

Occurrence of subacute thrombosis: *'atomic bomb' vs 'sniper rifle'*

Brachytherapy is analogous to an 'atomic bomb' not only because it exerts radiation but also because it destroys everything within reach. This includes not only the smooth muscle cells but also the 'good actors' such as the endothelial cells.[27] Because of this collateral damage, healing following PTA and stenting is significantly delayed and has possibly contributed to the subacute thrombosis that has been observed.[28] Subacute thrombosis is a serious problem especially when stenting is used in conjunction with brachytherapy. Several randomized trials evaluating the efficacy of brachytherapy have shown clinical benefit. However, one must be careful in interpreting these results. Most of these studies have utilized major adverse cardiac events as their primary endpoint. These consist of death, myocardial infarction, and target vessel revascularization. Leon *et al.*, reported benefit of brachytherapy in the treatment of in-stent restenosis based on the decreased rate of major adverse cardiac events compared with control (28% vs 44%, brachytherapy vs control)[21] (Table 2). However, most of the benefit came from the decreased need for target vessel revascularization (31% vs 46%). Ironically, more patients receiving brachytherapy suffered subacute thrombosis (5.3% vs 0.8%) and death (3.1% vs 0.8%) but this was masked by the decreased target vessel revascularization. Thus, prevention of restenosis was accomplished at the cost of increased subacute thrombosis and death.[16] This paradox was also observed in the PREVENT trial.[18] Avoiding stenting and longer administration of antiplatelet agents has been recommended. In addition, aneurysm formation following brachytherapy has been reported as early as 5-6 months following intervention.[19,29] This is another phenomenon due to collateral damage caused by the 'atomic bomb' effect.

In both drug-eluting stents trials, neither subacute thrombosis nor aneurysm formation has been observed despite the fact that antiplatelet therapy was discontinued at 1 month.[12,13] Drug-eluting stents function like a 'sniper rifle' and attack primarily the 'bad actors' minimizing collateral damage.

Edge effect and geographic miss

Both edge effect and geographic miss are other unique phenomena following brachytherapy. Edge effect is accelerated intimal hyperplasia (more than control) occurring within the dose fall-off zone (proximal and distal edges of the radiated segment) triggered by a sub-therapeutic dose (<7Gy), or dose transition.[30] This is due to the fact that radiation stimulates intimal hyperplasia at doses lower than 7 Gy. Since the dose of radiation wears off with distance, there will always be a region at both ends which will be subjected to inadequate doses of radiation. Edge effect was not seen in drug-eluting stent trials.

Geographic miss is any injury that occurs within a sub-therapeutic zone (within the dose-fall off zone or beyond) usually due to inadequate coverage.[30] It can be caused by misplacement or inaccurate placement of the source catheter. While careful technique may minimize geographic miss, since the source delivery catheter is known to move longitudinally with each beat of the heart, it will be difficult to eliminate geographic miss and this may be considered an inherent limitation along with edge effect.[31] For femoropopliteal lesions, a gamma-emitting source will be utilized and thus the need for a patient to be transferred to the radiation oncology suite further increases the chance of geographic miss. Since the drug-eluting stent can be deployed at the target site under fluoroscopic guidance and since the drugs are attached directly to the stent, geographic miss will not occur unless the stent is misplaced.

Chemistry between stents

The fact that lesions that require stenting are a relative contraindication to brachytherapy must be viewed as a disadvantage.[18,21,26,28] This is due to the increased risk of subacute thrombosis with the simultaneous use of stent and brachytherapy. This has been termed 'unhappy marriage'. As mentioned earlier, stenting has been proved to be effective by providing greater initial gain, fixing dissections and virtually eliminating abrupt closure following PTA and resisting against negative remodelling. To give up such a proven technology for the sake of using brachytherapy is not comprehensible.

Drug-eluting stent is a very 'happy marriage' between a stent that needs prevention of intimal hyperplasia and a drug that needs a large and smooth lumen to work on as well a platform in which it can be delivered.

One shot deal vs persistent strikes

Naturally, it is not possible to apply brachytherapy repeatedly to the target site and this, therefore, makes it a one-shot deal. The opportunity for brachytherapy effectively to inhibit intimal hyperplasia is only at the time of the procedure. This narrow window leads to 'overkill' as well an inability to recover from geographic miss. In addition, intimal hyperplasia is a complex event where numerous cells play various roles over a substantial time period. Brachytherapy has no control of events taking place after the intervention and this may be responsible for some late failures that have been reported.[32] On the other hand, drug-eluting stents can be programmed so that various drugs will be released at various times over a substantial period coordinating drug release with cell specific intimal hyperplasia process.[10,11] In fact, the sustained effect of rapamycin-eluting stent up to 12 months has recently been reported.[33] Although current drug-eluting stent technology may result in some late failures, there are an infinite number of possible combinations available for the future.

A word about brachytherapy trials in the femoropopliteal lesions

Following the seminal work by the Frankfurt group,[23,34] several randomized trials have been conducted comparing the efficacy of brachytherapy with control (PTA or stenting) in the treatment of femoropopliteal lesions[24-26, 35] (Table 3). Although both randomized trials showed improved patency rates compared with control, there is not enough data to conclude that brachytherapy is a worthwhile modality. The control arm consisted of PTA (with or without stenting) which is not the gold standard therapy. Despite the fact that these trials predominantly treated patients with claudication (80-85%) with good run-off, the restenosis rate and patency rate at 6 months for the control PTA arm were dismal and were in the range of 30–54%. (Table 3) This is clearly inferior to the results with femoropopliteal bypass which is the gold standard and provides patency rates ranging from 80 to 90% at 6 months.[36]

Recently, the preliminary result of the SIROCCO trial was presented by Duda.[37] This randomized trial compared the efficacy of Sirolimus-coated SMART stent (Cordis) and standard SMART stent for the treatment of femoropopliteal lesions. As shown in Table 3, this trial showed that the promising results shown in the coronary lesions could be reproduced in the peripheral vasculature utilizing self-expanding Nitinol stents. The restenosis rate for the control arm (standard SMART stent) was 23% at 6 months whereas it was 0% for the Sirolimus-coated group.[37]

It is essential that both PTA alone and PTA with brachytherapy or with drug-eluting stent be compared with femoropopliteal bypass before further clinical application to these lesions are utilized.

Table 3. Results of brachytherapy, drug-eluting stent and surgical bypass for femoropopliteal artery

Trial/Author	VIENNA-2[25]	Wolfran RM[26]	PARIS[35]	SIROCCO[37]	Green RM[36]
Type of trial	Randomized	Feasibility	Feasibility	Randomized	Randomized
Treatment modality	Gamma + PTA vs PTA	Gamma + PTA	Gamma + PTA	Sirolimus coated stent vs standard stent	Prosthetic bypass
Number treated (no. controls)	113 (57)	33 (NA)	40 (NA)	36 (18)	240 (NA)
Claudicants	77%	85%	100%	53%	59%
Primary patency at 6 months (12 months)	72% (63%)	79% (?)	83% (NA)	100%	88% (75%)
Primary patency at 6 months for control (12 months)	45% (35%)	NA	NA	94%	NA

NA: not applicable

Conclusion: the future of brachytherapy

Based on the evidence provided above, we believe that brachytherapy will have a limited role in preventing restenosis after peripheral interventions. Some theoretical advantages include its application to small vessels (passing a stent may be a challenge), in-stent restenosis, and relatively long lesions (multiple drug-eluting stents may not be cost-effective). These questions will be answered when results of ongoing clinical trials become available. The Boston Scientific's Taxus-3 study will compare brachytherapy with the TAXUS stent in patients with in-stent restenosis, while Taxus-4 will evaluate the efficacy in small vessels, long lesions and in patients with diabetes. The ultimate role for drug-eluting stents in the treatment of peripheral vascular disease will be determined by results of randomized comparison with surgical bypass procedures and not with brachytherapy.

Summary

Drug-eluting stent is preferable to brachytherapy to reduce peripheral artery restenosis because:

- Zero restenosis, near zero late gain, sustained effect (up to 12 months).

- No subacute thrombosis, no aneurysm formation.

- Selective inhibition ('sniper rifle') vs 'atomic bomb' approach.

- User-friendliness.

References

1. Johnston KW. Femoral and popliteal arteries: reanalysis of results of balloon angioplasty. *Radiology* 1992; **183**: 767-771.
2. Murray RR Jr, Hewes RC, White RI Jr *et al.* Long-segment femoropopliteal stenoses: is angioplasty a boon or a bust? *Radiology* 1987; **162**: 473-476.
3. Capek P, McLean GK, Berkowitz HD. Femoropopliteal angioplasty. Factors influencing long-term success. *Circulation* 1991; **83**(Suppl): 170-180.
4. Fischman DL, Leon MB, Baim DS *et al.* A randomized comparison of coronary-stent placement and balloon angioplasty in the treatment of coronary artery disease. Stent Restenosis Study Investigators. N Engl J Med 1994; **331**: 496-501.
5. Serruys PW, de Jaegere P, Kiemeneij F *et al.* A comparison of balloon-expandable-stent implantation with balloon angioplasty in patients with coronary artery disease. Benestent Study Group. *N Engl J Med* 1994; **331**: 489-495.
6. Cejna M, Thurnher S, Illiasch H *et al.* PTA versus Palmaz stent placement in femoropopliteal artery obstructions: a multicenter prospective randomized study. *J Vasc Interv Radiol* 2001; **12**: 23-31.
7. Vroegindeweij D, Vos LD, Tielbeek AV, Buth J, Bosch HC. Balloon angioplasty combined with primary stenting versus balloon angioplasty alone in femoropopliteal obstructions: A comparative randomized study. *Cardiovasc Intervent Radiol* 1997; **20**: 420-425.
8. Casterella PJ, Teirstein PS. Prevention of coronary restenosis. *Cardiol Rev* 1999; **7**: 219-231.
9. Ross R. The pathogenesis of atherosclerosis—an update. *N Engl J Med* 1986; **314**: 488-500.

10. De Scheerder IK. Phosphorylcholine coated stents as a drug delivery platform. Presented at the 12ᵗʰ Transcatheter Cardiovascular Theraputics, Washington DC, 11–16 September 2001.
11. Litvack F. The Conor Medsystems Stent: A programmable drug delivery device. Presented at the 12ᵗʰ Transcatheter Cardiovascular Theraputics, Washington DC, 11–16 September 2001.
12. Grube E. Preliminary report of the BSC TAXUS-1 trial. Boston Scientific Corp. Annual analyst meeting, 17 September 2001.
13. Morice MC, Serruys PW, Sousa JE et al. A Randomized double-blind study with the Sirolimus-eluting Bx Velocity Balloon expandable stent in the treatment of patients with de novo native coronary artery lesions. (RAVEL) Presented at the 12ᵗʰ Transcatheter Cardiovascular Theraputics, Washington DC 11–16 September 2001.
14. Rogers C. Paclitaxel and Taxane derivatives structure, mechanisms, and delivery considerations. Presented at the 12ᵗʰ Transcatheter Cardiovascular Theraputics, Washington DC, 11–16 September 2001.
15. Bouchey D. Industry Update: Drug eluting stents and prevention of restenosis in coronary arteries. In WWW.unterberg.com 12 March 2001.
16. Axel DI, Kunert W, Goggelmann C, Oberhoff M et al. Paclitaxel inhibits arterial smooth muscle cell proliferation and migration in vitro and in vivo using local drug delivery. Circulation 1997; 96: 636–645.
17. Verin V, Popowski Y, de Bruyne B et al. The Dose-Finding Study Group. Endoluminal beta-radiation therapy for the prevention of coronary restenosis after balloon angioplasty. The Dose-Finding Study Group. N Engl J Med 2001; 344: 243–249.
18. Raizner AE, Oesterle SN, Waksman R et al. Inhibition of restenosis with beta-emitting radiotherapy: Report of the Proliferation Reduction with Vascular Energy Trial (PREVENT). Circulation 2000; 102: 951–958.
19. Condado JA, Waksman R, Calderas C, Saucedo J, Lansky A. Two-year follow-up after intracoronary gamma radiation therapy. Cardiovasc Radiat Med 1999; 1: 30–35.
20. King SB 3rd, Williams DO, Chougule P et al. Endovascular beta-radiation to reduce restenosis after coronary balloon angioplasty: results of the beta energy restenosis trial (BERT). Circulation 1998; 97: 2025–2030.
21. Leon MB, Teirstein PS, Moses JW et al. Localized intracoronary gamma-radiation therapy to inhibit the recurrence of restenosis after stenting N Engl J Med 2001; 344: 250–256.
22. Nag S, Cole PE, Crocker I et al. The American Brachytherapy Society perspective on intravascular brachytherapy. Cardiovasc Radiat Med 1999;1(1):8-19.
23. Liermann D, Kirchner J, Bauernsachs R, Schopohl B, Bottcher HD. Brachytherapy with iridium-192 HDR to prevent from restenosis in peripheral arteries. An update. Herz 1998; 23: 394–400.
24. Minar E, Pokrajac B, Maca T et al. Endovascular brachytherapy for prophylaxis of restenosis after femoropopliteal angioplasty: results of a prospective randomized study Circulation 2000; 102: 2694-2699.
25. Pokrajac B, Potter R, Maca T et al. Intraarterial (192)Ir high-dose-rate brachytherapy for prophylaxis of restenosis after femoropopliteal percutaneous transluminal angioplasty: the prospective randomized Vienna-2-trial radiotherapy parameters and risk factors analysis. Int J Radiat Oncol Biol Phys 2000; 48: 923–931.
26. Wolfram RM, Pokrajac B, Ahmadi R, Endovascular brachytherapy for prophylaxis against restenosis after long-segment femoropopliteal placement of stents: initial results. Radiology 2001; 220: 724–729.
27. Ohki T, Baitler J, Marin ML, Yuan JG, Veith FJ. Endoluminal irradiation fails to reduce pre-established anastomotic intimal hyperplasia. Annual Meeting of the American Radium Society, New York, 1-3 May 1997.
28. Costa MA, Sabat M, van der Giessen WJ et al. Late coronary occlusion after intracoronary brachytherapy. Circulation 1999; 100: 789–792.
29. Vandergoten P, Brosens M, Benit E. Coronary aneurysm five months after intracoronary beta-irradiation. Acta Cardiol 2000; 55: 313–315.
30. Sabate M, Costa MA, Kozuma K et al. Geographic miss: a cause of treatment failure in radio-oncology applied to intracoronary radiation therapy. Circulation 2000; 101: 2467–2471.
31. Giap HB, Bendre DD, Huppe GB, Teirstein PS, Tripuraneni P. Source displacement during the cardiac cycle in coronary endovascular brachytherapy. Int J Radiat Oncol Biol Phys 2001;49(1):273–7.
32. Teirstein PS, Massullo V, Jani S et al. Three-year clinical and angiographic follow-up after intracoronary radiation : results of a randomized clinical trial. Circulation 2000; 101: 360–365.
33. Sousa JE, Costa MA, Abizaid AC et al. Sustained suppression of neointimal proliferation by sirolimus-eluting stents: one-year angiographic and intravascular ultrasound follow-up. Circulation 2001; 104: 2007–2011.

34. Liermann D, Bottcher HD, Kollath J *et al.* Prophylactic endovascular radiotherapy to prevent intimal hyperplasia after stent implantation in femoropopliteal arteries. *Cardiovasc Intervent Radiol* 1994; **17**: 12–16.

35. Waksman R, Laird JR, Jurkovitz CT *et al.* Intravascular radiation therapy after balloon angioplasty of narrowed femoropopliteal arteries to prevent restenosis: results of the PARIS feasibility clinical trial. Peripheral Artery Radiation Investigational Study (PARIS) Investigators. *J Vasc Interv Radiol* 2001; **8**: 915–921.

36. Green RM, Abbott WM, Matsumoto T *et al.* Prosthetic above-knee femoropopliteal bypass grafting: five-year results of a randomized trial. *J Vasc Surg* 2000; **31**: 417–425.

37. Duda S. A clinical investigation of the Sirolimus coated Cordis SMART™ nitinol self-expandable stent for the treatment of obstructive superficial femoral artery disease. Presented at the International Symposium on Endovascular Therapy, 20–24 Jan 2002, Miami, FL, USA.

Vascular brachytherapy is preferable to drug–eluting stents to reduce peripheral artery restenosis

Charing Cross Editorial Comments towards Consensus

This is a truly new topic and bursting with possibilities. Much of the experience and effort to reduce restenosis has been achieved within the coronary circulation but the peripheral vascular specialist has great interest in restenosis also. There is evidence of restenosis occurring after angioplasty, after surgery, and even after stent with persuasive demonstrations of intimal hyperplasia appearing to grow through the interstices of stents. The question of how to reduce this process has been a matter of great interest for decades.

These two methods are now the great hopes. Persuasive arguments are made for brachytherapy with careful referencing and then drug elution of stents suddenly becomes the rage also. It is fair to say that there is very little experience in the peripheral circulation and little or none in terms of large series of major centres let alone comparisons between the methods. Therefore in the history of this struggle we are at the point where the rationale for methodology is being justified and we are appropriately enthused to see the possibility of advance at last. Eventually comparisons will be made and random controlled trials but it is early days. However, some extravagant claims were made in the Veith New York meeting of 2001 which implied that drug elution of stents could completely wipe out restenosis. Indeed stretching further, if one paints the appropriate fluid on the inside of any artery this could have miraculous effects, etc, etc. We hope that this proves to be correct. Only time will tell. Nevertheless it is an exciting moment for this subject.

Roger M Greenhalgh
Editor

Mild to moderate intermittent claudication is benefited by angioplasty

For the motion
Dierk Vorwerk

Introduction

There is a long-standing concensus that a vascular surgical approach to peripheral vascular disease requires major clinical symptoms such as severe claudication or rest pain. Using the European classification of Fontaine, an advanced II b or III stage is therefore accepted as mandatory for invasive management. Endovascular treatment, however, has been proved to cause a low morbidity and even a lower mortality being followed by a satisfactory outcome. Thus, it is fair to reconsider why an endovascular approach should be reserved only for those with major clinical symptoms.

Furthermore, occlusive arterial disease tends to occur earlier in life due to changed smoking and dietary habits among the population, hitting those still in the active phase of their professional life.

On the other hand, intermittent claudication is not likely to worsen over time and only about 5% of claudicants are at risk of developing critical limb ischaemia if no important co-morbidity factors such as diabetes are present.

Problems of definition

To classify intermittent claudication is not an easy task if standardized methods are not used. Patients are poor at defining their true walking distance, blaming mainly their general physical abilities (e.g. co-existing pectorial angina) and lifestyle. For an exact definition of walking distance a standardized treadmill test is needed.

In the Fontaine classification, stage IIa defines a walking distance of more than 200m and stage IIb a walking distance of less than 200m. The Rutherford system divides between category 1 (mild claudication), 2 (moderate) and 3 (severe). Comparing both systems stage IIa is equivalent to category 1 while stage IIb combines categories 2 and 3.

Both systems try to work as an objective framework of guidelines for treatment and are very useful tools for scientific reporting although they largely fail to meet the individual needs of a patient.

Life-style limiting claudication

Intermittent claudication may inflict a patient's life in a various degrees and different levels of suffering. It is obvious that a patient with co-existing major angina pectoris or severe emphysema may not have major deficits even from severe intermittent claudication since his co-existing diseases will limit his walking distance anyway. An 85-year old patient with severly limited physical abilities certainly suffers less than a young and active patient of 45 years. However, in an amputated patient, even mild claudication in the remaining leg may cause major restrictions of his lifestyle since the patient is full dependent on his claudicant limb. People living in a flat area may not have major problems compared with those living in a mountain area or on the seventh floor with no access to a lift. A younger individual previously used to an active sports life will hardly accept mild claudication since it is preventing him from returning to activities that mean a lot to him.

Therefore, in each patient, the individual lifestyle circumstances should be taken into account before indication for an invasive treatment is turned down. For an individual decision, lifestyle limiting claudication is a very useful term and should be considered along with classical classifications.

Evidence

Endovascular vs surgical treatment

Endovascular therapy is known to be of low invasiveness with good technical success and a fair overall patency. In iliac PTA (taken from five publications reporting on 1264 procedures), an average complication rate of 3.6% with a 95% success rate shows a 61% patency after 5 years.[1] In iliac stenting for stenoses (taken from nine publications reporting on 1365 patients), the results are a little better with a 99% technical success and 72% 5-year patency. Weighted average complication rate was 6.3%.[1] In femoropopliteal endovascular interventions (taken from eight publications reporting on 1469 procedures), weighted average technical success was 90%, complication rate was 4.3% and 3-year patency rate was 51%. Stents do not improve patency showing a 3-year patency of 58% after 3 years.

Surgery offers a limb-based 5-year patency of 91% for aortobifemoral bypasses; weighted average mortality was 3.3%. For distal reconstruction, an average 5-patency of 80% for vein bypasses and 65-75% for ePTFE (expanded polytetrafluoroethylene bypasses has been reported. Combined mortality and amputation risk was calculated to be about 2.2 % for aortobifemoral reconstructions and 1.4% for femoropopliteal reconstructions.[1]

It has to be taken into account that life expectancy of patients with intermittent claudication is limited compared with a non-claudicant control group. Mortality rates after 5, 10 and 15 years are approximately 30%, 50% and 70% although most patients will not die from peripheral vascular but from cardiac, cerebral or non-vascular causes.[1]

Despite better clinical outcome for surgery, Trans Atlantic Society Concensus (TASC) recommendation 37, therefore, recommends surgery only as a treatment for intermittent claudication in cases where other forms of medical therapy have recommended but have either failed or been rejected for good reasons.[1] Furthermore there should be a high benefit-to-risk ratio given.[1]

This is difficult to achieve in patients with mild to moderate claudications. Thus, endovascular therapy appears to be the method of choice – if applicable – in this subgroup of patients with intermittent claudications.

Location of lesion

Mild to moderate claudication is mainly related to lesions in the aortoiliac or the femoropopliteal region. It is unlikely to be due to infrapopliteal lesions and there is general agreement that treatment below the knee is strictly limited to patients with critical limb ischaemia i.e. stage III and IV (Fontaine) or category 4 to 6 (Rutherford).

In the aortoiliac segment, a major part of lesions are amenable to percutaneous treatment with an acceptable outcome. In the femoropopliteal segment, overall success and long-term efficiency of percutaneous treatment is less beneficial and the type of a lesion becomes more important for success.

Thus, the location of a lesion and its type has to be taken into consideration before treatment is recommended. While in the aortoiliac segment, most lesions will be prone to an endovascular approach, this is not generally true for femoropopliteal lesions. In addition, the risk of treatment is related to its location and has to be addressed before recommending an endovascular approach.

Type of lesion

Morphology of a lesion treated will have an influence on the technical outcome, follow-up results and also risk of treatment. The TASC document therefore introduced a classification system that tries to categorize lesions with regard to their accessabil-ity to either percutaneous treatment or surgery with type A lesions ideal for percutaneous approach, type B lesions where percutaneous approach is still the pre-ferred technique, type C lesions where surgical approach should be preferred and type D lesions where surgery is the option of choice. The TASC classification overrules older classifications since it takes into account all available and published techniques including stent technology which offers a much wider variation of treatment and also an effective tool to deal with current acute complications of balloon angioplasty such as occluding dissection or vascular rupture.

If we consider percutaneous therapy as the preferred method to deal with those patients presenting with mild or moderate claudications, treatment might be offered to those presenting with type A and B lesions but should be discussed in depth with patients with type C lesions since the risk and the potential benefit of treatment will be related to the underlying morphology.

For iliac lesions, single stenoses up to 3 cm in length both in the common (CIA) and external iliac artery (EIA) are classified as type A lesions while single stenoses of 3 to 10 cm (not involving the common femoral artery), double stenoses not longer than 5 cm each and unilateral occlusions of the common iliac artery are classified as type B lesions.

As type C, bilateral long stenoses (5-10 cm in lengths), unilateral EIA occlusions not extending into the common femoral artery (CFA) and unilateral EIA stenoses extending into the CFA are classified. More advanced lesions are classified as type D.

Using this classification, many iliac lesions will meet the A and B group opening a potentially growing field for endovascular procedures if applied on mild to moderate claudicants. Even in some type C lesions, our own experience let us feel that percu-taneous treatment has no more major technical concern, complication risk or compromised outcome. This is in particular the case for EIA occlusions not extending into the CFA. However, published data are lacking to back this experience.

In the femoropopliteal field, type A lesions are single stenoses up to 3 cm in length not involving the very proximal superficial femoral and the distal popliteal artery. Type B lesions are stenoses 3–5 cm in length, heavily calcified stenoses, multiple

Figure 1.   Unilateral occlusion in a young patient with active sports life and moderate claudications.

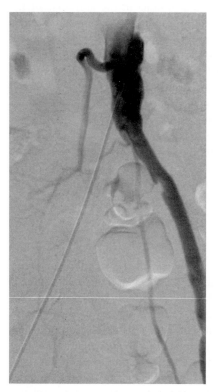

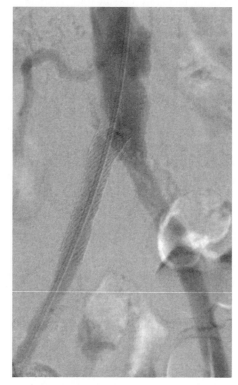

Figure 1a.   Total occlusion of the common iliac artery at the level of the bifurcation (TASC B lesion).

Figure 1b.   After primary stenting, full patency is restored and the patient is asymptomatic enabling him to continue with his usual activities.

lesions (each up to 3 cm) and lesions with no sufficient tibial run-off (the latter are unlikely to meet the criteria of mild ore moderate claudication). Type C lesions are classified as stenoses or occlusions longer than 5 cm and multiple mid-size lesions (3–5 cm). Total common femoral, superficial femoral and popliteal occlusions are classified as type D lesions. There was some dissenting discussion on the definition of type B lesions since interventional radiologists represented by CIRSE wished to express their assumption that even longer lesions up to 10 cm may be justified to be classified as type B instead of type C claiming that the results reported are mainly due to underdeveloped techniques and instruments which have majorly improved in the meantime and no evidence exists comparing efficacy of PTA versus bypass surgery for lesions between 4 and 10 cm.

Other than in the iliac area, fewer lesions will meet the criteria of type A and B lesions especially if limited to 5 cm in length. Thus, fewer patients with mild and moderate claudications due to femoropopliteal lesions will become ideal candidates for percutaneous treatment. Moreover – without limiting the importance of the TASC document which certainly means a step forward in the joint approach to peripheral vascular disease – the morphological classification does not take into account some technical considerations that depend on the age and composition of a lesion. Particularly in femoral occlusions, the degree of organization of the occluding thrombus or the composition of the lesion with the original stenosis at the proximal and distal end, or in the middle, are factors which are not well predictable but may influence the technical outcome of the intervention or also its complication rate i.e. distal embolization which might cause a aggravation of symptoms. Other than in the iliac arteries, liberal use of stents and stent grafts may help to overcome a failed balloon angioplasty and to solve the technical outcome but do not achieve an improved long-term efficacy or may start up a life-time dependency on recurrent interventional or surgical procedures. These associated potential drawbacks have to be carefully balanced against the potential benefits and need to be discussed in depth with the patient before treatment is performed especially in association with mild or moderate claudication.

These considerations mainly restrict use of endovascular treatment in femoropopliteal lesions to stage IIa patients presenting with type A and less pronounced type B lesions.

Approach to multi-level disease

Even mild symptoms may be associated with multi-level disease i.e. with iliac stenosis and a well-collateralized femoropopliteal lesion. There is some chance that exclusive intervention in the iliac region may be sufficient to improve the clinical situation. If present, multi-level disease does not preclude treatment in those patients.

Ancillary activities

It is widely accepted that well-conducted physical exercise should precede any type of interventional treatment and cessation of smoking is mandatory. Nevertheless, it is also true that in many institutions it is most difficult to find an infrastructure that allows the teaching of state-of-the-art physical exercise in claudicants and as far as smoking is concerned, there is a major difference between willing and doing.

Moreover, even with state-of-the-art exercise a young patient will not recover completely from claudication in all activities including sport. The process will be longer and compromise his or her professional life. It might, therefore, be discussed whether especially young and active patients should be vigourously put under the axioma of 'physical exercise first' or whether in this group of patients, invasive treatment might be offered even as a first approach.

Conclusion

The decision for invasive treatment should be based on the individual circumstances of each patient. Age, social life, physical ability and professional requests have to be taken into consideration and simple administration of rigid classification systems should be avoided. Under these circumstances, patients with mild to moderate claudications might also become candidates for invasive treatment. Due to its lower morbidity and mortality, endovascular therapy should be considered as the method of choice unless morphological or other reasons oppose an endoluminal therapy.

The TASC consensus document backs this individualized therapeutic approach to patients with mild to moderate claudications by recommendation 21:

'Before offering a patient with intermittent claudication the option of any invasive treatment, endovascular or surgical, the following considerations must be taken into account:

1. A predicted or observed lack of adequate response to exercise therapy and risk factor modification.
2. The patient must have a severe disability, either being unable to perform normal work or having serious impairment of other activities important to the patient.
3. Absence of other diseases that would limit exercise even if the claudication was improved.
4. The individual's anticipated natural history and prognosis.
5. The morphology of the lesion must be such that the appropriate intervention would have low risk and high probability of initial and long-term success'.

Nothing more needs to be added.

Summary

- Current classifications give general guidelines for treatment but do not meet the individual situation in a patient.

- Life-style limiting claudication is a term that reflects more to the individual situation.

- Interventional radiological techniques offer a low morbidity and invasiveness thus justifying interventions even in patients with mild to moderate claudications under special circumstances.

- Type and location of a lesion determines the potential risk of a procedure that has to critically taken into account in mild to moderate claudicants.

Reference

1. The TASC Working Group. Management of peripheral arterial disease (PAD). Transatlantic inter-society consensus (TASC). *J Vasc Surg* 2000; 31: S1-S296.

Mild to moderate intermittent claudication is benefited by angioplasty

Against the motion
Paul Burns, Andrew Bradbury

Introduction

An assessment of the clinical and cost-effectiveness of infrainguinal percutaneous balloon angioplasty (PBA) for intermittent claudication depends upon weighing the risks and benefits of the procedure against the natural history of the condition. Intermediate clandication affects 5% of the middle-aged (55–75 years) population and is associated with a community-based limb loss rate of less than 1% per year.[1,2] Although the prognosis for the limb is extremely benign, the claudicant suffers a cardiovascular event rate of 5–10% per annum, some two to three times greater than an age and sex matched non-claudicant population.[3] There is overwhelming evidence that the institution of best medical therapy comprising predominantly of smoking cessation, (supervised?) exercise, cholesterol-lowering and anti-platelet therapy significantly reduces cardiovascular morbidity and mortality and increases exercise tolerance.[4] The fundamental question is whether PBA represents a useful adjuvant therapy. Across the world, millions of infrainguinal PBAs have been performed for intermittent claudication. Despite the complete lack of any evidence for its durable efficacy, the numbers of procedures appear to be increasing. This is an extremely unfortunate situation for the following reasons.

1. Infrainguinal PBA for intermittent claudication is not a risk-free procedure.
2. It is widely accepted that surgical bypass for intermittent claudication actually leads to an increased risk of limb loss in the long-term. There are no data to reassure us that this is not also the case with endovascular intervention.
3. Infrainguinal PBA for intermittent claudication almost certainly represents a gross misuse of health service funds that would be better spent elsewhere.
4. Focusing on the 'lesion' inevitably leads to suboptimal treatment of the patient as a whole.

The evidence

The quality of the literature regarding the efficacy of PBA for lower limb ischaemia is extraordinarily poor. Small, uncontrolled, biased studies with short and incomplete follow-up using clinically irrelevant end-points abound. Astonishingly, only two randomized controlled trials have been published; one from Oxford and one from Edinburgh.

In the Edinburgh trial, approximately 600 consecutive claudicants presenting to a vascular surgery clinic were assessed by means of duplex to determine whether they had a pattern of supra- or infrainguinal disease amenable to PBA.[5] Of these, only 94 patients were found to be suitable. Of these, only 62 were confirmed as suitable for PBA on the basis of angiography and were randomized to either best medical therapy alone (aspirin, smoking and exercise advice) or best medical therapy and PBA. Although there was some benefit for PBA at 6 months, at 2 years there was no difference between the two groups in walking distance, quality of life or the haemodynamic status of the limb (Fig. 1). So, despite the fact that only the most anatomically favourable lesions were submitted to PBA, and that the best medical therapy offered was suboptimal by today's standards, there was absolutely no clinically useful adjuvant benefit for PBA. The Oxford trial was similar, with 56 patients randomized to PBA or medical treatment.[6] Of these, 37 were available for follow-up at 6 years, at which time there was no difference in walking distance between the two groups.

Critics of these trials will argue that they are simply too small to be regarded as the last word on the subject. For this reason, we are about to embark upon a much larger study, the Exercise versus Angioplasty in Claudication Trial (EXACT). This UK-based, Health Technology Assessment funded, trial will randomize patients with intermediate claudication due to infrainguinal disease to best medical therapy only, best medical therapy plus supervised exercise, or best medical therapy plus PBA. The primary end-point will, of course, be walking distance but a wide range of clinically important secondary end-points, as well as a quality of life and a full economic analysis will be recorded. Others trials, both in the UK and elsewhere, are planned. Until such time as EXACT reports its findings, one has to conclude that infrainguinal PBA for intermediate claudication it should not be funded from the public purse or performed without the confines of a trial.

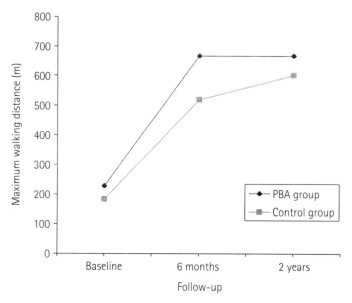

Figure 1. Maximum walking distance of patients with intermediate claudication randomized to PBA or control in Edinburgh study.

Why is PBA so popular?

One clearly has to look beyond science to explain the apparent popularity of infrainguinal PBA for intermittent claudication.

1. PBA involves the use of expensive, disposable equipment, and is therefore subject to intense marketing pressures.
2. Referring the clinic patient for PBA is easier and quicker than trying to institute best medical therapy. PBA can be the vascular surgery equivalent of the lazy GP's prescription pad.
3. In a proportion of patients PBA leads to an immediate, but almost always very short-lived, improvement in walking distance. Patients like this 'quick fix', not least because it is usually interpreted by them as meaning that they can ignore all this nonsense about quitting smoking and improving their diet etc.
4. Interventionalists like the quick fix too; especially if the patient is still improved by the time it comes to pay the bill!
5. Patients are happiest if they feel the treatment they are being offered is 'high-tech', 'keyhole' intervention that unlike 'low-tech' best medical therapy requires no personal commitment on their part.

Why doesn't PBA work?

If we accept, as we must, that infrainguinal PBA for intermediate claudication is ineffective, we must next ask – why? The reasons fall into three main areas; patient selection; misunderstanding of the pathophysiology of intermittent claudication, and failure of the technique itself (Fig. 2).

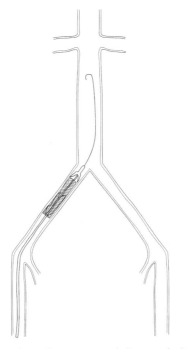

Figure 2. Diagram of the technique of percutaneous balloon angioplasty. Reproduced with permission from Ref. 7.

Patient selection

Intermittent claudication affects 5% of the population but only a small (unknown) proportion of those affected seek medical advice; only a proportion (again unknown) of those are referred to secondary care; and only a (highly variable) proportion of those are referred for PBA. It seems reasonable to assume, although there is no evidence to support this and it may not be true, that those with the worst symptoms are more likely to be referred and to be offered PBA. It also seems reasonable to assume that those individuals will have more extensive arterial disease; as well as other co-morbidity. So the great majority of patients (90% in the Edinburgh experience) presenting to vascular surgeons do not have a pattern of disease that invites PBA. While a short stenosis in an otherwise pristine superficial femoral artery (SFA) with normal inflow and run-off may remain patent for many years following PBA, the fact is that this sort of patient is unlikely to present to a vascular surgeon or radiologist (at least in the UK). Identifying the 10% or so of claudicants with a disease pattern that suggests durable angioplasty is simply too cost-ineffective. As shown in the Edinburgh study, duplex may be found wanting as a screening test for endovascular suitability. The non-invasive alternative, magnetic resonance angiography, raises even greater issues of affordability and availability. Would it be reasonable to go out in to primary care and actively seek these sorts of claudicants with limited disease? Even if that were logistically and financially possible, which it never will be, it is likely that these patients will also do very well with best medical therapy alone. And, unlike PBA, best medical therapy will deal with the real problem, the excess cardio-vascular morbidity and mortality.

The pathophysiology of claudication

The fact is that genuine short-distance claudication is due to either widespread arterial disease that responds badly to PBA, or to limited arterial disease that is part of a constellation of other morbidity that restricts mobility. PBA in a patient with significant cardiorespiratory and/or neuro-muscular-skeletal disease is unlikely to improve walking distance even if haemodynamically successful. There is ample evidence to show that there is a poor relationship between anatomic patency, the overall haemo-dynamic status of the leg(s) as determined by ankle:brachial pressure index (ABPI), and walking distance.[5] And, of course, most patients have bilateral disease – interventional 'double jeopardy'! A treatment such as PBA whose sole purpose is to relieve arterial blockage is always going to be found wanting as a treatment for a multi-factorial condition like intermittent claudication that requires a 'holistic' approach.

The technique

Although infrainguinal PBA for intermittent claudication is undoubtedly safer than surgical bypass, it is not risk free. For example in the senior author's previous institution (Edinburgh), 238 primary infrainguinal PBAs were performed for intermittent claudication between 1989 and 1997 and this was associated with a 6% major morbidity rate. This included acute limb ischaemia, haematoma and false aneurysm requiring urgent surgical intervention. Furthermore, there was a 7% technical and

11% immediate clinical failure rate. In other words almost one in five patients submitted to femoral angioplasty for intermediate claudication had an unsuccessful procedure and a quarter of those suffered a clinically significant complication. These data do not appear to be atypical and are unlikely to improve in the future. Although there was no associated mortality, this complication rate must be viewed in the context of the natural history of the condition.

Conclusions

After almost 40 years, PBA for intermittent claudication disease remains a contentious issue. Clinical experience suggests that it may have a place somewhere in our armamentarium for highly selected patients. However, critically appraisal of literature shows the evidence base to be severely deficient. On-going and proposed randomized control trials will provide, for the first time, level I evidence of clinical and cost-effectiveness (or the lack of it). The authors would encourage all European vascular surgeons and radiologists to enter their patients in to such trials so that we can, at last, move forward.

Summary

- Percutaneous balloon angioplasty (PBA) is used commonly in the treatment of intermittent claudication.

- There is a surprising lack of adequate studies investigating the use of PBA in intermittent claudication.

- The evidence that is available shows no long-term benefit of PBA over best medical therapy.

- This is unsurprising given that the nature of intermittent claudication makes it unsuitable for PBA.

- Randomized controlled trials currently taking place will help define the role, if any, of PBA in intermittent claudication.

References

1. Leng GC, Lee AJ, Fowkes FGR *et al.* Incidence, natural history and cardiovascular events in symptomatic and asymptomatic peripheral arterial disease in the general population. *Int J Epidemiol* 1996; **25**: 1172–1181.
2. Fowkes FGR, Housley E, Cawood EHH, MacIntyre CAA, Ruckley CV, Prescott RJ. Edinburgh Artery Study: prevalence of asymptomatic and symptomatic peripheral arterial disease in the general population. *Int J Epidemiol* 1991; **20**: 384–391.
3. Bainton D, Sweetnam P, Baker I, Elwood. Peripheral vascular disease: consequence for survival and association with risk factors in the Speedwell prospective heart disease study [see comments]. *Br Heart J* 1994; **72**: 128–132.
4. Davies A. The practical management of claudication. *B Med J* 2000; **321**: 911–912.

5. Whyman MR, Fowkes FG, Kerracher EM *et al.* Is intermittent claudication improved by percutaneous transluminal angioplasty? A randomised controlled trial. *J Vasc Surg* 1997; *26*: 551–557.

6. Perkins JM, Collin J, Creasy TS, Fletcher EW, Morris PJ. Exercise training versus angioplasty for stable claudication. Long and medium term results of a prospective randomised trial. *Eur J Vasc Endovasc Surg* 1996; **11**: 409–413.

7. Buckenham TM. The complications of iliac and subclavian artery stenting. In *Vascular and Endovascular Surgical Techniques* 4th edn. Greenhalgh RM (ed). London: WB Saunders, 2001: 409–413.

Mild to moderate intermittent claudication is benefited by angioplasty

Charing Cross Editorial Comments towards Consensus

The mild to moderate intermittent claudication (MIMIC) trial has been designed to settle this question

The referral of patients with this condition to a specialist is variable across Europe and within countries. Some patients think intermittent claudication occurs naturally when they get older and thus do not seek any medical advice at all. It is impossible to know how many people get an ache in the calf when they walk as they get older. It is likely to be much more common than we imagine. Whether the patient complains or not is a fascinating theme but not the one before us here.

The current thoughts about intermittent claudication are that the symptom is the mildest for peripheral arterial disease and is a pointer to atherosclerosis elsewhere in the body and cardiovascular events such as future heart attack or stroke are much more important than the outcome of the management of intermittent claudication. However, it is intermittent claudication which is the complaint before us.

There has been a vogue to measure peripheral arterial disease objectively and to ignore the patient's subjective cries. At last there are specific measures of health-related quality of life for the symptom in question. So-called symptom specific questionnaires actually address the problem from the patient's viewpoint.

Without question it emerges that best medical treatment should be offered to all in the interests of reduction of cardiovascular events as far as possible. Best medical treatment will include control of hypertension, diabetes, cigarette cessation, lipid lowering as well as platelet inhibitory therapy.

Exercise is an old chestnut and the evidence for the type of exercise emerges more recently. It would appear that supervised exercise of at least 30 minutes at least once per week is absolutely essential for patients with mild intermittent claudication and this seems to have a marked impact over and above exercise advice. The question of the MIMIC trial and of these chapters is whether angioplasty is of adjuvant benefit or not. There could easily be a different result for the aortoiliac segment as opposed to the femoral–popliteal segment. Practitioners are not agreed whether a stent should be used in the aortoiliac segment and with present knowledge the best would seem to be to allow practitioners the use of stent in the aortoiliac segment if they believe that it is necessary. There are some who use pull-through pressures to check the result of angioplasty at the time of the procedure (see pp. 277–288). Pull-through pressures are not well regarded for the femoral popliteal segment nor is the use of stenting except in the bail-out situation. The current predominating view would appear to be that the angioplasty is likely to show adjuvant benefit in the aortoiliac segment but may not in the femoral–popliteal segment. It is, therefore, entirely possible that a different result will emerge for aortoiliac as for the femoral–popliteal. In terms of angioplasty patients with mild to moderate intermittent claudication currently large numbers of angioplasties are being performed and evidence for the procedure is slim.

Then comes the question of luminal as opposed to subintimal angioplasty and that is raised pp. 327–343.

Roger M Greenhalgh
Editor

Superficial femoral subintimal angioplasty beats luminal PTA

For the motion
Amman Bolia

Introduction

The treatment of peripheral vascular disease has been transformed following the introduction of percutaneous transluminal angioplasty (PTA) after the early pioneering works of Dotter in 1964[1] and Gruntzig in 1974.[2] It is widely used for stenotic and occlusive disease of the iliac, femoral and tibial arteries in the treatment of intermittent claudication and critical limb ischaemia. However, the primary success rates and long-term outcomes of recanalization of long occlusions have been poor.[3,4] Conventionally, occlusions of the superficial femoral artery, popliteal artery of more than 10cm, or flush occlusions of the superficial femoral artery have been treated by a surgical bypass. Since the development of the technique of subintimal angioplasty, the majority of occlusions, whether they are full length of the superficial femoral artery or flush occlusions can be treated.[5-7] Tibial artery occlusions in patients with critical ischaemia have been successfully treated by subintimal angioplasty.[8-11]

Intentional subintimal angioplasty is practised for two main reasons:

1. To extend the scope of treatment of a large number of femoropopliteal occlusions.[5-7,12]
2. To extend long-term patencies.[13]

The procedure is simple, inexpensive, offers low complication rates, good primary success rates and long-term results. It has made a significant impact on the treatment of chronic critical limb ischaemia.[14, 15] The technique offers a number of advantages to conventional surgical bypass and is applicable in patients who are poor candidates for general anaesthesia or have inadequate vein for distal bypass.

Technique and illustration

The technique of subintimal angioplasty involves the creation of a dissection intentionally throughout the whole length of an occlusion, in order to achieve a clean disease-free lumen with a possibility of improved long-term patency.

Following an antegrade puncture, a Van Andel catheter (Cook, Letchworth, UK) is introduced and advanced up to the level of the occlusion. The occlusion is entered with the help of a hydrophilic curved guidewire (Terumo, Japan) which is directed towards the wall of the artery, away from any important collaterals. The tip of the

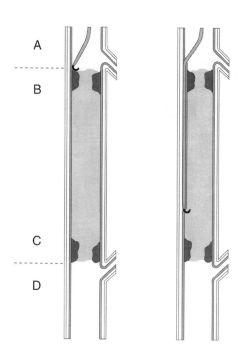

Figure 1. The dissection space is entered with a curved hydrophilic guidewire pointing away from the collateral. Reproduced with permission from Ref. 20.

wire, supported with the Van Andel catheter is advanced eccentrically into the occlusion. This normally results into a dissection, because the wire takes the path of least resistance, which is in the dissection plane. Once the wire is in a dissection (Fig. 1) the catheter is advanced and the position of the dissection may be confirmed with a small amount of dilute contrast medium. Most of the length of the occlusion is then traversed using a combination of the Van Andel catheter and a large loop made in the hydrophilic guidewire (Fig. 2). It is this large loop of the guidewire, which allows re-entry into the lumen to be achieved (Fig. 3). Sometimes the dissection has to be extended beyond the occlusion particularly when there is diffuse disease before re-entry may be achieved. Having crossed the lesion, the entire length of the dissection is dilated with a balloon catheter. The balloon normally used is 5mm in diameter, 4cm long and able to take high pressures. Short inflations of 5–10 seconds duration and approximately 12 atmospheres of pressure are used to balloon dilate the dissection channel.

When a successful outcome has been achieved, any contrast injection done beyond the level of the occlusion will show rapid clearance of the contrast. Any reluctance in the washout of the contrast should be carefully assessed and corrected. Further inflations, possibly using even higher pressures, may be necessary in order to remove any residual stenoses. The success of the procedure is judged on how rapidly the contrast clears from the angioplastied artery (haemodynamic success) rather than the anatomical appearances of the recanalized segment.

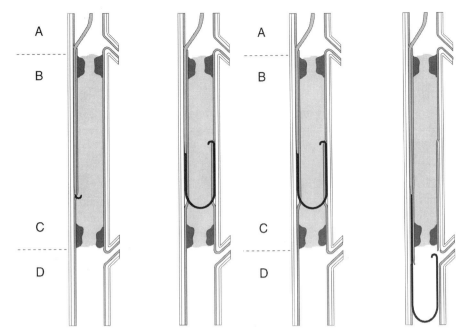

Figure 2. The length of occlusion is crossed, usually with the hydrophilic wire in a large loop, one limb of which is supported with a Van Andel catheter. Reproduced with permission from Ref. 20.

Figure 3. Re-entry into the true lumen is achieved with the help of the hydrophilic wire in a large loop. Reproduced with permission from Ref. 20.

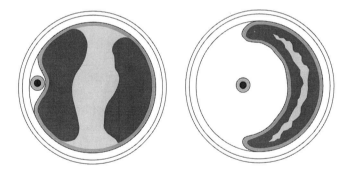

Figure 4. following subintimal angioplasty the occluding material is displaced eccentrically providing a disease free channel for blood flow. Reproduced with permission from Ref. 20.

Evidence

There are two main reasons why subintimal angioplasty is practised, in favour of conventional intraluminal angioplasty. First of all, there are <u>extended indications</u> in the treatment of femoropopliteal occlusive disease. Second, we believe that <u>improved long-term patencies</u> can be achieved compared with the conventional intraluminal approach.

Extended indications

There are very many indications where subintimal angioplasty is applicable where intraluminal angioplasty would not work

Long occlusions

When a long occlusion is present, it is very unlikely that the guidewire / catheter could be maintained intraluminally, hence dissection is likely to ensue, allowing subintimal approach to be pursued.

Occlusions in diffuse disease

When there is underlying diffuse disease and an occlusion is present, it is unlikely that the guidewire will be able to negotiate the true lumen throughout the length of the occlusion. Therefore, dissection is likely to ensue and subintimal angioplasty becomes appropriate.

Occlusion in a moderately calcified vessel

The presence of calcification implies long-standing disease. The occlusion is hard and therefore it is unlikely that intraluminal angioplasty would be successful. Dissection is likely to ensue. Subintimal angioplasty offers a better chance of success.

Perforation during an attempted PTA

When a perforation occurs during subintimal angioplasty, an alternative dissection is usually possible and a successful outcome can be achieved.

A large proximal collateral

When a large proximal collateral is present, the resultant anatomy may not allow the guidewire/catheter to engage into the origin of an occlusion. In such cases an intraluminal approach would fail. Subintimal angioplasty allows a dissection to be initiated above the level of the occlusion using the hard end of a standard Teflon guidewire. Once an intimal flap has been lifted, it is possible to continue the dissection, which usually follows the main vessel rather than the collateral and in this way, a collateral entry can be avoided.

Occlusions extending into bifurcations or trifurcations

Subintimal angioplasty allows an occlusion to be recanalized into two or three vessels, assuming they are patent distally. For example a popliteal occlusion that extends into the trifurcation may be recanalized into all the three run-off vessels, or a common femoral bifurcation may be recanalized into the superficial femoral artery and the profunda artery.

Long stenoses

Conventional intraluminal angioplasty of long stenoses produces poor results due to high incidence of recurrence of disease. Subintimal angioplasty may be applicable in these situations where the predominantly diseased segment can be dissected resulting into a smooth disease free channel with the possibility of improved long-term patency.

Flush superficial femoral artery occlusion

Subintimal angioplasty is applicable in occlusions that start from the origin of the superficial femoral artery where no stump is available for guidewire / catheter entry. This is made possible by the fact that the guidewire has a number of positions from which to enter the plane of weakness into a dissection. With the conventional intra-luminal approach, the wire has to be gently manipulated into the 'lumen' of the occlusion, which for a flush superficial femoral artery occlusion and an ipsilateral puncture, is difficult.

Tibial artery occlusions

Full length occlusion of the tibial artery can be recanalized using subintimal angio-plasty, which is particularly useful in the treatment of patients with critical limb ischaemia.

Iliac artery occlusions

During attempted retrograde recanalization of an iliac occlusion, dissection fre-quently ensues and re-entry back into the lumen proximally is often difficult, possibly because of the relatively thick and tough intima that is present as the wire approaches towards the aorta. In such situations subintimal angioplasty is possible by the crossover approach, effecting antegrade dissection from the proximal part of the occlusion.

Improved long-term patency

During conventional intraluminal recanalization, the atheroma and occluding mate-rial is cracked, disrupted and concentrically displaced by the balloon. This would encourage platelet adhesion and recurrence of disease encroaching into the lumen.

The rationale behind subintimal angioplasty is that the subintimal space, which is disease-free, forms the new lumen, having displaced the atheroma and occluding materials eccentrically to one side. Making use of this new disease-free lumen would delay the formation of atheroma for a long time.

Results

There has been extensive experience of the technique of subintimal angioplasty at the Leicester Royal Infirmary, from where most of the publications have originated. Since the development of the technique in 1987, many procedures have been carried out in the femoropopliteal segment but the technique has also been extended to other terri-tories, particularly in the tibial artery occlusions, the treatment of which has made a substantial impact on the management of chronic critical limb ischemia. In the past few years, a number of papers have appeared from other centres, broadly achieving similar results to those from the Leicester Royal Infirmary.[6, 16–18]

The first study involved 200 procedures in 176 patients over a 64-month period, carried out between 1987 and 1992.[13] For a mean length of occlusion of 11cm, there was a technical success rate of 80% (159/200) and there were no significant differ-ences between the technical success and failure group with respect to the incidence of diabetes, critical ischaemia, claudication, occlusion site and occlusion length. The technical success rate of occlusions less than 10cm was 81%, for occlusions 11-20 cm was 83% and for occlusions more than 20 cm was 68%, with no significant statistical difference in terms of ability to cross a short or long occlusion.

Two major complications (1%) were puncture-site related haematomas and there were 13 minor complications (6.5%).

A further analysis of the subsequent 275 procedures gave a primary success rate of 89%, with mean length of occlusion of 15 cm.

There were 13 failures (11%) which were due to failed re-entry distally in 15 (5%), heavy calcification in six (2%), perforation in four (1.5%), fresh occlusion in two (1%) and damage to important collaterals without reconstitutional flow in four (1.5%). In these four cases, emergency by-pass surgery was required. There were ten embolic complications of which eight were aspirated percutaneously and the other two were haemodynamically not significant. Surgical embolectomy was not required in any case.

A study by Berengoltz-Zlochin comparing subintimal angioplasty and intraluminal laser-assisted recanalization of occluded femoropopliteal arteries was conducted in 63 patients.[16] Their primary success rate in the subintimal angioplasty group of 17 patients was 85%. The angiographic cumulative primary patency rate at 1 year was 93% in the subintimal angioplasty group and their conclusion from the study was that the 1 year clinical and angiographic results of subintimal and intraluminal recanalizations were comparable and that subintimal route *per se* should not be regarded as a failure of the procedure. However, laser angioplasty is now obsolete and used to be much more expensive compared with the inexpensive technique of subintimal angioplasty.

Reekers reported their 2-year experience in 40 chronic long occlusions.[6] He reported an 85% primary success rate, and a secondary clinical patency of 71% at 1 year.

A more recent study by McCarthy included 69 procedures in 66 patients, of whom 38% were claudicants and 62% had critical limb ischaemias.[17] The mean occlusion length was 10cm and the primary technical success rate was 74%. At 6 months, the cumulative symptomatic and haemodynamic primary patency for the successful procedures were 80% and 77% respectively.

More recently, Vraux *et al.* reported their experience of subintimal angioplasty in tibial occlusions.[18] Whilst tibial occlusions is not a subject of this article, some very encouraging results have been shown, particularly in the treatment of chronic critical limb ischaemia.

The impact of subintimal angioplasty on critical limb ischaemia

Subintimal angioplasty has made a major impact on the treatment of chronic critical limb ischaemia at the Leicester Royal Infirmary. A prospective survey of all critical limb ischaemia patients who presented at the Leicester Royal Infirmary was carried out during a 12-month period in 1994.[14] There were 222 referrals in 188 patients. This survey showed that the majority of the patients were treated with angioplasty (42%), 6% of the patients had a combined treatment of angioplasty and surgery (minor amputations) and 24% of the patients has reconstructive surgery; 17% of the patients were treated conservatively and 10% had primary amputation. The mean (range) hospital stay for patients treated by surgery was 16 (3-97) days, for angioplasty 4.5 (1-73) days, and for amputation 18 (7-91) days. The in-hospital mortality rate was 10% with a limb salvage rate of 79%. The complication rate of angioplasty requiring surgery was 5.5%.

A further prospective 12-month study was carried out as a continuation of this previous study.[15] The aim of the study was to assess and compare the efficacy of angioplasty and surgery in the treatment of severe lower limb ischaemia. Of the 188 patients (222 critically ischaemic limbs) complete 12-month follow-up data could be obtained in 180 patients (187 limbs).

The overall 12-month patient survival was 75%. The 12-month survival rates for surgery and angioplasty were significantly higher (91% and 78% respectively). Compared with those of primary amputation and conservative management (57% and 52% respectively).

The overall 12-month limb salvage rate was 71%. The limb salavage for patients treated with either angioplasty or surgery was 76%.

The policy to attempt angioplasty whenever possible enabled 46% of the patients in the study to be revascularized by this modality compared with a national average of 22%.[19] Furthermore, the limb salvage rates for angioplasty compare favourably with surgery.[15]

The data from this study strongly supports the use of angioplasty as first-line treatment for severe lower limb ischaemia with no major evidence that angioplasty is detrimental to subsequent surgery if required. In the context of a 12-month survival of 75% and a 3-year survival of only 50-60%, a long-term solution is not what many of these elderly frail patients require. This study highlights that as a minimally invasive procedure, PTA and subintimal angioplasty serves the majority of patients very well, with a short hospital stay, and 12-month limb salvage rates that equate with those achieved by surgery.

Summary

- Subintimal angioplasty is effective in femoropopliteal occlusions.

- Intentional subintimal angioplasty extends the scope of treatment to include a large number of femoropopliteal occlusions.

- We believe subintimal angioplasty provides extended long-term patency, though large prospective studies are required to prove this.

- Subintimal angioplasty makes a substantial impact on the treatment of chronic critical limb ischaemia.

References

1. Dotter CT, Judkins MP. Transluminal treatment of arterio-sclerotic obstruction: Description of a new technique and preliminary report of its application. *Circulation* 1964; **30**: 654-670.

2. Gruntzig A, Hopff H. Percutane rekanlisation chronischer arterieller verschlusse mit einem neuen dilatationskatheter: modifikation der Dotter Technik. *Deutsch Med Wochenschr* 1974; **99**: 2502-2511.

3. Johnston KW, Rae M, Hogg Johnston SA *et al*. Five year results of a prospective study of percutaneous tranluminal angioplasty. *Ann Surg* 1987; **206**: 403-413.

4. Johnston KW. Femoral and popliteal arteries: reanalysis of results of balloon angioplasty. *Radiology* 1992; **183**: 767-771.

5. Bolia A, Miles KA, Brennan J, Bell PRF. Percutaneous transluminal angioplasty of occlusions of the femoral and popliteal arteries by subintimal dissection. *Cardiovasc Intervent Radiol* 1990; 13: 357-363.

6. Reekers JA, Kromhout JG, Jacobs MJHM. Percutaneous intentional extraluminal recanalization of the femoropopliteal artery. *Eur J Vasc Surg* 1994; 8: 723-738.

7. Reekers JA, Bolia A. Percutanous intentional extraluminal (subintimal) recanalization: how to do it yourself. *Eur J Radiology* 1998; 28:192-198.

8. Nydahl S, London NJM, Bolia A. Technical report: recanalization of all three infrapopliteal arteries by subintimal angioplasty. *Clin Radiol* 1996;51:366-367.

9. Nydahl S, Hartshorne T, Bell PRF, Bolia A, London NJM. Subintimal angioplasty of infrapopliteal occlusions in critically ischaemic limbs. *Eur J Vasc Endovasc Surg* 1997; 14: 212-216.

10. Bolia A, Sayers RD, Thompson MM, Bell PRF. Subintimal and intraluminal recanalization of occluded crural arteries by percutaneous balloon angioplasty. *Eur J Vasc Surg* 1994; 8: 214-219.

11. Bolia A. Percutaneous intentional extraluminal (subintimal) recanalization of crural arteries. *Eur J Radiol* 1998; 28: 199-204.

12. Bolia A, Bell PRF. Femoropopliteal and crural artery recanalization using subintimal angioplasty. *Semin Vasc Surg* 1995; 8: 253-264.

13. London NJM, Srinivasan R, Sayers RD, *et al.* Subintimal angioplasty of femoropopliteal artery occlusion: the long-term results. *Eur J Vasc Surg* 1994; 8: 148-155.

14. Varty K, Nydahl S, Butterworth P, *et al.* Changes in the management of critical limb ischaemia. *Br J Surg* 1996; 83: 953-956.

15. Varty K, Nydahl S, Nasim A, Bolia A, Bell PRF, London NJM. Results of surgery and angioplasty for the treatment of chronic severe lower limb ischaemia. *Eur J Vasc Endovasc Surg* 1998; 16: 159-163.

16. Berengoltz-Zlochin SN, Mali WP, Borst C, *et al.* Subintimal versus intraluminal laser assisted recanalization of occluded femoropopliteal arteries: one year clinical and angiographic follow-up. *J Vasc Intervent Radiol* 1994; 15: 689-696.

17. McCarthy RJ, Neary W, Roobottom C, Tottle A, Ashley S. Short-term results of femoropopliteal subintimal angioplasty. *Br J Surg* 2000; 87: 1361-1365.

18. Vraux H, Hammer F, Verhelst R, Goffette P, Vandeleene B. Subintimal angioplasty of tibial vessel occlusions in the treatment of critical limb ischaemia: mid-term results. *Eur J Vasc Endovasc Surg* 2000; 20: 441-446.

19. The Vascular Surgical Society of Great Britian and Ireland. Critical limb ischaemia: management and outcome. Report of a national survey. *Eur J Vasc Endovasc Surg* 1995; 10: 108-113.

20. Bolia A. Techniques in subintimal angioplasty. In *Vascular and Endovascular Surgical Techniques* 4th edn. Greenhalgh RM (ed). London: WB Saunders, 2001: 415-420.

Superficial femoral subintimal angioplasty beats luminal PTA

Against the motion
James T Lee, Mauricio Heilbron Jr,
Rodney A White

Foreword

The following analysis supports percutaneous transluminal angioplasty (PTA) over subintimal angioplasty (SAP). We caution the reader that preprocedural angiographic morphology of the lesion, quality of the distal vasculature, and the indication for intervention, are essential when comparing SAP with PTA.

Introduction to PTA

First described by Dotter and Judkins in 1964, PTA has been established as an effective therapeutic modality in the treatment of peripheral arterial occlusive disease.[1] The technique is practised worldwide and is well described in numerous journals and textbooks.[2-4]

Although fairly standardized, varying nuances exist between endovascular specialists regarding the application of this intervention. Preferences differ with respect to access (antegrade femoral, contralateral femoral, or retrograde popliteal), heparinization, choice of vasodilating agent, and post-procedural antiplatelet therapy.

Technically, traversing the lesion is the most critical component of the entire intervention. Typically a soft or floppy-tip guidewire is used to cross a concentric lesion. This is often exchanged for either a J-tipped or hydrophilic-coated wire for eccentric plaques. A low-compliance balloon with sufficient length and a diameter equivalent to the adjacent normal vessel (usually oversized by 10-20%), is selected. Duration of inflation approximates 30 to 120 seconds until the lesion is effaced.[4]

Non-invasive vascular laboratory measurements (i.e. pulse volume recordings, ankle-brachial pressure index (ABI), segmental Doppler pressures) are obtained at appropriate time intervals for surveillance. A decrease in pulse volume waveforms of 5mm or a mean ABI decrease of 0.15 (range, 0.1–0.2) did prompt angiographic evaluation in most investigative centres.[5-9] Interestingly, no significant difference in prognosis between primary and secondary interventions was demonstrated.[6,10]

Evidence for PTA

PTA is the most commonly applied percutaneous intervention in the superficial femoral arteries. The application of this intervention to femoropopliteal disease has become widely accepted due to its low complication rate and high technical success as recently published by the TransAtlantic Inter-Society Consensus (TASC).[11]

Since the inception of PTA, multiple studies have been conducted in order to determine objective clinical data for long-term success. Patient presentation and specific angiographic anatomical criteria were found to influence short and long-term patency. Utilizing a Cox proportional hazards regression model, predictive factors influencing durable success were evaluated. Eight studies cited in the TASC document, and data obtained from the STAR registry were included.[5-8,10] Primary patency and intergroup analyses were determined with the use of the Kaplan-Meier method and log rank test, respectively (Fig. 1, Table 1).

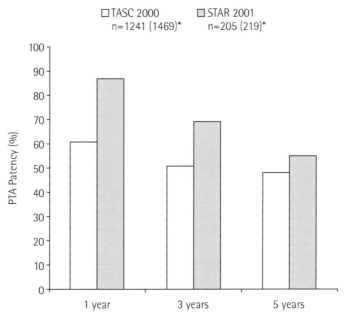

Figure 1. Collective PTA patency rates over time; *n* = patients (limbs)*.

Over time, greater patency was established in patients with claudication as an indication, stenoses, short lesions, good distal run-off, and the absence of residual stenosis on completion angiography. The presence of diabetes, renal failure, and an eccentric plaque negatively influenced overall results (Table 2).[2]

In the STAR Registry no statistically significant difference was seen in primary patency between AHA Category 2 and 3 lesions.[5] This suggests indications for femoral angioplasty can be extended to include longer and more complex Category 3 lesions. By far the most consistent determinant of long-term clinical success among the studies listed in Table 1 is the status of run-off circulation below the knee.[7,10,12,13,15]

An epidemiological study conducted on the natural history of lower extremity peripheral vascular disease reported 27% of patients with intermittent claudication, developed symptomatic progression; 11% eventually required either bypass surgery

Table 1. PTA of femoropopliteal arteries

	Study design	Patients (limbs)	Claudicants (%)	Primary Patency Rate (%)		
				1 year	3 years	5 years
Gallino et al.,[12] 1984[a]	R	280 (329)	61	62[c]	60[c]	58[c]
Krepel et al.,[13] 1985[a]	R	129 (164)	90	71	62	62
Jeans et al.,[14] 1990[a]	P	190 (190)	51	50	45	41
Capek et al.,[6] 1991[a]	R	152 (217)	74	81	61	58
Johnston,[7] 1992[a]	R	236 (254)	80	63	51	38
Hunnick et al.,[8] 1993[a]	P	106 (131)	58	57	45	45
Matsi et al.,[10] 1994[a]	P	106 (140)	100	47	42	NA
Murray et al.,[15] 1995[a]	P	42 (44)	89	86	53	NA
Clark et al.,[5] 2001[b]	P	205 (219)	58	87[c]	69[c]	55[c]

R: retrospective; P: prospective.

[a] Study included in the TransAtlantic Inter-Society Consensus.

[b] Study included in SCIVR Transluminal Angioplasty and Revascularization Registry. Patency reported for all limbs on an intent-to-treat basis.

[c] Adjusted for inclusion of technical failures.

Table 2. Factors affecting patency

Favourable	Unfavourable
Claudication[a]	Critical ischaemia
Stenosis (AHA 1, 2)[b]	Occlusion (AHA 3, 4)
Short lesion < 3cm	Long lesion >10cm
Good run-off (score 0-4)[c]	Poor run-off (score 5-6)
Concentric lesion	Eccentric lesion
No residual stenosis	Residual stenosis
Palpable pulse after PTA	No palpable pulse after PTA

[a] Symptom severity was graded according to the Society for Vascular Surgery (SVS) International Society of Cardiovascular Surgery (ICVS) / SCVIR classification.

[b] American Heart Association (AHA) Task Force categories of femoropopliteal lesions characterized lesions based on presence and length of stenoses or occlusion.

[c] Stratified run-off score is based on severity of stenoses and patency of the distal vasculature.

or amputation.[16] PTA has been applied with increasing success to this subset of patients.[3] A prospective randomized Veteran's Affairs Cooperative Study compared standard operative bypass with PTA. In a similar group of patients with equivalent stages of arterial insufficiency, the durability of haemodynamic improvement was not statistically different (Fig. 2).[9]

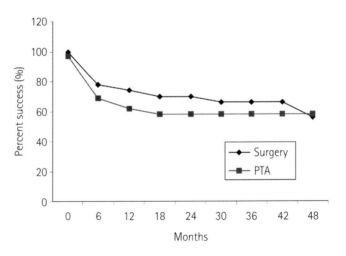

Figure 2.   Life-table analysis for patients with femoral lesions (p=0.3723).

Future perspectives for PTA

As a therapeutic modality, PTA continues to evolve and advance in conjunction with the manufacturing of new device designs as well as refining technical expertise. Criteria once thought to limit the technical success and long-term results of PTA have recently been challenged. PTA of femoral occlusions has improved, and acceptable patency in patients with diabetes or presenting with severe to critical limb ischaemia, has been established (Table 3).

Patient selection is critical, but with appropriate anatomic criteria documented on angiography combined with the presence of clinical symptoms, the place of PTA in the management of specific lesions is proven. As long as this evolutionary process continues, prospective, standardized trials will be necessary.[6]

Table 3.   Clinical predictors of long-term success addressed

Study	Patients (limbs)	Limiting factor challenged	Results	
Morgenstern *et al.*,[17] 1989	116	Femoral occlusion	1977–1980: 1981–1988:	74% 91%
Stokes *et al.*,[18] 1990	97 (127)	Diabetes	5 year patency: (equivalent to non-diabetics)	60 %
London *et al.*,[19] 1995	(54)	Critical limb ischaemia	2 year patency: 2 year limb salvage:	78% 89%
Murray *et al.*,[20] 1995	(44)	≥ 10cm stenosis	Technical success: 2 year patency:	93% 69%
Varty *et al.*,[21] 1998	82	Critical limb ischaemia	1 year limb salvage:	75%

SAP: clearly a minority option

Since its first description in 1990, SAP has undergone minimal evolution.[22] Relatively few centres have demonstrated proficiency and have published data. Reported satisfactory results have not been duplicated by other expert centres nor has the technique been embraced by other institutions compared with PTA. There are no specific indications for SAP as first-line therapy, nor do clinical predictors of prolonged patency exist. Although technical success was acceptable, more procedural complications and a high early occlusion rate was experienced (Table 4).

Table 4. SAP of femoropopliteal arteries

Study	Technical success (%)	Patency (%) 1 year	2 years	3 years	Complications (%)	Early occlusion (within 7 days)
London et al.,[23] 1994	159/200 (80)	71	62	58	15/200 (8)	5/159 (3)
Reekers et al.,[24] 1994	34/40 (85)	59	59	–	8/40 (20)	5/34 (15)
McCarthy et al.,[25] 2000	51/69 (74)	6 months: 51			11/69 (16)	NA
Yilmaz et al.,[26] 2001	32/39 (82)	62	–	–	2/39 (5)	3/39 (8)

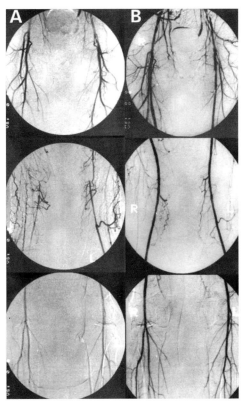

Figure 3. Results of operative subintimal angioplasty of the superficial femoral artery at 3 months. Reproduced with permission from Ref. 28.

In the two larger groups, the majority of patients presented with moderate claudication and would not normally have been candidates for surgery.[27] Recently, open SAP has been combined with a common femoral endarterectomy and patch angioplasty in a minority of patients with again anecdotal short-term success (Fig. 3).[28]

Comparison of complications of PTA and SAP

Overall morbidity including major complications from eight single centres in the TASC document averaged 4.3% (range, 2.5–6.3) in 1469 procedures.[11] The average procedural complication rate for SAP from the four largest series was 11% (range 7.5–20) in 348 procedures.[23–26] Chi-square analysis determined a significant difference did exist between the complication rates of the two procedures (χ^2=18.2, p ≤ 0.001). In a series of 3784 patients who underwent PTA, morbidity was largely attributed to the puncture site.[29] Other associated adverse events are presented in Table 5.

Groin haematomas and distal embolization were the more common adverse events in SAP. Procedure specific complications included vessel perforation and collateral branch vessel occlusion (Table 4, Fig. 4).

Table 5. Technical complications of PTA

Description	Incidence (%)
Groin puncture site	
(retroperitoneal haemorrhage, pseudoaneurysm, anteriovenous fistula)	4
PTA site (thrombosis, vessel rupture)	3.5
Distal vessel (embolization, dissection)	2.3
Unrelated events (myocardial infarction, renal failure, cerebrovascular accident)	0.95

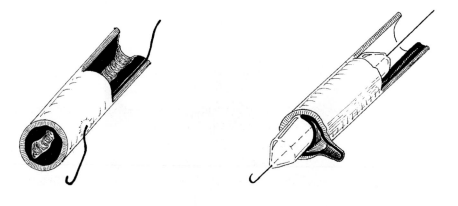

(a) (b)

Figure 4. (a) Perforation of the femoral vessel with a hydrophilic glidewire can also predispose to the creation of an arteriovenous communication. (b) Dissection initiated above the origin of a major collateral vessel can result in inadvertent occlusion necessitating emergent bypass surgery for limb salvage.

Technical success of PTA over SAP

In reviewing the TASC report and Society of Cardiovascular and Interventional Radiology (SCVIR) Transluminal Angioplasty and Revascularization Registry (STAR), a greater impact on technical success was seen in more recent studies when compared with SAP (Fig. 5).

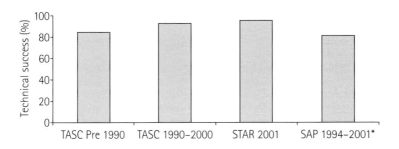

Figure 5. Overall technical success (%) of PTA vs subintimal angioplasty.
*Compilation of the four largest series of SAP reported, n=348 procedures.

Therefore, the current indications for SAP remain speculative and the benefits theoretical, without adequate substantiation.

Random controlled trial?

The limited results of SAP must be compared with those obtained with surgical treatment, which is considered the gold standard for patients who have femoropopliteal occlusive disease. At present the optimal choice for conduit is autologous vein which portends a 5-year patency rate of 85%.[30,31]

Summary

- PTA is a safe and durable therapeutic modality in the treatment of femoropopliteal occlusive disease.
- Published technical success, log-term patency, and decreased complication rates are superior following PTA in appropriately selected patients.
- In a similar cohort, haemodynamic success did not statistically differ between PTA and conventional surgical intervention.
- Negative clinical predictors continue to be addressed in order to provide PTA to a wider patient population.
- Results of SAP are not reproducible and no data exist to indicate success is comparable with peripheral revascularization.
- There is no role for SAP in the treatment of moderate claudication.

Acknowledgement

The authors would like to thank Colleen L Brayack for her timely assistance in preparing the illustrations for this chapter.

References

1. Dotter CT, Judkins MP. Transluminal treatment of arteriosclerotic obstruction: description of a new technique and a preliminary report of its application. *Circulation* 1964; **30**: 654-670.
2. Stock X, Lawrence PF, Oderich G *et al.* Interventions in the femoropopliteal arteries. In *Textbook of Endovascular Procedures.* Dyet JF, Nicholson AA, Ettles DF, Wilson SE (eds). Philadelphia, PA: Churchill Livingstone, 2000: 100-125.
3. Martin EC, Fankuchen EI, Karlson KB *et al.* Angioplasty for femoral artery occlusion: comparison with surgery. *AJR* 1981; **137**: 915-919.
4. Kidney, DD, Kafie FE, Deutsch LS *et al.* Balloon angioplasty in infrainguinal arterial occlusive disease. In *Endovascular Surgery* 3rd edn. Moore WS, Ahn SS (eds). Philadelphia, PA: WB Saunders, 2001: 285-297.
5. Clark TW, Groffsky JL, Soulen MC. Predictors of long-term patency after femoropopliteal angioplasty: results from the STAR registry. *J Vasc Interv Radiol* 2001; **12**: 923-933.
6. Capek P, McLean GK, Berkowitz HD. Femoropopliteal angioplasty: factors influencing long-term success. *Circulation* 1991; **83** (Suppl I): I-70 I-80.
7. Johnston KW. Femoral and popliteal arteries: reanalysis of results of balloon angioplasty. *Radiology* 1992; **183**: 767-771.
8. Hunnick MG, Donaldson MC, Meyerovitz MF *et al.* Risks and benefits of femoropopliteal percutaneous balloon angioplasty. *J Vasc Surg* 1993; **17**: 183-194.
9. Wilson SE, Wolf GL, Cross AP. Percutaneous transluminal angioplasty versus operation for peripheral arteriosclerosis. *J Vasc Surg* 1989; **9**: 1-9.
10. Matsi PJ, Manninem HI, Vanninen RL *et al.* Femoropopliteal angioplasty in patients with claudication: primary and secondary patency in 140 limbs with 1-3 year follow-up. *Radiology* 1994; **191**: 727-733.
11. Rutherford RB, Dormandy JA, Heeck L *et al.* TransAtlantic Inter-Society Consensus: Management of peripheral arterial disease. *J Vasc Surg* 2000; **31**: Pt 2: S103-S107.
12. Gallino A, Mahler F, Probst P *et al.* Percutaneous transluminal angioplasty of the arteries of the lower limbs: a 5 year follow-up. *Circulation* 1984; **70**: 619-623.
13. Krepel VM, van Andel GJ, van Erp WF *et al.* Percutaneous transluminal angioplasty of the femoropopliteal artery: initial and long term results. *Radiology* 1985; **156**: 325-328.
14. Jeans WD, Amstrong S, Cole SE *et al.* Fate of patients undergoing transluminal angioplasty for lower limb ischemia. *Radiology* 1990; **177**: 559-564.
15. Murray JG, Apthorp LA, Wilkins RA. Long-segment (≥10cm) femoropopliteal angioplasty: improved technical success and long-term patency. *Radiology* 1995; **195**: 158-162.
16. Weitz JI, Byrne J, Clagett GP *et al.* Diagnosis and treatment of chronic arterial insufficiency of the lower extremities: a critical review. *Circulation* 1996; **94**: 3026-3049.
17. Morgenstern BR, Getrajdman GI, Laffey KJ *et al.* Total occlusions of the femoropopliteal artery: high technical success rate of conventional balloon angioplasty. *Radiology* 1989; **172**: 937-940.
18. Stokes KR, Strunk HM, Campbell DR *et al.* Five-year results of iliac and femoropopliteal angioplasty in diabetic patients. *Radiology* 1990; **174**: 977-982.
19. London NJ, Varty K, Sayers RD *et al.* Percutaneous transluminal angioplasty for lower-limb critical ischaemia. *Br J Surg* 1995; **82**: 1232-1235.
20. Murray JG, Apthorp LA, Wilkins RA. Long-segment (10cm) femoropopliteal angioplasty: improved technical success and long term patency. *Radiology* 1995; **195**: 158-162.
21. Varty K, Nydahl S, Nasim A *et al.* Results of surgery and angioplasty for treatment of chronic severe lower limb ischemia. *Eur J Vasc Endovasc Surg* 1988; **16**: 159-163.
22. Bolia A, Miles KA, Brennan J *et al.* Percutaneous transluminal angioplasty of occlusions of the femoral and popliteal arteries by subintimal dissection. *Cardiovasc Intervent Radiol* 1990; **13**: 357-363.
23. London NJ, Srinivasan R, Naylor AR *et al.* Subintimal angioplasty of femoropopliteal artey occlusions: The long-term results. *Eur J Vasc Surg* 1994; **8**: 148-155.
24. Reekers JA, Kromhout JG, Jacobs MJ. Percutaneous intentional extraluminal recanalisation of the femoropopliteal artery. *Eur J Vasc Surg* 1994; **8**: 723-728.

25. McCarthy RJ, Neary W, Roobottom C *et al.* Short-term results of femoropopliteal subintimal angio-plasty. *Br J Surg* 2000; **87**: 1361-1365.
26. Yilmaz S, Sindel T, Ceken K *et al.* Subintimal recanalization of long superficial femoral artery occlusions through the retrograde popliteal approach. *Cardiovasc Intervent Radiol* 2001; **24**: 154-160.
27. Bolia A, Bell PR. Subintimal angioplasty. In *Textbook of Endovascular Procedures*. Dyet JF, Nicholson AA, Ettles DF, Wilson SE (eds). Philadelphia, PA: Churchill Livingstone, 2000: 126-138.
28. Balas P, Pangratis N, Ioannou N *et al.* Open subintimal angioplasty of the superficial femoral and distal arteries. *J Endovasc Ther* 2000; **7**: 68-71.
29. Pentecost MJ, Criqui MH, Dorros G *et al.* Guidelines for peripheral percutaneous transluminal angioplasty of the abdominal aorta and lower extremity vessels. *Circulation* 1994; **89**: 511-531. 1994
30. Veith FJ, Gupta SK, Ascer E *et al.* Six-year prospective multicenter randomized comparison of autologous saphenous vein and expanded polytetrafuoroethylene grafts in infrainguinal arterial reconstructions. *J Vasc Surg* 1986; **3**: 104-114.
31. Abbott WM. Prosthetic above-knee femoro-popliteal bypass: Indications and choice of graft. *Semin Vasc Surg* 1997; **10**: 3-7.

Superficial femoral subintimal angioplasty beats luminal PTA

Charing Cross Editorial Comments towards Consensus

Who would ever have believed that subintimal angioplasty would catch on? Was it not a mistake in the first place? Did it not all happen by chance? This would not be the first time that a major advance in vascular surgery took place in this way! It is suggested that Cid dos Santos in Lisbon was under orders from his father, the professor, to remove a clot from a femoral artery when Cid pulled a little hard and tugged out half of the artery wall and produced a thrombendarterectomy. What his father said is not recorded in history, but it is known that this occurred in the late 1940s and by 1953 Dr Michael DeBakey had used thrombendarterectomy for the carotid artery successfully. News travelled fast.

What of subintimal angioplasty? Dr Amman Bolia established that the plane between the artery wall and the atheroma forms a smooth channel which can be turned into a tube by the use of a balloon angioplasty. He simply claims that the artery wall on the one side and the back of the atheroma on the other side forms smoother surfaces and are more suitable than the lumen itself. Certainly subintimal angioplasty has been attempted for long lesions where few radiologists would consider balloon angioplasty within the lumen to be an option. Is it only one centre that can do it? Certainly Peter Bell and the surgeons in Leicester are also doing it and have learned it from radiological colleagues: they all swear by it. Several groups have taken it on now and it has crossed the Atlantic and received some acclaim by those who have taken the trouble to learn the technique.

Naturally, there is doubt about it. These two chapters bring head to head the two sides of the argument. The problem seems to be that subintimal angioplasty can take on problems which interluminal angioplasty cannot attempt and thus proper comparisons cannot really be made. The question perhaps should have been to compare subintimal angioplasty with surgery which is perhaps the real alternative for long lesions. The technique is used mainly for the superficial femoral artery segment and reaches down to the popliteal and even the tibial. The anatomical appearance at the end of it can be dreadful occasionally but Dr Bolia argues that it is the functional result that really matters.

Everyone thought that Dr Dotter was crazy and hard things have been said about Dr Bolia. It could yet be that subintimal angioplasty establishes a place which superficial femoral luminal angioplasty fails to achieve. Who would ever have believed that a few years ago?

Roger M Greenhalgh
Editor

Prosthetic bypass should never cross the knee joint

For the motion

Christos D Liapis, John D Kakisis

Introduction

Patency rate of infragenicular bypasses has been the focus of interest for several studies. The choice of conduit has been unanimously recognized as one of the most important determinants of long-term patency. However, there is only one randomized study by Veith *et al.*[1] back in the 1980s comparing vein with prosthetic grafts crossing the knee, with results undoubtedly in favour of autologous material. This paucity of controlled randomized trials is reflected in the complete lack of data on the subject from the Cochrane Library.[2]

Continuous efforts are being made in order to develop durable grafts and configurations that would ensure high patency and limb salvage rates. Knitted, woven, velour Dacron; carbon, fluoride polytetrafluoroethylene (PTFE), externally supported or not; prosthetic-biological composition grafts such as Dacron-reinforced umbilical vein; cryopreserved arterial allografts and preshaped grafts are some of the options that technologic advances have made available to us. Various interventions at the distal anastomosis have been invented, aiming at the improvement of long-term patency. Miller collars, Linton patches, Taylor patches and composite grafts have all been employed to improve the compliance difference between graft and artery. The limb salvage rates undoubtedly increased but vascular surgeons became confused about which graft and which technique of distal anastomosis is more effective and durable. In this changing world of continuous progress and revision, there is, however, a constant value, a graft which, 50 years after its initial use as a vascular conduit, remains the conduit of choice and the standard against which newer graft materials must be compared. This graft is the autologous saphenous vein and although Parsons *et al.*[3] went as far as evaluating the use of prosthetic grafts for infrapopliteal bypasses as an alternative to primary amputation, a more rational comparison should be between prosthetic and autologous grafts crossing the knee joint.

Technique

Surgical technique of both reversed and *in situ* saphenous vein harvest has been well established, with the only debate focusing on the technique of valvulotomy. Potential advantages of the *in situ* method include the smooth tapering of the vein, reduced

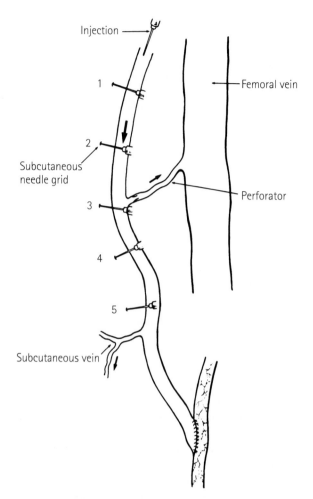

Figure 1. Completion arteriogram of an *in situ* saphenous vein bypass, identifying remaining fistulae and demonstrating technical accuracy of the distal anastomosis. A subcutaneous needle grid allows rapid location of the fistulae. Reproduced with permission from Ref. 26.

size disparity at the anastomotic sites between vein and arteries, avoidance of trauma, vasoconstriction and rotation associated with removal and reversal of the vein, maintenance of the vasa vasorum and preservation of a normally functioning endothelium. On the other hand, criticism of the operation is based on the risk of incomplete valvulotomy, intimal laceration by valvulotomes and residual arteriovenous fistulae (Fig. 1). Despite extensive clinical investigation, no clear benefit from either one or the other technique has been proven.

Evidence

Level I evidence of the superiority of the autologous saphenous vein over prosthetic grafts, particularly for below-knee reconstructions, has been available since 1986.[1] In a classic, prospective multicentre randomized study, which stands as a model of integrity and application of the scientific method, Veith *et al.*[1] showed that primary

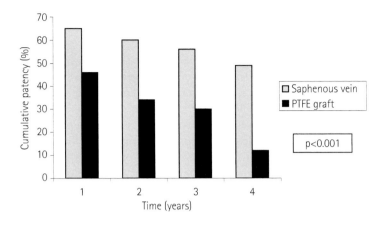

Figure 2. Cumulative primary patency rates for randomized bypasses to infrapopliteal arteries with autologous saphenous vein and polytetrafluoroethylene (PTFE) grafts.[1]

patency of femoropopliteal below-knee bypasses at 1,2,3 and 4 years was 86%, 84%, 84% and 76%, respectively, for vein grafts compared with 87%, 81%, 54% and 54%, respectively, for PTFE grafts (p<0.05). In femoroinfrapopliteal bypasses, primary patency at 1,2,3 and 4 years was 65%, 60%, 56% and 49%, respectively, for vein grafts compared with 45%, 33%, 30% and 12%, respectively, for PTFE grafts (p<0.001) (Fig. 2). These data constitute a clear and indisputable argument against the preferential use of PTFE grafts for bypasses crossing the knee joint.

Opposition to this statement could be based on the finding that there was no significant difference in limb salvage rates between patients with randomized autologous saphenous vein femoropopliteal or distal grafts and those with randomized PTFE femoropopliteal or distal bypasses respectively. Nevertheless, the authors clearly state that this was achieved at a cost of more frequent reoperation for graft failure in patients with PTFE bypasses. A quantification of this higher incidence of reoperation was given by a retrospective study of 932 infrainguinal bypass procedures, in which Rafferty et al.[4] found that PTFE grafts required reoperations at three times the rate of vein grafts to maintain limb salvage.

Except for the study of Veith et al.,[1] there is no other randomized trial comparing the outcome of vein and prosthetic grafts in infragenicular revascularization. Several comparative, non-randomized studies have been performed, in all of which saphenous vein was the preferred conduit, with prosthetic grafts being reserved for those patients in whom the saphenous vein was not available or was of poor quality. All of these studies,[5–13] except for one,[14] verified the superiority of the saphenous vein for infragenicular bypasses, with the advantage being even more pronounced in infrapopliteal bypasses. There is only one study, performed by Allen et al.,[14] which did not show any difference between vein and PTFE grafts. The peculiarity of the study is that it included claudicants only, while in all of the other studies the majority of the patients had critical ischaemia. In addition, the patency rate of vein grafts in this study was surprisingly low (5-year primary patency: 60.3%). This figure is the lowest in the literature and inexplicably lower than the 85% patency rate, which was reported by the same group for *in situ* saphenous vein grafts performed for limb salvage.[15]

The main argument against the results of these non-randomized studies is that the outcome of prosthetic grafts is prejudiced negatively by their placement in an unfavourable circumstance. This is due to the fact that prosthetic grafts were often used in reoperations, where the ipsilateral saphenous vein had already been used in the primary procedure, or in cases of previous coronary artery bypass grafting, which is indicative of severe atherosclerosis. However, it is exactly in the situations associated with a high risk of failure where the advantages of vein grafts are most marked. Indeed, several authors have shown that the superiority of vein grafts is more evident in cases of poor distal run-off,[4,12] secondary reconstructions,[10] distal grafting[5] and critical ischaemia.[16]

In order to explore the 'unfair bias' against prosthetic grafts, Panayiotopoulos and Taylor[17] compared the outcome of vein and prosthetic grafts in patients with poor, moderate or excellent inflow and run-off conditions separately. While vein grafts were superior to PTFE when the whole cohort was included, there was no significant difference when the patients were stratified for inflow and run-off status. However, it should be noted that, after such stratification, there were only five patients left in the group of PTFE grafts with good inflow and outflow conditions, leading to a standard error of 21.65. Furthermore, in the group of moderate inflow and run-off conditions, follow-up of patients with PTFE grafts was limited to 21 months. A larger number of patients, followed for longer periods of time, is needed in order to draw definite conclusions after such stratification.

In order to summarize the currently available evidence on patency of various grafts in infragenicular bypasses, we reviewed the leading vascular literature (impact factor >1.5) of the past 20 years. We identified 80 studies, reporting on a total of 10 492 patients, which contained sufficient data regarding the type of graft and the site of distal anastomosis. A meta-analysis of these data would be desirable but cannot be performed, mainly due to inconsistent reporting practices, which make data difficult to assess and compare. Therefore, the estimated average patencies should not be considered as evidence but as an indication of what is currently available. These estimates are shown in Tables 1 and 2 and are graphically depicted in Figs 3 and 4. It can be seen that autologous veins have the best reported patency in all the bypasses that cross the knee joint, while the prosthetic grafts have a dismal 5-year patency of 38% and 22% for below-knee femoropopliteal and femorodistal bypasses respectively.

The clear superiority of the autologous saphenous vein over prosthetic grafts is even more evident in the treatment of popliteal aneurysms. Patency rates of as high as 94% at 10 years have been reported with the saphenous vein compared with 27% with other bypasses.[18] There is no question that the autologous saphenous vein graft is the material of choice for popliteal artery aneurysm replacement.[19]

Several secondary issues regarding infragenicular revascularization should also be addressed. In the study of Veith *et al.*,[1] patency difference between randomized autologous saphenous vein and PTFE infrapopliteal bypasses became apparent within 1 month of operation and increased progressively thereafter. On the contrary, patency rates with the two grafts in the femoropopliteal position remained similar for 2 years after operation and only diverged thereafter. Thus, the use of PTFE grafts as femoropopliteal bypasses could be justified in poor-risk patients with a life expectancy of 2–3 years or less. However, life expectancy cannot be predicted so accurately, so there is no justification for not offering the best available graft to all patients instead of making precarious predictions about life expectancy.

The preservation of the long saphenous vein for possible future use as a coronary artery bypass is an argument often put forward by surgeons advocating the preferential use of prosthetic grafts in lower limb revascularization. This argument is reinforced by the fact that 45–56%[5,9] of patients undergoing infrainguinal bypass surgery have coronary artery disease and 9–21%[5,6,14] have already been submitted to coronary artery revascularization. However, the question of vein preservation for coronary artery surgery does not stand up to close scrutiny.[20] First, it applies only to

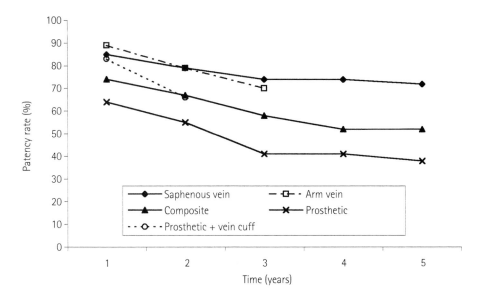

Figure 3. Average patency rates for various types of grafts in below-knee femoropopliteal reconstructions.

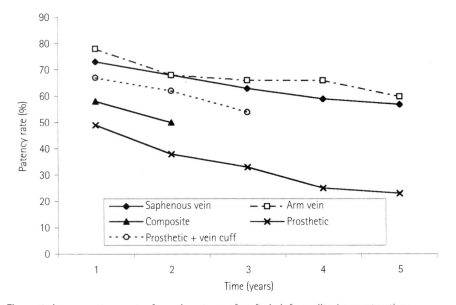

Figure 4. Average patency rates for various types of grafts in infrapopliteal reconstructions.

operations on the second leg and only a minority of patients will require revascularization of both legs. Second, as Houser et al.[21] showed, only 5% of patients who are submitted to femoral outflow reconstruction will undergo subsequent aortocoronary bypass. Conversely, among patients who are submitted to aortocoronary bypass, only 1.4% have a history of prior femoral outflow reconstruction. Based on these data, there should be little concern about the possibility of future cardiac surgery and little hesitation regarding the use of the greater saphenous vein to revascularize the leg, when indicated. Moreover, in case of coronary artery bypass grafting, the lack of a greater saphenous vein due to prior use for limb revascularization is unlikely to be encountered as a major problem, taking into account the availability of satisfactory alternative autologous conduits such as the internal mammary arteries, the lesser saphenous and the arm veins, the right gastroepiploic artery, the inferior epigastric artery and the radial or the splenic artery. The radial artery in particular is being used with increasing frequency instead of the saphenous vein in coronary artery bypass grafts and is currently considered by most cardiac surgeons as the graft material of second choice after the internal mammary arteries, with the saphenous vein being the third.[22,23]

The elimination of complications of vein harvest is another argument in favour of the preferential use of prosthetic grafts. Nevertheless, it is of utmost importance to categorize wound complications with regard to the degree of severity, since an erythema of the surgical wound can hardly be compared with an exposed graft infection. In this context, Johnson et al.[24] showed that the type of graft material used (vein vs PTFE) was the only factor predictive of severe wound complications after infrainguinal bypass. The incidence of wound breakdown was 26% after PTFE bypass compared with 13% after vein grafts (p=0.04), while 86% of the infected wounds and all of the graft infections occurred in patients with PTFE grafts (p=0.017). This finding provides a compelling argument for the routine use of autologous grafts, if possible, even when equivalent patency rates are expected with prosthetic graft use.

Undoubtedly, the time and effort needed for vein harvest cannot be compared with the rapidity and ease of a graft taken 'off the shelf' but there are no data confirming that this leads to any increase in perioperative morbidity or mortality. In any case, the reduced risk of infection of an autologous graft outweighs the risk ensuing from the longer operative time.

The remaining question is what graft to use in the absence of an autologous saphenous vein. A review of the literature, shown in Tables 1 and 2 and graphically depicted in Figs 3 and 4, justifies an 'all autologous reconstruction' policy, with the use of the arm veins in any case where the autologous saphenous veins, ipsilateral and contralateral, are not suitable or available. Alternative autologous vein grafting is, of course, tedious and time consuming. It involves additional incisions and usually

Table 1. Average patency rates for various types of grafts in below-knee femoropopliteal reconstructions

	No of patients	Year				
		1	2	3	4	5
Autologous saphenous vein	3051	85	79	74	74	72
Arm vein	83	89	79	70		
Prosthetic + vein cuff	202	83	66			
PTFE-vein composite	171	74	67	58	52	52
Prosthetic	1406	64	55	41	41	38

Table 2. Average patency rates for various types of grafts in infrapopliteal reconstructions

	No of patients	Year				
		1	2	3	4	5
Autologous saphenous vein	3304	73	68	63	59	57
Arm vein	534	78	68	66	66	60
Prosthetic + vein cuff	267	67	62	54		
PTFE-vein composite	229	58	50			
Prosthetic	1245	49	38	33	25	23

requires general anaesthesia, but it still yields better long-term results than the prosthetic grafts and is comparable with those of the autologous saphenous vein.

Several techniques, such as composite prosthetic-vein grafts and vein interposition cuffs, have been employed in order to enhance the patency of prosthetic bypasses to infragenicular arteries.[25] Both of these techniques undoubtedly improve the outcome of prosthetic grafting but not to the point of autologous vein conduits (Figs 3 and 4). We therefore believe that PTFE-vein composite grafts are an acceptable form of distal revascularization only in the absence of sufficient autogenous material for in-line reconstruction. On the contrary, there is no justification for a prosthetic graft crossing the knee joint in any case.

Summary

- Level I evidence exists regarding the superiority of autologous saphenous vein over prosthetic grafts for infragenicular revascularization

- A review of all available literature of the last 20 years shows that autologous vein grafts have the best reported patency in all situations, with prosthetic grafts showing a dismal long-term outcome

- Reported potential advantages of prosthetic grafts cannot stand up to close scrutiny

- Randomized controlled trials will be justified to evaluate newer prosthetic grafts and distal anastomotic configurations only if their track record improves

- Autologous saphenous vein remains the graft material of choice for bypasses crossing the knee joint, with alternative autologous veins being the second choice and composite configurations the third

- Prosthetic grafts should never cross the knee joint

References

1. Veith FJ, Gupta SK, Ascer E *et al.* Six-year prospective multicenter randomized comparison of autologous saphenous vein and expanded polytetrafluoroethylene grafts in infrainguinal arterial reconstructions. *J Vasc Surg* 1986; 3: 104–114.
2. Mamode N, Scott RN. Graft type for femoro-popliteal bypass surgery (Cochrane Review). *The Cochrane Library*, 2001: Issue 3.

3. Parsons RE, Suggs WD, Veith FJ *et al.* Polytetrafluoroethylene bypasses to infrapopliteal arteries without cuffs or patches: a better option than amputation in patients without autologous vein. *J Vasc Surg* 1996; 23: 347–356.

4. Rafferty TD, Avellone JC, Farrell CJ *et al.* A metropolitan experience with infrainguinal revascularization. Operative risk and late results in northeastern Ohio. *J Vasc Surg* 1987; 6: 365–371.

5. Veterans Administration Cooperative Study Group 141. Comparative evaluation of prosthetic, reversed, and *in situ* vein bypass grafts in distal popliteal and tibial-peroneal revascularization. *Arch Surg* 1988; 123: 434–438.

6. Archie JP. Femoropopliteal bypass with either adequate ipsilateral reversed saphenous vein or obligatory polytetrafluoroethylene. *Ann Vasc Surg* 1994; 8: 475–484.

7. Jackson MR, Belott TP, Dickason T *et al.* The consequences of a failed femoropopliteal bypass grafting: comparison of saphenous vein and PTFE grafts. *J Vasc Surg* 2000; 32: 498–505.

8. Edwards WH, Mulherin JL Jr. The role of graft material in femorotibial bypass grafts. *Ann Surg* 1980; 191: 721–726.

9. Cranley JJ, Hafner CD. Revascularization of the femoropopliteal arteries using saphenous vein, polytetrafluoroethylene, and umbilical vein grafts. *Arch Surg* 1982; 117: 1543–1550.

10. Londrey GL, Ramsey DE, Hodgson KJ, Barkmeier LD, Summer DS. Infrapopliteal bypass for severe ischemia: comparison of autogenous vein, composite, and prosthetic grafts. *J Vasc Surg* 1991; 13: 631–636.

11. Yeager RA, Hobson II RW, Jamil Z *et al.* Differential patency and limb salvage for polytetrafluoroethylene and autogenous saphenous vein in severe lower extremity ischemia. *Surgery* 1982; 91: 99–103.

12. Hall RG, Coupland GAE, Lane R, Delbridge L, Appleberg M. Vein, Gore-tex or a composite graft for femoropopliteal bypass. *Surg Gynecol Obstet* 1985; 161: 308–312.

13. Panayiotopoulos YP, Tyrrell MR, Owen SE, Reidy JF, Taylor PR. Outcome and cost analysis after femorocrural and femoropedal grafting for critical limb ischaemia. *Br J Surg* 1997; 84: 207–212.

14. Allen BT, Reilly JM, Rubin BG *et al.* Femoropopliteal bypass for claudication: vein vs PTFE. *Ann Vasc Surg* 1996; 10: 178–185.

15. Anderson CB, Stevens SL, Allen BT, Sicard GA. *In situ* saphenous vein for lower extremity revascularization. *Surgery* 1992; 112: 6–10.

16. Bennion RS, Williams RA, Stabile BE, Fox MA. Patency of autogenous saphenous vein versus polytetrafluoroethylene grafts in femoropopliteal bypass for advanced ischemia. *Surg Gynecol Obstet* 1985; 160: 239–242.

17. Panayiotopoulos YP, Taylor PR. A paper for debate: vein versus PTFE for critical limb ischaemia – an unfair comparison? *Eur J Vasc Endovasc Surg* 1997; 14: 191–194.

18. Anton GE, Hertzer NR, Beven EG, O'Hara PJ, Krajewski LP. Surgical management of popliteal aneurysms. Trends in presentation, treatment, and results from 1952 to 1984. *J Vasc Surg* 1986; 3: 125–134.

19. Davidovic LB, Lotina SI, Kostic DM *et al.* Popliteal artery aneurysms. *World J Surg* 1998; 22: 812–817.

20. Michaels JA. Choice of material for above-knee femoropopliteal bypass graft. *Br J Surg* 1989; 76: 7–14.

21. Houser SL, Hashmi FH, Jaeger VJ *et al.* Should the greater saphenous vein be preserved in patients requiring arterial outflow reconstruction in the lower extremity? *Surgery* 1984; 95: 467–472.

22. Weinschelbaum EE, Macchia A, Caramutti VM *et al.* Myocardial revascularization with radial and mammary arteries: initial and mid-term results. *Ann Thorac Surg* 2000; 70: 1378–1383.

23. Tatoulis J, Buxton BF, Fuller JA, Royse AG. Total arterial coronary revascularization: techniques and results in 3,220 patients. *Ann Thorac Surg* 1999; 68: 2093–2099.

24. Johnson JA, Cogbill TH, Strutt PJ, Gundersen AL. Wound complications after infrainguinal bypass. *Arch Surg* 1988; 123: 859–862.

25. Bastounis E, Georgopoulos S, Maltezos C, Alexiou D, Chiotopoulos D, Bramis J. PTFE-vein composite grafts for critical limb ischaemia: a valuable alternative to all-autologous infrageniculate reconstructions. *Eur J Vasc Endovasc Surg* 1999; 18: 127–132.

26. Leather RR, Shah DM, Chang BB, Darling RC. The *in situ* sephenous vein arterial bypass by valve incision. In *Vascular and Endovascular Surgical Techniques* 4th edn. Greenhalgh RM (ed). London: WB Saunders, 2001: 347–352.

Prosthetic bypass should never cross the knee joint

Against the motion

Jean-Pierre Becquemin, Bertrand Poussier

Introduction

In patients with severe limb ischaemia and femoropopliteal obstructive disease, the saphenous vein is the conduit of choice.[1] Veins of the arm and the lesser saphenous vein are also valuable alternatives. However, there are circumstances when veins are not available because they have been previously removed or because they are of poor quality. In these cases a prosthetic graft is the only alternative to amputation. Unfortunately, the results of prosthetic grafts are not rewarding, and the relatively high rates of postoperative complications including of thrombosis, but also infection, and false aneurysm restrain most vascular surgeons from performing a below-knee revascularization with a prosthetic graft.[2] We do think with others[3] that a number of legs and life can be saved by disobeying the proposition 'prosthetic bypass should never cross the knee joint'. In the following text, these arguments will be developed.

Prosthetic below-knee bypass: a poor reputation, which is not deserved

Prosthetic grafts have a poorer patency when they are used below the knee than above the knee.[4] However, most series reported a mixture of different situations including best and worst cases scenario. Unfortunately, the data are pooled and analysed together preventing a fair comparison and there are many variables other than the site of the distal anastomosis, which may influence the results.

The site of distal anastomosis

In many reports, grafts implanted on the distal popliteal artery are pooled with grafts implanted on the crural arteries. The high failure rate of the latter contributes to an over-exaggeration of poor results of the former. When crural artery grafts are left apart, the patency as well as the limb salvage rate is quite similar in the above- and below-knee positions. The randomized study of Stonebrige *et al.*[5] showed a similar patency of 73% at 2 years of above- and below-knee anastomosis. The classic randomized study by Veith *et al*,[6] comparing autologous saphenous vein and expanded polytetrafluoroethylene (PTFe) grafts in infra-inguinal arterial reconstruction has shown that the patency rates of below-knee prosthetic grafts was even superior to the patency of above-knee grafts (54% vs 38% at 4 years).

The inflow and outflow status

This is a key issue.[4,7] Most series of below-knee prosthetic grafts have included patients with good and poor outflow, contributing to the expression of globally poor results. Taylor[3] has shown that patients with a prosthetic graft and a good run-off have similar results to patients in whom a vein has been used. The 3-year patency rate was 80% in both groups. So there is absolutely no reason for denying a chance of saving a leg in a patient with two or three patent crural arteries on the grounds that he has no vein, and that the knee joint should be crossed. Conversely it is very questionable to perform a crural bypass even with a vein, in patients with an occluded popliteal artery and a severely diseased runoff.

The grade of ischaemia

All series showed that the patency is much better in claudicants than in patients with critical limb ischaemia. Surgeons are not reluctant to perform an above-knee prosthetic bypass for claudication. Conversely, they tend to attempt prosthetic below-knee grafts in the worst cases, which are critical limb ischaemia and no vein. Then when comparing above- and below-knee bypasses, more patients of the former are claudicants and more of the latter have a critical ischaemia.

First vs secondary procedure

In many series, 14–27%[6] infrapopliteal prosthetic grafts have been performed after a failed venous graft or a failed above-knee graft. Conversely only between 6% and 13% above-knee prosthetic graft are performed after a failed attempt.[6] Secondary procedures have a poorer outcome. Schweiger *et al.*[8] reported that the 4-year patency of femorotibial bypasses was 42% for primary procedure and 14% for repeated grafts.

The technique of grafting

There is no question that crural artery grafting offers poorer results than popliteal grafting. However, the patency of crural prosthetic grafts have been improved by the use of vein patch, FAV and composite grafts.[9,10] Unfortunately again, most series

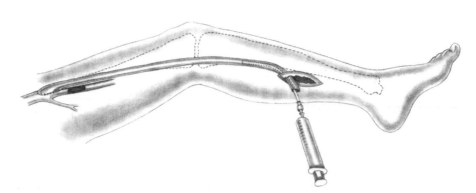

Figure 1. Care of the graft and prevention of clotting. Reproduced with permission from Ref. 27.

reported patients operated upon using a great variety of techniques, making conclusions uncertain.

The risk of amputation at a higher level

Acute prosthetic occlusion may lead to the propagation of clot into the native artery which may worsen the situation.[11] The risk is to shift what would have been a below-knee amputation had the patient not been operated upon for a transfemoral amputation.[12] Is the risk greater with a below- or an above-knee bypass? There is no clear answer to this question. Of note also is that in all series, the limb salvage rate even with a prosthetic graft is higher than the occlusion rate. Furthermore, Whittaker et al.[13] have shown that multiple amputations were not frequent in patients who were submitted to aggressive vascular attempts for critical ischaemia.

The risk of death

The postoperative death rate following a bypass in the leg is between 1% and 8%. The high mortality rate is linked to the co-morbidities of patients who need a femoropopliteal bypass. These patients are in their 70s or 80s; most of them have a coronary heart disease, or are diabetic or have an end-stage renal failure. For the current debate, there is no evidence that above-knee and below-knee grafts have a different mortality rate.

We do think that in patients with a limited life expectancy, reasonable risks can be taken. Following a below-knee or above-knee amputation, the mortality in the following days and months is very high, the probability of self-sufficiency and return to a normal walk is very low, the psychological and physical stress is high and the burden for the family and the society may be unbearable. Cheshire[14] has shown that 1-month mortality after reconstruction was <1% but was 10% after amputation. At 3 years, 20% of both groups were dead.

The quality of life

In all cases, the proposal should be placed in the clinical context where no other proper solution is available. And the true question, which is developed elsewhere in the book is: is it better to have a graft at high risk of failure or to have a primary amputation? Or is it better to have a primary amputation immediately or delayed after some months or years? The answer is not so simple and a sound reasoning is necessary for a fair decision. Of note is that in the Cheshire series,[14] 70% of amputated patients were confined to the home vs 9% of patients who underwent reconstruction. Again crossing the knee joint with a prosthetic graft improves the quality of life even if it is for a limited period of time.

What is the evidence

Operative techniques

Operative details are well known; however we will underline some technical details:

1. *Choice of upper anastomosis site*   It could be the common femoral artery generally in case of occlusive disease or at the distal part of the femoral artery when it is an aneurismal disease. The main advantage in the latter option is a shorter length of graft, which is less prone to occlusion.

2. *Choice of distal anastomosis site*   We tend to choose the distal popliteal artery even slightly diseased rather than a crural artery.
3. *Outflow improvement*   In cases of stenosis downstream of the anastomosis, we attempt to improve the run-off by combined balloon angioplasty.
4. *Choice of the most appropriate route*   The graft can be placed superficially in an extra-anatomical position, or anatomically. We prefer the first option because the surveillance of the graft is easier and also in case of redo-operation the access to the graft is much simpler. Also when bending the knee, the risk of kink and stenosis are reduced by the extra-anatomical route. However, in order to prevent skin erosion by the fabric, the graft is placed in the sub-facial space.
5. *Choice of the graft*   We routinely use thin-wall carbon-coated PTFe-ringed grafts. They are easy to suture, resistant to external compression and less thrombogenic.[15]
6. *Tricks to improve the results*

   • At the popliteal level, the angle between the graft and the recipient artery must be carefully checked.[16] With end-to-side anastomosis an acute angle may be created between the graft and the artery. Thus the flow distribution is not optimum. The graft can also be compressed by the bone structure, especially when the graft has been cut a little too short. To prevent these complications, we divide the popliteal artery above the suture line, when necessary.
   • At the crural level, we routinely perform the distal anastomosis with a vein cuff.[17]

Results

Results of prosthetic grafts to the popliteal artery below the knee

Patency

Authors	No of patients	2 years	3 years	4 years
Faries	29	83%	55%	
Harris		51%		
Stonebridge	48 (cuff)		82%	
Veith	57	85%		54%
Taylor			80%	

Refs 2, 3, 5, 6, 18.

Limb salvage

Authors	No of patients	1 year	2 years	3 years	4 years
Faries	29	91%		75%	
Stonebridge	48	86%	83%		
Veith	57				62%

Refs 5, 6, 18.

Results of prosthetic grafts to the crural arteries

Patency

Authors	No of patients	Adjunct	1 year	2 years	3 years	4 years	5 years
Faries	105	–	58%		41%		
Eagleton	24	–		44%			
Cavillon	31		53%				21%
Parsons	63	–			55%		43%
Eagleton	33	FAV		65%			
Jacobs	30	FAV	71%	71%			
Eagleton	16	Vein patch		35%			
Stonebridge	89	Vein patch	50%	32%			
Neville	79	Vein patch				62%	
Fichelle	149	Mixed			41%		35%

Refs 5, 18–24.

Limb salvage

Authors	No of patients	Adjunct	1 year	2 years	3 years	4 years	5 years
Faries	105	–	69%		63%		
Bastounis	60	–					80%
Cavillon	31		48%				41%
Parsons	63	–			71%		66%
Ascer	68	FAV			78%		
Jacobs	30	FAV	75%	75%			
Neville	79	Vein patch				79%	
Stonebridge	89	Vein patch	53%	44%			
Fichelle	149	mixed			68%		65%

Refs 5, 18, 20–26.

The alternatives are doubtful

Above-knee prosthetic graft bypass

1. Few patients with a critical limb ischaemia have a fully patent distal superficial femoral artery or a non-diseased popliteal artery. When choosing the site for the distal anastomosis one must bear in mind the resistance to flow which may be higher in the above-knee vessels than in the below-knee vessels.
2. During follow-up the graft is threatened by the evolution of the atherosclerotic disease on the popliteal artery distal to the anastomosis.
3. Sequential bypass may have a role in this situation.

Endovascular technique

Endoluminal angioplasty is generally not indicated due to the length of the lesions. Subintimal angioplasty may have a role, which is not fully evaluated yet. In our experience the procedure is do-able but not durable.

Summary

- Below-knee prosthetic grafts have an undeservedly poor reputation.

- Limiting prosthetic grafts to above-knee popliteal arteries indicates timidity rather than wisdom.

- In selected patients with critical limb ischaemia and no vein, a below-knee prosthetic graft is a better choice than amputation.

- Outflow and status of health are the main criteria for the decision of performing a below-knee prosthetic bypass.

- Adjunct procedures such as vein cuff and/or FAV improve the patency of crural vessels grafting.

- Below-knee prosthetic grafts should be avoided in claudicants.

- There is no, and probably there never will be a, randomized study comparing prosthetic grafts above and below the knee.

References

1. Mamode N, Scott RN. Graft ype for femoro-popliteal bypass surgery. *Cochrane Database Syst Rev* 2000: CD001487.
2. Harris PL, Campbell H. Femoro-distal bypass for critical ischaemia: is the use of prosthetic grafts justified? *Ann Vasc Surg* 1986; 1: 66–72.
3. Panayiotopoulos YP, Taylor PR. A paper for debate: vein versus PTFE for critical limb ischaemia – an unfair comparison? *Eur J Vasc Endovasc Surg* 1997; 14: 191–194.
4. Budd JS, Brennan J, Beard JD, Warren H, Burton PR, Bell PR. Infrainguinal bypass surgery: factors determining late graft patency. *Br J Surg* 1990; 77: 1382–1387.
5. Stonebridge PA, Prescott RJ, Ruckley CV. Randomized trial comparing infrainguinal polytetrafluoroethylene bypass grafting with and without vein interposition cuff at the distal anastomosis. The Joint Vascular Research Group. *J Vasc Surg* 1997; 26: 543–550.
6. Veith FJ, Gupta SK, Ascer E *et al.* Six-year prospective multicentre randomized comparison of autologous saphenous vein and expanded polytetrafluoroethylene grafts in infrainguinal arterial reconstructions. *J Vasc Surg* 1986; 3: 104–114.
7. Ljungman C, Ulus AT, Almgren B *et al.* A multivariate analysis of factors affecting patency of femoropopliteal and femorodistal bypass grafting. *Vasa* 2000; 29: 215–220.
8. Schweiger H, Klein P, Lang W. Tibial bypass grafting for limb salvage with ringed polytetrafluoroethylene prostheses: results of primary and secondary procedures. *J Vasc Surg* 1993; 18: 867–874.
9. Stonebridge PA, Naidu S, Colgan MP, Moore DJ, Shanik DG, McCollum PT. Tibial and peroneal artery bypasses using polytetrafluoroethylene (PTFE) with an interposition vein cuff. *J R Coll Surg Edinb* 2000; 45: 17–20.
10. Sayers RD, Raptis S, Berce M, Miller JH. Long-term results of femorotibial bypass with vein or polytetrafluoroethylene. *Br J Surg* 1998; 85: 934–938.
11. Jackson MR, Belott TP, Dickason T *et al.* The consequences of a failed femoropopliteal bypass grafting: comparison of saphenous vein and PTFE grafts. *J Vasc Surg* 2000 32: 498–504.
12. Van Niekerk LJ, Stewart CP, Jain AS. Major lower limb amputation following failed infrainguinal vascular bypass surgery: a prospective study on amputation levels and stump complications. *Prosthet Orthot Int* 2001; 25: 29–33.
13. Whittaker L, Wijesinghe LD, Berridge DC, Scott DJ. Do patients with critical limb ischaemia undergo multiple amputations after infrainguinal bypass surgery? *Eur J Vasc Endovasc Surg* 2001; 21: 427–431.
14. Cheshire NJ, Wolfe JH, Noone MA, Davies L, Drummond M. The economics of femorocrural reconstruction for critical leg ischaemia with and without autologous vein. *J Vasc Surg* 1992; 15: 167–174.

15. Bacourt F. Prospective randomized study of carbon-impregnated polytetrafluoroethylene grafts for below-knee popliteal and distal bypass: results at 2 years. The Association: Universitaire de Recherche en Chirurgie. *Ann Vasc Surg* 1997; **11**: 596–603.

16. Ruckert RI, Kruger U, Heise M, Settmacher U, Scholz H. [Femoro-distal ePTFE bypass grafting using femoro-crural patch prosthesis (FCPP). Results of a prospective clinical study]. Femoro-distale ePTFE-Bypassrekonstruktionen mittels femoro-kruraler Patchprothese (FCPP). Ergebnisse einer prospektiven klinischen Studie. *Zentralbl Chir* 2001; **126**: 144–150.

17. Raptis S, Miller JH. Influence of a vein cuff on polytetrafluoroethylene grafts for primary femoropopliteal bypass. *Br J Surg* 1995; **82**: 487–491.

18. Faries PL, Logerfo FW, Arora S *et al*. A comparative study of alternative conduits for lower extremity revascularization: all-autogenous conduit versus prosthetic grafts. *J Vasc Surg* 2000; **32**: 1080–1090.

19. Eagleton MJ, Ouriel K, Shortell C, Green RM. Femoral-infrapopliteal bypass with prosthetic grafts. *Surgery* 1999; **126**: 759–764.

20. Neville RF, Tempesta B, Sidway AN. Tibial bypass for limb salvage using polytetrafluoroethylene and a distal vein patch. *J Vasc Surg* 2001; **33**: 266–271.

21. Cavillon A, Melliere D, Allaire E *et al*. Are femoro-infrapopliteal bypasses worthwhile for limb salvage? *J Cardiovasc Surg (Torino)* 1998; **39**: 267–272.

22. Parsons RE, Suggs WD, Veith FJ *et al*. Polytetrafluoroethylene bypasses to infrapopliteal arteries without cuffs or patches: a better option than amputation in patients without autologous vein. *J Vasc Surg* 1996; **23**: 347–354.

23. Jacobs MJ, Gregoric ID, Reul GJ. Prosthetic graft placement and creation of a distal arteriovenous fistula for secondary vascular reconstruction in patients with severe limb ischaemia. *J Vasc Surg* 1992; **15**: 612–618.

24. Fichelle JM, Marzelle J, Colacchio G, Gigou F, Cormier F, Cormier JM. Infrapopliteal polytetrafluoroethylene and composite bypass: factors influencing patency. *Ann Vasc Surg* 1995; **9**: 187–196.

25. Bastounis E, Georgopoulos S, Maltezos C, Alexiou D, Chiotopoulos D, Bramis J. PTFE-vein composite grafts for critical limb ischaemia: a valuable alternative to all-autogenous infrageniculate reconstructions. *Eur J Vasc Endovasc Surg* 1999; **18**: 127–132.

26. Ascer E, Gennaro M, Pollina RM *et al* Complementary distal arteriovenous fistula and deep vein interposition: a five-year experience with a new technique to improve infrapopliteal prosthetic bypass patency. *J Vasc Surg* 1996; **24**: 134–143.

27. Miller JH. The use of the vein cuff and polytetrafluoroethylene. In *Vascular and Endovascular Surgical Techniques* 4th edn. Greenhalgh RM (ed). London: WB Saunders, 2001: 353–365.

Prosthetic bypass should never cross the knee joint

Charing Cross Editorial Comments towards Consensus

The arguments are carefully rehearsed by the authors of these two chapters and it emerges that prosthetic bypass is certainly superior in the suprageniculate position. It has been argued that the prosthetic bypass in the thigh is even equivalent to vein. Clearly the problem comes when a prosthetic material crosses the knee. This is not new information. Perhaps the first prosthetic to be used to any extent in the femoral popliteal segment was Dacron and it rapidly became plain that Dacron had much better results when attached above the knee than below the knee. Subsequently polytetrafluoroethylene (PTFE), and other prosthetic materials were shown to have good results in the suprageniculate position. Therefore surgeons developed a preference for using vein to cross the knee. The problem arises of what to do when there is inadequate vein; whether prosthetic should be used at all. Prosthetic bypass to tibial vessels has produced a universally poor outcome but outcomes are better when anastamosis is made to the infrageniculate popliteal but even these are poor. This has accounted for the development of the modification of anastomosis such as the patch and the vein cuff. The argument for the use of these was to alter the compliance mismatch and to alter the shape of the anastomosis. More recently prosthetic bypasses are being fashioned in order to have a wider opening but it is too recent a concept to know if this is going to make any difference.

Is there an answer to this debate? No there is not! Certainly from the evidence, it is plain that vein is a preferable material to cross the knee joint and from this there is a logic to search for vein not only in the limb in question but in the other limb and the upper limbs also. Surgeons who distrust prosthetic material crossing the knee will go to inordinate lengths to cross the knee with a portion of vein found in one part of the body or another. Composite bypasses have had poor outcome and sequential bypasses, for example prosthetic to the suprageniculate position and vein crossing the knee, have improved outcome compared with composite grafts.

Should prosthetic ever cross the knee? Yes of course. One should be aware that the risks of failure are much greater than the vein. Research goes on for a prosthetic material to do the job satisfactorily when there is no other possibility.

Against all of this subintimal angioplasty has become available. This procedure was treated with great suspicion when first introduced but now is finding favour in more centres and could lead to substantial reduction of femoropopliteal bypasses to the infrageniculate position.

Roger M Greenhalgh
Editor

Balloon embolectomy is the first-line treatment for acute limb ischaemia

For the motion
Bradley B Hill, Thomas J Fogarty

Introduction

By the early 1960s, treatment for acute limb ischaemia involved various techniques for removing thrombus including retrograde flushing, suction catheter aspiration and direct operative exploration of the occluded vessel. Despite what seemed to be heroic efforts limb salvage rates were typically between 30 and 50% even in the best hands. After introduction of the Fogarty® balloon embolectomy catheter, limb salvage rates increased to approximately 90%.[1] Initial experience with balloon thromboembolectomy usually involved emboli of cardiac origin. Onset of symptoms was abrupt and clot retrieval was simple because emboli and propagated thrombus were usually loosely adherent. As the incidence of atherosclerosis has increased with the aging population, more *in situ* thrombosis has been responsible for native arterial and bypass graft occlusion. In response to this aetiological change, improved tools have been developed to remove adherent clot and treat the underlying arterial pathology. Technology to treat this condition is continually evolving and consequently current methods involve minimally invasive or percutaneous procedures for restoring limb perfusion quickly with limited associated morbidity.

The physiological effects of acute arterial occlusion are fairly consistent and depend primarily on the magnitude and duration of ischaemia. Necrosis of tissue occurs uniformly in the setting of acute ischaemia lasting more than 6 to 12 hours with nerve tissue being most sensitive. Reperfusion of profoundly ischaemic tissue may not always successfully salvage the limb and the resulting systemic toxicity can have devastating consequences. Systemic hyperkalaemia and acidosis, myoglobinaemia, and liberation of oxygen-free radicals may cause lethal arrhythmias, precipitate renal failure and incite a systemic inflammatory state producing multisystem organ dysfunction.

The primary indication for urgent or emergent balloon thromboembolectomy is arterial insufficiency with an associated abrupt onset of symptoms. Embolectomy alone will often facilitate rapid and complete tissue reperfusion and recovery of function. The procedure is best performed in the operating room or angiography suite without delay. Patients with normal pulses and arterial pressure in the contralateral limb usually do not require preoperative angiography. Completion angiography is useful, however, for evaluation of the arterial outflow and to document arterial patency. The acute onset of worsening symptoms in the setting of chronic arterial ischaemia is more complicated and arteriography becomes a critical part of the revascularization procedure.

Technique and illustrations

Treatment for acute limb ischaemia is determined by the patient's presenting symptoms and physical examination findings. Patients who have loss of motor or sensory function at the time of initial evaluation have limb-threatening ischaemia and are at high risk for loss of limb or life. The most expeditious treatment is necessary and the standard procedure is operative thromboembolectomy in a surgical setting where adjunctive procedures such as arteriography and arterial bypass can be performed as part of the definitive procedure.

The patient is fully anticoagulated immediately after making the diagnosis. The treating surgeon facilitates prompt transport of the patient to the operating room without delay. If preoperative angiography is indicated, delays must avoided. Intraoperative angiography can be performed instead if necessary. The technique of balloon thromboembolectomy is routine and most surgeons are familiar with it. In most circumstances local anaesthesia is effective and small incisions provide good exposure. For iliofemoral thrombus, a vertical groin incision is made and the distal common femoral artery is opened by transverse arteriotomy. This provides easy access to the iliac system, femoropopliteal and profunda femoris arteries. Fogarty® arterial embolectomy catheters (Edwards Lifesciences, Irvine, CA) are available in sizes from 2 F to 7 F to accommodate all peripheral vessel diameters (Fig. 1). When

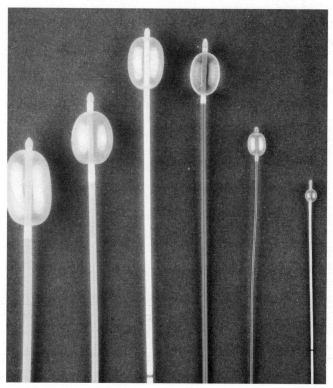

Figure 1. Fogarty® arterial embolectomy catheters in sizes ranging from 2 F to 7 F utilized to clear occlusive clot from in the peripheral vasculature.

working from the common femoral artery 3 F to 5 F catheters are typically used. Thru-lumen Fogarty® catheters are guidewire compatible and can be used to extract tibial artery thrombus with enabling fluoroscopic guidance and angiography. Directly approaching the tibial arteries through a popliteal incision is sometimes required and direct pedal artery thromboembolectomy may even be required in rare instances. Local delivery of thrombolytic agents into thrombosed distal vascular beds can be effective in restoring tissue perfusion at the time of surgery.

Additional adjunctive devices and methods can be utilized for difficult cases with *in situ* thrombosis and adherent clot. The Adherent Clot Catheter is often useful in native arteries while the Graft Thrombectomy Catheter (Edwards Lifesciences, Irvine, CA) has proven efficacious for prosthetic grafts to remove tenacious thrombus and fibrinous material from the luminal surface (Figs 2 and 3).

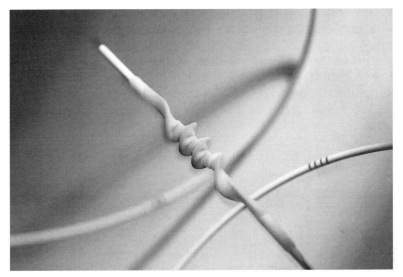

Figure 2. Working end of the Adherent Clot Catheter's latex covered corkscrew tip used to extract tenacious material from native vessels.

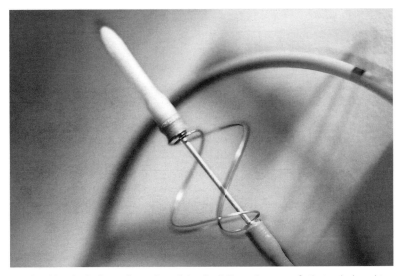

Figure 3. Double wire helix configuration of the Graft Thrombectomy Catheter designed to remove adherent thrombus from synthetic grafts.

Numerous percutaneous mechanical thrombectomy devices are also available. An extensive review of this technology is provided by Sharafuddin and Hicks.[2] These devices can be classified by their principles of action:

1. *Percutaneous aspiration thrombectomy* involves removal of thrombus by aspiration through a large lumen catheter or sheath. (SPAT/Balt Extrusion, Montmonrency, France; Stark catheter/Angiomed Bard, Covington, GA)
2. *Pullback thrombectomy and trapping* utilizes a balloon catheter or basket to collect thrombus which is then removed with a retrievable trapping device. (Greenfield pulmonary embolectomy/ Boston ScientificVascular,Quincy, MA; Syntel embolectomy and Latis graft cleaning catheter/Applied Medical Resources, Santa Margarita, CA)
3. *Rotational and hydraulic recirculation thrombectomy* involves microfragmentation of thrombus by the action of a hydrodynamic vortex (Helix Clot Buster/MicroVena, White Bear Lake, MN; Kensey Trac-Wright catheter/Dow Corning Wright Theratek International, Miami, FL; Angiojet/Possis Medical, Minneapolis, MN; Oasis/Boston Scientific Vascular, Quincy, MA, Hydrolyser/Cordis, Miami, FL)
4. *Non-recirculating mechanical thrombectomy* uses low speed rotation or cutting blades to break up the clot with or without aspiration (Arrow Trerotola PDT basket/Arrow International, Redding, PA: Atherotrack atherectomy catheter/Mallinckrodt, St. Louis, MO; Cragg and Castaneda brushes/Micro Therapeutics, Irvine, CA; Gelbfish Endo-Vac/NeoVascular Technologies, NYC, NY)

While balloon extraction thromboembolectomy continues to be the most widely used method to remove clot, percutaneous thrombectomy and thrombolysis, techniques are improving and becoming increasingly popular. Improvements in device design and techniques continue to be made in an attempt to minimize arterial trauma. Two new devices, the Solera Thrombectomy Catheter (Fig. 4) and Trellis System (Fig. 5) (Bacchus Vascular, Santa Clara, CA) are examples of new technology that may improve percutaneous treatment and shorten the time required for thrombolytic therapy.

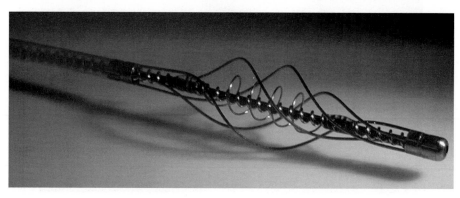

Figure 4. A close up view of the percutaneous Solera Device tip used to macerate and aspirate thrombus.

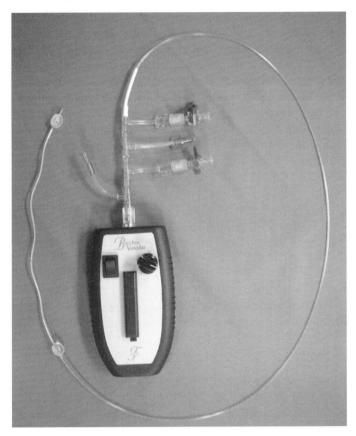

Figure 5. The Bacchus Vascular Trellis system's vibratory pharmacomechanical platform provides localized dissolution of blood clots using low doses of thrombolytic agents over a short time.

Evidence

Thrombolysis for treatment of acute limb ischaemia has typically had a high failure rate and many patients progressed to subsequent amputation or bypass surgery. In a review of 100 consecutively treated patients, Korn and found that 9% underwent major amputation and 20% required surgical revascularization after initial thrombolysis.[3]

Long-term outcome is better with surgical treatment and thrombolyis has a higher associated risk of haemorrhagic complications. The Cochrane Review Group on Peripheral Vascular Diseases reviewed all randomized studies comparing thrombolysis and surgery in the management of acute limb ischaemia. Patients with native vessel thrombosis of less than 14 days duration had a more favourable outcome with initial surgery than with thrombolysis at 1 year due to persistent ischaemia and higher amputation rate in the thrombolysis group (64% and 10% vs 35% and 0% respectively, p<0.0001). Mortality rate was equal in both groups (STILE: Surgery versus Thrombolysis for Ischaemia of the Lower Extremity; n=393). The review also revealed a higher overall risk of haemorrhagic complications, including stroke, with the thrombolysis-treated patients than with the surgical cohort.[4]

Persistent foot ischaemia after thromboembolectomy is usually related to residual thrombus in the distal runoff bed. Intraoperative use of fibrinolytic agents after catheter embolectomy has been described by numerous authors after this technique was initially reported by Quinones-Baldrich and associates in 1985.[5-9] These studies suggest that local bolus infusion of thrombolytics during surgery, or over a 30-minute period with proximal arterial clamping, can be a useful adjunct when persistent ischaemia is present after re-establishing arterial inflow. Success rates range from 74 to 100%.

Summary

- Acute limb ischaemia with loss of function requires urgent and definitive treatment which is best accomplished with surgical balloon catheter treatment.

- When acute ischaemia is not limb-threatening, initial thrombolytic treatment may be indicated but:

  Initial thrombolysis is fraught with uncertainty and is usually time dependent.
  Initial thrombolysis is associated with a higher incidence of recurrent ischaemia and subsequent amputation than surgical treatment.
  Initial thrombolysis has a higher overall incidence of haemorrhagic complications (including stroke) than surgical treatment.

- In certain instances surgical treatment is required because of underlying stenosis which does not lend itself well to treatment using endoluminal techniques such as angioplasty with or without stenting.

- Surgical thromboembolectomy can be combined with adjunctive catheter-mediated therapies or local delivery of thrombolytic agents for a single definitive procedure.

- Percutaneous thrombectomy and thrombolysis techniques are improving and evolving and may change the 'standard of treatment' for acute arterial ischaemia management over time.

References

1. Green RM, DeWeese JA, Rob CG. Arterial embolectomy before and after the Fogarty catheter. *Surgery* 1975; **77**: 24–33.
2. Sharafuddin MJA, Hicks ME. Current status of percutaneous mechanical thrombectomy. Part II. Devices and mechanisms of action. *J Vasc Interv Radiol* 1998; **9**: 15–31.
3. Korn P, Khilnani NM, Fellers JC *et al*. Thrombolysis for native arterial occlusions of the lower extremities: clinical outcome and cost. *J Vasc Surg* 2001; **33**: 1148–1157.
4. Berridge DC, Kessel D, Robertson I. Surgery versus thrombolysis for acute limb ischemia: initial management. *Cochrane Database Syst Rev 4*, 2000; CD002784.
5. Quinones-Baldrich WJ, Zierler RE, Hiatt JC. Intraoperative fibrinolytic therapy: an adjunct to catheter thromboembolectomy. *J Vasc Surg* 1985; **2**: 319–326.
6. Norem RF II, Short DH, Kerstein MD: Role of intraoperative fibrinolytic therapy in acute arterial occlusion. *Surg Gynecol Obstet* 1988; **167**: 87–91.
7. Gonzalez-Fajardo JA, Perez-Buckhardt JL, Mateo AM. Intraoperative fibrinolytic therapy for salvage of limbs with acute arterial ischemia: an adjunct to thromboembolectomy 1995; **9**: 179–186.
8. Parent FN III, Bernhard VM, Pabst TS III *et al*. Fibrinolytic treatment of residual thrombus after catheter embolectomy for severe lower limb ischemia. *J Vasc Surg* 1989; **9**: 153–160.
9. Comerota AJ, White JV, Grosh JD. Intraoperative intra-arterial thrombolytic therapy for salvage of limbs in patients with distal arterial thrombosis. *Surg Gynecol Obstet* 1989; **169**: 283–289.

Balloon embolectomy is the first-line treatment for acute limb ischaemia

Against the motion
Kenneth Ouriel

Introduction

The acute occlusion of a peripheral artery is a catastrophic event. Whether from *in situ* thrombosis of a native artery or bypass graft or from embolization, the acute limb ischaemia threatens both the patient's limb and life (Table 1). A now classic study by Blaisdell, published over 20 years ago, documented amputation and mortality rates in excess of 25% each following open surgical repair for acute leg ischaemia.[1] Despite improvements in operative technique and postoperative patient care, more recent series continue to verify unacceptably high rates of morbidity. Jivegård *et al.* observed a 20% mortality rate in patients treated operatively.[2] Even the more recent prospective studies of selected patients with recent peripheral arterial occlusions observed rates of limb loss and death that exceed desired targets.[3–6]

Table 1. Early (in-hospital or 30-day) rates of amputation and death in selected series of patients with recent peripheral arterial occlusion, treated with primary open surgical intervention

Study	Year	Amputation rate (%)	Mortality rate (%)
Blaisdell[1]	1978	25%	30%
Jivegård[2]	1988	–	20%
Rochester[7]	1994	14%	18%
STILE[5]	1994	5%	6%
TOPAS[13]	1998	2%	5%

Thus, the risk of morbidity and mortality following open surgical intervention remains at an unacceptably high level. What factors explain this finding? Clearly, the baseline medical status of the patients that present with acute peripheral arterial occlusion underlie the observation. Patients are frequently elderly, with a high rate of cardiac and other co-morbidities. They are ill equipped to tolerate the insult of ischaemia of an extremity, let alone an invasive surgical intervention to relieve the obstruction. A multivariable analysis of the data from the Rochester series uncovered several variables that were predictive of poor outcome, irrespective of the type of treatment instituted.[7] A summary of available literature would appear to confirm that individuals who present with acute, limb threatening ischaemia comprise one of the sickest subgroup of patients that the peripheral vascular practitioner is asked to treat.[8]

Evidence

There is some evidence to confirm the impression that a less invasive intervention is better tolerated in this very ill group of patients who develop acute limb ischaemia. Poor technique, inadequate devices and inferior agents coloured the initial experiences with catheter-directed thrombolytic therapy. For instance, the now well-accepted principle of ensuring infusion of the thrombolytic agent directly into the substance of the occluding thrombus was not always ardently adhered to. End-hole catheters were employed; it was not until the late 1980s that multi-sidehole catheters were available. Lastly, streptokinase was the most frequently used agent until the landmark article of McNamara in 1985 documented improved results with locally administered high-dose urokinase.[9]

There have been three well-controlled, randomized comparisons of thrombolytic therapy versus primary operation in patients with recent peripheral arterial occlusion. From the start, one must realize that thrombolytic therapy alone is seldom sufficient therapy. Successful pharmacological dissolution of thrombus must be followed by definitive therapy to address the underlying lesion that caused the occlusion. In fact, when no such lesion can be found, the risk of early rethrombosis is unacceptably high.[10] As testimony to this caveat, Sullivan observed post-thrombolytic 2-year patency rates of 79% in bypass grafts with flow-limiting lesions identified and corrected by angioplasty or surgery versus only 9.8% in those without such lesions.

The first study, the Rochester series, compared urokinase with primary operation in 114 patients presenting with what has subsequently been called 'hyperacute ischaemia.' Enrolled patients in this trial all had severely threatened limbs (Rutherford Class IIb) with mean symptom duration of approximately 2 days. This was a single-centre trial that was funded by the Thrombolysis and Thrombosis Program Project NIH grant at the University of Rochester. After 12 months of follow-up, 84% of patients randomized to urokinase were alive, compared with only 58% of patients randomized to primary operation (Fig. 1). By contrast, the rate of limb salvage was identical at 80%. A closer inspection of the raw data revealed that the defining variable for mortality differences was the development of cardiopulmonary complications during the periprocedural period. The rate of long-term mortality was high when such periprocedural complications occurred but was relatively low when they did not occur. It was only the fact that such complications occurred more commonly in patients taken directly to the operating theatre that explained the greater long-term mortality rate in the operative group.

The second prospective, randomized analysis of thrombolysis versus surgery was the Surgery or Thrombolysis for the Ischemic Lower Extremity (STILE) trial. Genentech (South San Francisco CA), the manufacturer of the Activase brand of rt-PA, funded the study. At its termination, 393 patients were randomized to one of three treatment groups, rt-PA, urokinase or primary operation. Subsequently, the two thrombolytic groups were combined for purposes of data analysis when the outcome was found to be similar. While the rate of the composite endpoint of untoward events was higher in the thrombolytic patients, the rate of the more relevant and objective endpoints of amputation and death were equivalent (Fig. 2). There appeared articles that comprised subgroup analyses of the STILE data, one relating to native artery occlusions[11] and one to bypass graft occlusions.[12] Thrombolysis appeared more effec-

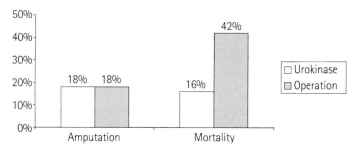

Figure 1. Rochester trial 12-month follow-up data. The rate of amputation was identical in the two treatment groups in the Rochester trial, but the mortality rate was significantly lower in patients assigned to the thrombolytic arm.

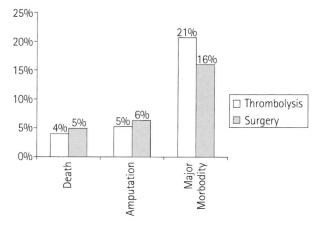

Figure 2. Outcome measures from the STILE data after 30 days of follow-up. Note that the rate of death and amputation are similar.

tive in patients with graft occlusions. The rate of major amputation was higher in native arterial occlusions treated with thrombolysis (10% thrombolysis vs 0% surgery at 1 year; p = 0.0024). By contrast, amputation was lower in patients with acute graft occlusions treated with thrombolysis (p = 0.026). These data suggest that thrombolysis may be of greatest benefit in patients with acute bypass graft occlusions of less than 14 days.

The third and final randomized comparison of thrombolysis and surgery was the Thrombolysis Or Peripheral Arterial Surgery (TOPAS) trial, funded by Abbott Laboratories (Abbott Park, IL). Following completion of a preliminary dose-ranging trial in 213 patients,[13] 544 patients were randomized to a recombinant form of uroki-nase or primary operative intervention. After a mean follow-up period of 1 year, the rate of amputation-free survival was identical in the two treatment groups, 68.2% and 68.8% in the urokinase and surgical patients, respectively (Table 2). While this trial failed to document improvement in survival or limb salvage with thrombolysis, fully 31.5% of the thrombolytic patients were alive without amputation with nothing more than a percutaneous procedure after 6 months of follow-up (Table 3). After one year, this number had decreased only slightly, with 25.7% alive, without amputation and with only percutaneous interventions. Thus, the original goal of the TOPAS trial, to generate data on which regulatory approval of recombinant urokinase would be

Table 2. Results of the TOPAS trial, demonstrating similar mortality rates and amputation-free survival rates in the thrombolytic and surgery groups

Intervention	Native-artery occlusions (n=242)			Bypass-graft occlusions (n=302)		
	Urokinase (n=122)	Surgery (n=120)	p value	Urokinase (n=150)	Surgery (n=152)	p value
Complete dissolution of clot on final angiogram – no./total no. of patients (%)	67/112 (60)	NA	–	100/134 (75)	NA	–
Increase in ankle – brachial index	0.44±0.04	0.52±0.04	0.15**	0.48±0.03	0.50±0.03	0.76**
Mortality – %						
6 months	20.8	15.9	0.33‡	12.1	9.4	0.45‡
1 year	24.6	19.6	0.36‡	16.2	15.0	0.77‡
Amputation-free survival – %						
6 months	67.6	76.1	0.15‡	75.2	73.9	0.79‡
1 year	61.2	71.4	0.10‡	68.2	68.8	0.91‡

*Plus-minus values are means ±SE. NA denotes not applicable.
**The p value was based on one-way analysis of variance.
‡The p value was based on Kaplan–Meier analysis.

Table 3. The thrombolytic group in the TOPAS trial achieved similar rates of limb-loss and mortality without the need for open surgical intervention in a significant number of patients

Intervention or outcome	Urokinase group (n=272)		Surgery group (n=272)	
	6 months	1 year	6 months	1 year
	no. of interventions			
Operative intervention				
Amputation	48	58	41	51
above the knee	22	25	19	26
below the knee	26	33	22	25
Open surgical procedures	315	351	551	590
major	102	116	177	193
moderate	89	98	136	145
minor	124	137	238	252
Percutaneous procedures	128	135	55	70
	% of patients			
Worst outcome				
Death	16.0	20.0	12.3	17.0
Amputation	12.2	15.0	12.9	13.1
above the knee	5.6	6.5	6.1	7.5
below the knee	6.6	8.5	6.8	5.6
Open surgical procedures	40.3	39.3	69.0	65.4
major	23.6	24.3	39.3	39.3
moderate	10.3	8.7	16.3	13.4
minor	6.4	6.3	13.4	12.7
Endovascular procedures	16.9	15.4	2.1	1.7
Medical treatment alone	14.6	10.3	3.7	2.8

based, was not achieved. Nevertheless, the findings confirmed that acute limb ischaemia could be managed with catheter-directed thrombolysis, achieving similar amputation and mortality rates but avoiding the need for open surgical procedures in a significant percentage of patients.

Summary

- The rate of amputation and death is much higher than expected when patients with acute limb ischaemia are treated by primary open surgical means.

- These rates remain high, in spite of technical improvements in the conduct of operative procedures and advances in perioperative patient care.

- The findings of prospective, randomized comparisons of thrombolytic therapy vs primary surgery are somewhat conflicting. Some observations appear valid, however:
    - mortality may be lower in medically compromised patients with very severe ischaemia when treated with thrombolysis (Rochester Trial),
    - patients with bypass graft thromboses fare better with thrombolysis than patients with native arterial occlusions (STILE Trial),
    - overall, thrombolysis offers the potential to achieve similar rates of mortality and limb salvage, avoiding the need for open surgical procedures in a significant proportion of patients (TOPAS Trial).

References

1. Blaisdell FW, Steele M, Allen RE. Management of acute lower extremity arterial ischemia due to embolism and thrombosis. *Surgery* 1978; **84**: 822–834.
2. Jivegård L, Holm J, Scherstén T. Acute limb ischemia due to arterial embolism or thrombosis: Influence of limb ischemia versus pre-existing cardiac disease on postoperative mortality rate. *J Cardiovasc Surg* 1988; **29**: 32–36.
3. Ouriel K, Shortell CK, DeWeese JA *et al.* A comparison of thrombolytic therapy with operative revascularization in the initial treatment of acute peripheral arterial ischemia. *J Vasc Surg* 1994; **19**: 1021–1030.
4. Ouriel K, Veith FJ, Sasahara AA. A comparison of recombinant urokinase with vascular surgery as initial treatment for acute arterial occlusion of the legs. *N Engl J Med* 1998; **338**: 1105–1111.
5. Anonymous. Results of a prospective randomized trial evaluating surgery versus thrombolysis for ischemia of the lower extremity. The STILE trial. *Ann Surg* 1994; **220**: 251–266.
6. Ouriel K, Kandarpa K, Schuerr DM *et al.* Prourokinase versus urokinase for recanalization of peripheral occlusions, safety and efficacy: the PURPOSE trial. *J Vasc Interv Radiol* 1999; **10**: 1083–1091.
7. Ouriel K, Veith FJ. Acute lower limb ischemia: determinants of outcome. *Surgery* 1998; **124**: 336–342.
8. Dormandy J, Heeck L, Vig S. Acute limb ischemia. *Semin Vasc Surg* 1999; **12**: 148–153.
9. McNamara TO, Fischer JR. Thrombolysis of peripheral arterial and graft occlusions: improved results using high-dose urokinase. *AJR* 1985; **144**: 769–775.
10. Sullivan KL, Gardiner GAJ, Kandarpa K *et al.* Efficacy of thrombolysis in infrainguinal bypass grafts. *Circulation* 1991; **83**(2:Suppl): 105.
11. Weaver FA, Comerota AJ, Youngblood M *et al.* Surgical revascularization vs thrombolysis for non-embolic lower extremity native artery occlusions: results of a prospective randomized trial. The STILE Investigators. Surgery vs Thrombolysis for Ischemia of the Lower Extremity. *J Vasc Surg* 1996; **24**: 513–521.
12. Comerota AJ, Weaver FA, Hosking JD *et al.* Results of a prospective, randomized trial of surgery versus thrombolysis for occluded lower extremity bypass grafts. *Am J Surg* 1996; **172**: 105–112.
13. Ouriel K, Veith FJ, Sasahara AA. Thrombolysis or peripheral arterial surgery: phase I results. TOPAS Investigators. *J Vasc Surg* 1996; **23**: 64–73.

Balloon embolectomy is the first-line treatment for acute limb ischaemia

Charing Cross Editorial Comments towards Consensus

Thomas Fogarty comes to town! Could we find anyone to oppose balloon embolectomy when Fogarty himself is proposing the motion and showing his balloon? Did he not revolutionize vascular surgical practice with this thought? Did he not give rise to the whole of endovascular surgery with balloon? Can we expect fireworks when he debates? Ken Ouriel is certainly up to it and he has given hard evidence comparing other treatments. The discussion by the surgeons who hear the debate will be crucial but it all probably hangs on the precise nature of the situation in question. For example, an acute-on-chronic situation was never best managed by balloon embolectomy and this brings the balloon into disrepute. On the other hand, lytic therapy can cause strokes unnecessarily in patients who can have a quick and easy balloon embolectomy even under local anaesthetic when it is plain that a single embolus needs to be fished out of a limb. The answer lies in the precise situation for which the procedures are required.

Roger M Greenhalgh
Editor

There is a place for primary amputation for critical ischaemia

For the motion

Hero van Urk

Amputation, one of the meanest, and yet one of the greatest operations in surgery: mean, when resorted to where better may be done – great, as the only step to give comfort and prolong life.

Sir William Fergusson, 1865

Introduction

The implicit aim of recommendation number 25 of the Second European Consensus Document on Chronic Critical Leg Ischaemia[1] is that attempts at reconstruction of a limb threatened by critical ischaemia should <u>not</u> be undertaken if there is a chance of less than 25% of saving the patient and his/her limb. In those cases primary amputation is one of the two options that are left, the other option being conservative treatment. Conservative treatment or 'tender loving care' can be an appropriate choice for elderly patients, with or without serious co-morbidity and not necessarily taking into consideration the probability of perioperative death. Refraining both from reconstruction and from amputation can be a wise decision for the patient as well as for the surgeon, thus avoiding a life-threatening or mutilating operation in the final phase of a patient's life. This option only underscores the fact that amputation is not always the inevitable consequence of not-attempting a vascular reconstruction. However, at the same time it stresses the importance of reliable assessment of the chances for a patient to survive a difficult operation <u>and</u> to save a useful limb, whilst being released of unbearable pain, taking into account that a relief that lasts only a short period usually only adds to the burden for the patient, as it ultimately still leads to amputation.

A reconstructive procedure should be attempted if there is a 25% chance of saving a useful limp for the patient for at least one year

Recommendation no. 25 [1]
Second European Consensus Document on
Chronic Critical Leg Ischaemia

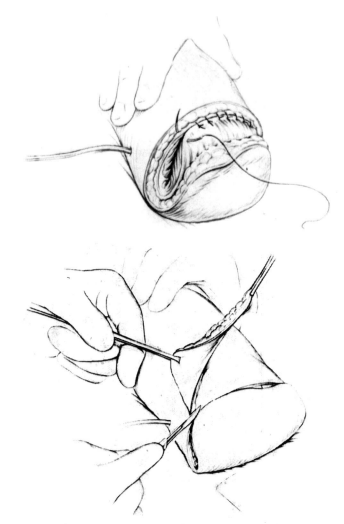

Figure 1. Posterior-flap below-knee amputation. Reproduced with permission from Ref. 31.

What are the drawbacks of arterial reconstruction?

Arterial reconstruction and percutaneous catheter interventions have become well-established procedures for peripheral arterial obstructive disease, particularly in advanced stages like chronic and acute critical ischaemia. The other side of the coin is that operations need repeating to maintain or restore patency of obstructed arteries or bypasses and the chances that a failed bypass operation may lead to a worsened local condition of the extremity, sometimes necessitating amputation at a higher level than might have been attainable initially.

The additional surgical or percutaneous procedures usually outnumber the original procedures. As a consequence, these repeated procedures contribute to the total costs of the initial procedure. This is reflected in the costs of healthcare, as extended and repeated hospital stays constitute a large proportion of these costs and hospital stays are inherently expensive.[2] These frequent hospital admissions reduce the quality of life whilst they are supposed to improve quality of life in the long run. In many cases the repeated major surgical procedures require general anaesthesia, which – for patients with increased cardiopulmonary risk – can put their lives at risk.

> The decision whether to reconstruct or amputate is always made clinically, and it is never possible to find absolute predictors for an adverse outcome; so there are no absolute contraindications to CLI surgery. Yet multiplying the estimated risk for known factors, when present, gives a clinical impression when not to perform infrapopliteal bypass surgery and, rather, to amputate.
>
> F Biancari *et al.*
> *World J Surg* 2000; 24: 727–738

In the case of an individual patient, the surgeon is faced with the question: 'is this patient likely to benefit from a vascular reconstruction or not?'. In other words: what are the chances of being able to perform a successful operation that keeps the patient alive and in possession of a useful limb for at least a period of one year? A 'successful reconstruction' is usually defined by its patency; patency, in turn, depends on many factors (in random order):[3,4]

1. the quality of the inflow tract,
2. the quality of the outflow tract, usually defined by the number of open crural vessels and availability of a patent pedal arch,
3. the availability of autologous (saphenous or other) veins of good quality,
4. the general condition of the patient – i.e. the presence or absence of serious co-morbidity measured as increased cardiac, pulmonary or renal risk[5]
5. the experience of the surgical/radiological/anaesthesiological team, including the quality of medical care available in the pertaining hospital,[6]
6. serum concentration of C-reactive protein,[4]
7. renal failure requiring long-term dialysis,[4]
8. patient gender.[7]

> Surgeons with lower annual experience of patients with vascular disease tended to undertake fewer revascularisation and more amputations then those treating larger numbers. The mean limb salvage rate achieved by surgeons with a lower throughput of vascular operations was significantly lower than that achieved by other groups of surgeons.
>
> National Survey on Critical Limb Ischaemia:
> VSSGBI[6]

Patency rates quoted in various publications vary widely from series to series and from hospital to hospital.[8] The number of variations and improvements of technique, materials and adjunctive procedures and medication seems endless.[9,10] Caution is needed to interpret the various ways of reporting, despite clear standards for reporting. Over the past decade general consensus seems to exist about the patency rates of various reconstructions and interventions (Table 1) for patients with critical ischaemia.

Table 1. Approximate patency rates of surgical reconstructions for critical leg ischaemia[11]

	1-year patency rate
Aortofemoral	90%
Femoropopliteal AK (vein)	75%
Femoropopliteal AK (prosthetic)	65%
Femoropopliteal BK (vein)	70%
Femoropopliteal BK (prosthetic)	60%
Femorotibial (vein)	70%
Femorotibial (prosthetic)	40%
Femoropedal (vein)	45%

For prosthetic bypasses impressive patency rates have been reported using various modifications of the 'vein cuff' principle, as introduced by Miller and further refined by Tyrell and Wolfe, or the use of a 'vein patch' as devised by Taylor.

All these adjunctive procedures are only as good as the hands of those who perform them but, especially for femorocrural bypasses, the use of a venous cuff or patch seems generally accepted for those patients who do not have an adequate vein and the use of prosthetic material is unavoidable.

Primary amputation

Primary amputation is the only and unavoidable choice for treatment, if there is no run-off below the popliteal artery, including the pedal arch, when no bypass surgery is technically feasible. Subintimal balloon angioplasty has been advocated even in cases of extensive crural occlusions, but also this technique is not feasible when no patent run-off vessel (distal crural or pedal artery) is available. This procedure is technically demanding and the reported good results are not easily duplicated by others.[12] Long-term patency in these cases is limited and 1-year patency is obtained in only 46% even in the best of hands.

Primary amputation is not a 'safe' operation: postoperative mortality is cited as 10–13%, assuming that the 0% achieved by Malone et al. is exceedingly low and probably only achievable in centres that have specialized in perioperative care for amputees.[13] As randomized trials comparing reconstruction with primary amputation are ethically unacceptable, only non-randomized prospective and retrospective series are available for comparison.[14]

> In the surgical management of the ischaemic lower extremity, amputation must be looked on as a prosthetic reconstruction.
>
> Burgess and Marsden (1974)[15]

In this regard, it is interesting to note that bypass surgery, just like for example laparoscopic surgery, was introduced and generally accepted as being beneficial without any formal evaluation. The Cochrane Library concluded in 2001 that the evidence for the effectiveness of bypass surgery is limited, and therefore no clear implications for practice can be drawn.[16] Nevertheless, most vascular surgeons intuitively agree that arterial reconstruction, even to crural vessels, is better and cheaper than amputation.[17] Gupta et al. (1988),[18] Callow and Mackey (1988)[19] and Bruijnen et al. (1989)[20] independently all concluded that primary arterial reconstruction using autologous vein in the ischaemic lower limb is substantially cheaper than amputation, a view that was supported in a prospective series by Cheshire and Wolfe in 1992.[21] However, when polytetrafluoroethylene (PTFE) grafts were used, secondary procedures were much more frequent, reducing the difference in costs to a mere 6% compared with amputation (including community care costs). These secondary operations accounted for 56% of the overall costs of arterial reconstructions to all levels in the leg.[2,21]

> Failed grafts have poor long-term patency and moderate limb salvage rates, and our data do not justify secondary procedures to attempt save failed grafts in patients with renal insufficiency.
>
> Rhodes *et al.*[22]

The high number of reoperations after reconstruction do not always reflect an improved outcome: one out of every three amputations was performed after failure of the primary graft without attempted revision. Aggressive secondary intervention has been advocated by Veith, claiming a reduction in secondary amputation rate from 41% to 14%.[22,23]

Several authors have voiced their concern that, if the primary graft and the secondary interventions fail, the level of amputations might have to be raised. Stirnemann retrospectively found that 30% of patients with failed reconstructions required above-knee amputations as opposed to 13% in patients with primary amputations.[24] Primary wound healing was achieved in 68% of primary amputations as opposed to only 39% in amputations after reconstruction. The ultimate measurement to judge this phenomenon is probably the degree of rehabilitation and quality of life.[25]

> Few vascular surgeons fail to remember at least one patient whose limb became more ischaemic after closure of a graft
>
> Warren (1974)[26]

Quality of life

Data on quality of life after either vascular reconstruction or primary amputation are scarce. Most published series are retrospective in design. The results of these series should be considered with caution.

Thompson *et al.* analysed a self-assessment postal questionnaire and found that 1) infragenicular surgical reconstruction led to a higher quality of life than primary amputation, and 2) repeated interventions to maintain graft patency did not adversely affect the quality of life of patients following infragenicular reconstruction. In addition they demonstrated that quality of life scores of patients undergoing secondary amputation after failed reconstructions were similar to those of patients undergoing primary amputation.[27] Other authors came to the same conclusion. Based on these findings they recommended that, to attain the maximum quality of life in patients with critical ischaemia, femorodistal bypass should be performed wherever feasible. Johnson *et al.* were much more reserved, based on a part retrospective, part prospective open study.[28] They observed no difference in pain in the study groups, whereas mobility was – not surprisingly – better after limb salvage than after amputation. However, they also found increased anxiety among patients with limb salvage procedures and depression was significantly higher in this group compared with amputees. They concluded that, although limb salvage may be the most cost-effective way of managing limb-threatening ischaemia, up to 22% of vascular reconstructions are doomed to failure; the ultimate outcome in quality of life of patients undergoing amputation after failed attempts at limb salvage is almost as good as that of patients whose limbs are saved but at an overall cost which is greater than if primary amputation had been performed initially.[28]

> More accurate prediction of the likelihood of success of surgical reconstruction in CLI could lead to marked savings in human and financial terms.
>
> Johnson et al. (1995)[28]

The real problem in the management of the individual patient with limb-threatening ischaemia lies in our inability to calculate the chances of success of a limb salvage procedure.[29] The various factors that will affect outcome of a reconstructive procedure are known, but we don't know how to use them to calculate a risk profile for a given patient, both concerning the chances of surviving the operation and concerning the chances of long-term patency of the reconstruction.[3,17] When primary amputation seems the best option we still have difficulty to assess the chances of survival, primary woundhealing and good rehabilitation with a useful prosthesis.[30]

Since the cost of surgical reconstruction compared with primary amputation is not a decisive argument in either direction, the quality of life for the patient should play a major role. Here too, we fail to accurately predict the likelihood of being able to attain the highest quality for our patients. Until we have the tools to better predict our patients' future, primary amputation will play an important, but otherwise undetermined, role in the management of patients with limb-threatening arterial disease.

Summary

- In patients with chronic critical ischaemia of the lower limbs surgical reconstruction can usually be attempted, but will lead to failure within 1 year in about one-third of the cases.

- The cost of primary amputation is higher than the cost of vascular reconstruction. However, the cost of amputation after a failed vascular reconstruction is the highest of all.

- Several factors are known to have a negative effect on outcome of vascular reconstruction, but it is not possible to accurately predict a negative outcome.

- Quality of life after primary amputation is similar to quality of life after secondary amputation, but the latter is obtained at higher costs.

References

1. Second European Consensus Document on Chronic Critical Leg Ischaemia. *Circulation* 1991; **84**(4) (Suppl); *Eur J Vasc Surg* 1992; 6(Suppl A).
2. Jansen RMG, de Vries SO *et al*. Cost-identification analysis of revascularization procedures on patients with peripheral arterial occlusive disease. *J Vasc Surg* 1998; **28**: 617–623.
3. Panayiotopoulos YP, Edmondson RA *et al*. A scoring system to predict the outcome of long femorodistal arterial bypass grafts to single calf or pedal vessels. *Eur J Vasc Endovasc Surg* 1998; **15**: 380–386.

4. Biancari F, Kantonen I *et al*. Limits of infrapopliteal bypass surgery for critical leg ischaemia: when not to reconstruct. *World J Surg* 2000; **24**: 727–733.

5. Kwolek CJ *et al*. Peripheral vascular bypass in juvenile-onset diabetes mellitus: are aggressive revascularization attempts justified? *J Vasc Surg* 1992; **15**: 394–401.

6. VSSGBI. Critical limb ischaemia: management and outcome. Report of a national survey. *Eur J Vasc Endovasc Surg* 1995; **10**: 108–113.

7. Troeng T. Swedish Vascular Registry: National adverse outcomes following distal revascularization for critical limb ischaemia. *Vascular Symposium on Critical Limb Ischaemia, Rigshospitalet Copenhagen* 1996; **6**: 7–8.

8. Califf RM, Eisenstein EL. Critical concepts in cost-effectiveness for cardiovascular specialists. *AHJ* 2000; **140**: 143–147.

9. Connors JP, Walsh DB *et al*. Pedal branch artery bypass: A viable limb salvage option. *J Vasc Surg* 2000; **32**: 1071–1079.

10. Kalra M, Gloviczki P *et al*. Limb salvage after successful pedal bypass grafting is associated with improved long-term survival. *J Vasc Surg* 2001; **33**: 6–16.

11. Branchereau A, Myhre HO *et al*. When to attempt a reconstructive procedure. Second European Consensus Document on Chronic Critical Leg Ischaemia. *Eur J Vasc Surg* (1992; **6** (Suppl.)

12. Muradin GSR, Hunink MGM. Cost and patency rate targets for the development of endovascular device to treat femoropopliteal arterial disease. *Radiology* 2001; **218**: 464–469.

13. Malone JM, Moore WS *et al*. Therapeutic and economic impact of a modern amputation program. *Ann Surg* 1979; **189**: 798–802.

14. Dormandy J *et al*. Major amputations: clinical patterns and Predictors. *Semin Vasc Surg* 1999; **12**: 154–161.

15. Burgess EM, Marsden FW. Major lower extremity amputations following arterial reconstruction. *Arch Surg* 1974; **108**: 655–660.

16. Leng GC, Davis M, Baker D. Bypass surgery for chronic lower limb ischaemia (Cochrane Review). In: *The Cochrane Library* Issue 4, 2001

17. Panayiotopoulos YP, Tyrell MR *et al*. Outcome and cost analysis after femorocrural and femoropedal grafting for critical limb ischaemia. *Br J Surg* 1997; **84**: 207–212.

18. Gupta S, Veith F, Ascer E, Flores S, Gliedman M. Cost factors in limb threatening ischaemia due to infrainguinal arteriosclerosis. *Eur J Vasc Surg* 1988; **3**: 151–154.

19. Callow A, Mackey W. Costs and benefits of prosthetic vascular surgery. *Int Surg* 1988; **73**: 237–240.

20. Bruijnen H, Loeprecht H. Kosten-Nutzen Analyse der Beinerhaltung. *Lagenbecks Arch Chir* Suppl II.

21. Cheshire NJW, Wolfe JHN *et al*. The economics of femorocrural reconstruction for critical leg ischaemia with and without autologous vein. *J Vasc Surg* 1992; **15**: 167–175.

22. Rhodes JM, Gloviczky P *et al*. The benefits of secondary interventions in patients with failing or failed pedal bypass grafts. *Am J Surg* 1999; **178**: 151–155.

23. Veith F, Gupta S, Wengetter K *et al*. Changing arteriosclerotic disease patterns and management strategies in lower-limb threatening ischaemia. *Ann Surg* 1990; **212**: 402–414.

24. Stirnemann P, Walpoth B *et al*. Failed vascular reconstruction may place patients at increased risk for higher levels of amputation. *Surgery* 1992; **111**: 363–368.

25. Luther M. Surgical treatment for chronic critical leg ischaemia: a 5 year follow-up of socio-economic outcome. *Eur J Vasc Endovasc Surg* 1997; **13**: 452–459.

26. Warren R. Editorial comment. *Arch Surg* 1974; **108**: 660.

27. Thompson MM, Sayers RD *et al*. Quality of life following infragenicular bypass and lower limb amputation. *Eur J Vasc Endovasc Surg* 1995; **9**: 310–313.

28. Johnson BF, Evans L *et al*. Surgery for limb threatening ischaemia: A reappraisal of the costs and benefits. *Eur J Vasc Endovasc Surg* 1995; **9**: 181–188.

29. Tyrrell MR, Wolfe JHN. Critical leg ischaemia: an appraisal of clinical definitions. *Br J Surg* 1993; **80**: 177–180.

30. Fowl RJ, Kempczinski RF. Success rates and failure rates, and causes of failure for common arterial reconstructive procedures. *Semin Vasc Surg* 1994; **7**: 132–138.

31. McCollam CN. Posterior-flap below-knee amputation. In *Vascular and Endovascular Surgical Techniques* 4th edn. Greenhalgh RM (ed). London: WB Saunders, 2001: 439–443.

There is a place for primary amputation for critical ischaemia

Against the motion
Jan D Blankensteijn

Introduction

Two legs are better than one. Unfortunately, an amputation for ischaemia cannot always be avoided. That is not the argument, as evidenced by a major lower limb amputation incidence of about 15–20 per 100 000.[1] The argument defended here is that, with the exception of the hopelessly non-ambulatory, neurologically impaired and institutionalized patients, revascularization always must be attempted, by any means, for any combination of risk factors, and in any given situation, no matter how extensive or difficult the proposed operative procedure might seem. In other words, if a leg is potentially salvageable, primary amputation is a bad choice. Case closed, as this is almost the exact wording of one of the recommendations on critical limb ischaemia made by the TransAtlantic Inter-Society Consensus (TASC) working group.[2]

Unfortunately, there is no clear definition of 'potentially salvageable'. This is where some surgeons take the easy way out, combining several arguments to label a leg beyond salvage and trying to convince the patient of being better off with an amputation. It maybe true for a subpopulation of all patients with critical limb ischaemia, but as long as very strong predictors of failure of revascularization are unavailable, it cannot and should not be suggested to the individual patient.

As will be recapitulated in this chapter, most arguments once used to give up on a leg primarily have been proven wrong. In addition, the disastrous consequences of major amputation will be reiterated to support the position of always trying to salvage a critically ischaemic limb.

Despite dramatic improvement in infrainguinal arterial reconstructive surgery over the past decades, many physicians persist in the belief that limb salvage should not be attempted in many patients with critical leg ischaemia. They continue to recommend primary amputation even though numerous reports on large patient groups have documented a dismal prognosis after ischaemic limb loss.

In the past, many reasons have been given for not taking the time and effort to revascularize. Diabetics, patients without any adequate autogenous vein, patients requiring a very long bypass to ankle or foot, and patients with large soft-tissue defects and renal insufficiency have been offered primary amputation as limb salvage was not considered worthwhile.

Citing a *Lancet* Editorial from 1992:[3]

> Success frequently depends on surgical skill and painstaking microsurgical technique. Preoperative and intraoperative advanced imaging modalities are required and postoperative graft surveillance with appropriate action in case of problems is necessary. Bypass surgery may take 2 hours or as long as 8 hours and it commits the surgeon to long-term responsibility. An amputation only takes 30–60 minutes and afterwards the surgeon can quickly devolve responsibility to the limb fitter and rehabilitation specialist.

If patients are denied an attempt at limb salvage for critical leg ischaemia it must be based on evidence that revascularization in certain patient subgroups is inferior to results achieved by primary amputation. This in turn may be based on anticipation of unacceptably high operative risk of revascularization, low revascularization patency, failure of successful revascularisation to achieve limb salvage, or an inferior cost-benefit ratio of revascularization compared with amputation.[4]

There are no randomized studies on the issue. As can be expected, most retrospective series on limb salvage for critical ischaemia seem to justify the selection criteria for revascularization used over the reporting period. Some authors have taken a very aggressive approach conceding to primary amputation only rarely (<5%),[4] while others have taken a more conservative attitude opting for revascularization in just over half of the cases.[5] Apart from the surgeon's attitude many other factors including hospital setting, geography and referral pattern play an important role in determining how large is the proportion of patients suitable for revascularization.

In the absence of randomized controlled trials on the subject, the level 3 and 4 evidence that is presented to challenge the title motion will attest to the statements in our **Summary** on page 385.

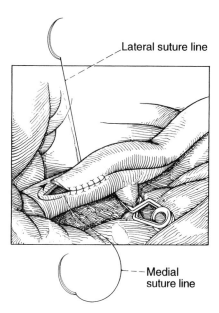

Lateral suture line

Medial
suture line

Figure 1. *In situ* saphenous vein arterial bypass by valve incision. After placement of as many sutures as the length of suture material allows, the vein is drawn down to the artery. Reproduced with permission from Ref. 40.

Evidence

Quality of life studies

It must be remembered that those patients who require limb salvage have high rates of other co-morbid diseases, including coronary disease, cerebrovascular disease, and diabetes, which may also influence the patient's quality of life.

Furthermore, all available evidence comparing quality of life after revascularization and amputation suffers from an important selection bias, as the quality of life at presentation itself may well be one of the most important determinants of the decision to revascularize or not.

Finally, in most amputation follow-up studies, rehabilitation is evaluated only in terms of mobility. Assessment of the overall quality of life after lower limb amputation also requires a more complex evaluation of social and psychological effects.

In a prospective study by Johnson,[6] various domains were prospectively studied: pain, mobility, anxiety, depression, self-care and life-style at presentation, and 6 and 12 months thereafter. The prospective design and the preoperative quality of life assessments for a large part ruled out differences at presentation between the revascularized and amputated patients. In Fig. 2, pain scores, mobility scores, Barthel ADL index and Frenchay lifestyles scores measured preoperatively, at 6 months and 1 year postoperatively are summarized.

Pain was improved in all patient groups but mobility was better in patients after limb salvage than after primary amputation. The patients' abilities for independent ADL (Barthel index) were maintained at high levels in both outcome groups with a surprising improvement in the amputation group but not quite as good as after bypass. Lifestyle was maintained at high levels only after revascularization and not after amputation. The authors concluded that limb salvage resulted in a better-maintained overall quality of life than amputation. Others have also found quality of life indices in patients with critical leg ischaemia to be improved if major amputation could be avoided.[8,9] In keeping with this, improved rehabilitation and mobility has been demonstrated after arterial revascularization in comparison with primary amputation.[5] Additional evidence is supplied by a large prospective study on the

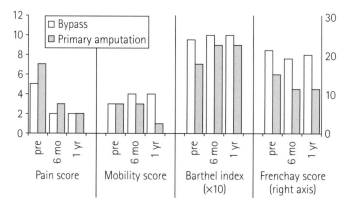

Figure 2. Various quality of life related scores as measured preoperatively (pre), 6 months (6 mo) and 1 year (1 yr) postoperatively, for bypass revascularization and primary amputation. Except for pain, higher scores represent improved outcome. Adapted from Johnson *et al.*[7]

effectiveness of oral anticoagulant therapy.[10] Revascularization enhanced quality of life and amputation seemed to be the worst possible outcome.

In octogenarians, improvement of quality of life was also found for successful revascularization but not for amputation.[11] Two-thirds of patients with salvaged limbs were able to return to their own home compared to only one-third after primary amputation. In addition, survival after 3 years was better for revascularized patients (60%) than for amputees (30%).

The walking ability has been demonstrated to be better after revascularization than after amputation.[12] In a prospective cohort study, Pernot et al.[1] studied the outcome of 191 major lower limb amputations. They found that after 1 year the majority of amputees have poor walking skills and the walking distance is limited. They are often ADL-dependent and their amputation greatly limits their daily function.

After an amputation, only about one-third of patients were able to walk with a prosthesis.[13] As many as 24%–50% of amputees are unable to leave their home even with assistance.[13]

In a retrospective study of the ambulatory status of patients initially presenting with critical limb ischaemia, at follow-up examination (1–7 years after the initial procedure), 65% of patients were walking independently after limb salvage compared with only 36% in patients who had undergone an amputation.[14]

In conclusion, limb salvage results in a better maintained overall quality of life, better overall survival, better rehabilitation and better chances of independent mobility than primary amputation.

High operative risk

Operative risk modifiers such as coronary disease, cerebrovascular disease, and diabetes are common among patients who require limb salvage. This has been used to oppose aggressive revascularization but it must be remembered that major limb amputation carries an operative mortality at least as high as limb salvage procedures.

Because a selective policy for bypass surgery tends to exclude patients with high operative risks, only series describing a very aggressive limb salvage policy would be representative for the operative mortality after surgical revascularization. In a large series of aggressive limb salvage in which fewer than 3% of all patients referred for limb-threatening ischaemia were treated with primary amputation, the operative mortality of revascularization was 2.3%.[4] In octogenarians the operative mortality for revascularization was 11% and 45% for primary amputees.[11]

In one study,[5] risk stratification was attempted retrospectively to minimize the natural bias associated with the tendency to perform revascularization in well patients and amputation in ill patients. Treatment modalities were compared in groups of patients categorized for the severity of concurrent medical illness. Operative mortality, ambulatory abilities, length of hospital stay and long-term survival were better for revascularized patients compared with amputees in all categories. Paradoxically, these differences were most significant as the degree of medical compromise increased. They conclude that an aggressive approach towards lower-extremity vascular reconstruction is warranted irrespective of medical status. In fact, the patients who benefit most from attempts at limb salvage are precisely those patients with the poorest operative risks.

In conclusion, the operative risks of primary amputation are at least as high as if not higher than those of revascularization.

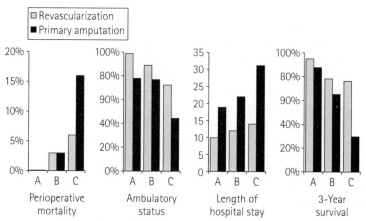

Figure 3. Perioperative mortality (%), ambulatory status (% of patients regaining full ambulatory status), mean length of hospital stay (days), 3-year cumulative survival after revascularization or primary amputation. Category A: ASA I or II; Category B: ASA III; Category C: ASA IV or V. Adapted from Ouriel *et al.*[5]

Low chance of success

There is a large variation in reported results of femorodistal bypass for critical limb ischaemia: from 30% 12-month patency[15] to almost 80% 5-year patency.[16] The European Consensus Document[17] suggested that patency rates for infrapopliteal grafts carried out for critical ischaemia should be about 70% at 12 months for vein grafts.

Reported limb salvage rates show a similar wide range reminiscent of the large variation of indications and selection criteria. Typical limb salvage rates are 70%–80% at 3 years,[4,18,19] even in the octogenarians.[20]

Adjunctive wound healing strategies such as free tissue transfer, vacuum devices, or topical growth factor therapies merit further investigation in an effort to augment limb salvage.

In summary, results of a low-threshold policy for limb revascularization justify an attempt at limb salvage in all but the exceptional patient.

Predicting failure of limb salvage

Saters *et al.*[18] tried to identify high-risk groups in the treatment of severe lower-limb ischaemia, but age, sex, presentation, diabetes, and ankle systolic pressure of 50 mmHg or less did not attain statistical significance as a predictor.

In two other studies, age was studied as an independent predictor of the outcome of limb revascularization. In a retrospective study, Hosie *et al.*[21] studied all patients over 70 years of age who were presented with lower-limb ischaemia over a given period of time. Of 214 patients, 46% had vascular reconstruction, 23% had primary amputation and 31% did not have a major operation. Mortality was high (31% at 6 months), but there was no significant difference between those having amputation and those having vascular reconstruction. However, the outcome of vascular reconstruction in surviving patients was better in terms of independent mobility (63/70 vs 16/38), long-term care (9/70 vs 22/38), use of hospital beds (27.2 vs 69.9 days) and was more acceptable to the patient. Nehler *et al.*[20] studied limb salvage in 88 octogenarians and concluded that an aggressive policy toward revascularization is appropriate in this age group. Although the percentage of institutionalized elderly patients increases with age, only 16% of men and 26% of women over the age of 85 reside in nursing homes.[22] On the other hand, rehabilitation potential in the elderly amputee is poor.[23] Very few learn to walk independently after amputation.

A few decades ago, several studies have reported higher mortality, amputation, and infection rates and lower limb salvage after peripheral arterial reconstruction in diabetics compared with non-diabetic patients.[24,25] More recent studies have shown similar salvage rates.[26,27]

End-stage renal disease has been associated repeatedly with bad outcome of infrainguinal revascularization.[28,29] These results have been challenged by others,[30-33] some authors reporting up to 84% limb salvage at 3 years in this patient group.[34] End-stage renal disease patients have poorer early morbidity due to a higher incidence of wound complications and lower overall survival rates.[35,36] Furthermore, analogous to non-end-stage renal disease patients, improved survival for patients with end-stage renal disease undergoing revascularization (44%) compared with primary amputation has been reported.[19] In one study of end-stage renal disease patients, no adequate predictors of failure of infrainguinal revascularization could be identified, although a heel ulcer of more than 4 cm may indicate an unsalvageable foot.[33] Yet others have demonstrated successful limb salvage in larger ulcers.[37]

In summary, the outcome of limb revascularization cannot be predicted by age, sex, presentation, ankle systolic pressure, or the presence of diabetes mellitus or end-stage renal disease. These factors cannot be used to give up on an ischaemically threatened limb.

Cost–benefit

In the UK National Health Service, a major amputation costs over £10 000 per patient while arterial reconstruction costs about half as much.[38,39] The mean total cost including long-term care is estimated around £33 000 for primary amputation vs £13 500 for the reconstructed patient.[11]

In conclusion, femorodistal bypass is more economic than primary amputation.

Summary

- The quality of life and ambulation after revascularization is substantially better than after amputation.
- The operative risks of primary amputation are at least as high as, if not higher than those of revascularization.
- A low chance of successful revascularization is not an argument not to try.
- Failure to revascularize a critically ischaemic limb cannot be predicted adequately to justify primary amputation.
- The cost-benefit ratios of primary amputation and revascularization support the latter.

References

1. Pernot HF, Winnubst GM, Cluitmans JJ, De Witte LP. Amputees in Limburg: incidence, morbidity and mortality, prosthetic supply, care utilisation and functional level after one year. *Prosthet Orthot Int* 2000; 24: 90–96.

2. Management of peripheral arterial disease (PAD). TransAtlantic Inter- Society Consensus (TASC). Section D: chronic critical limb ischaemia. *Eur J Vasc Endovasc Surg* 2000; 19 Suppl A: S144–S243.

3. Amputation or arterial reconstruction? *Lancet* 1992; 339: 900–901.

4. Taylor LM, Jr, Hamre D, Dalman RL, Porter JM. Limb salvage vs amputation for critical ischemia. The role of vascular surgery. *Arch Surg* 1991; 126: 1251–1257.

5. Ouriel K, Fiore WM, Geary JE. Limb-threatening ischemia in the medically compromised patient: amputation or revascularization? *Surgery* 1988; 104: 667–672.

6. Johnson BF, Singh S, Evans L *et al.* A prospective study of the effect of limb-threatening ischaemia and its surgical treatment on the quality of life. *Eur J Vasc Endovasc Surg* 1997; 13: 306–314.

7. Johnson BF, Evans L, Drury R *et al.* Surgery for limb threatening ischaemia: a reappraisal of the costs and benefits. *Eur J Vasc Endovasc Surg* 1995; 9: 181–188.

8. Chetter IC, Spark JI, Scott DJ *et al.* Prospective analysis of quality of life in patients following infrainguinal reconstruction for chronic critical ischaemia. *Br J Surg* 1998; 85: 951–955.

9. Albers M, Fratezi AC, De Luccia N. Assessment of quality of life of patients with severe ischemia as a result of infrainguinal arterial occlusive disease. *J Vasc Surg* 1992; 16: 54–59.

10. Tangelder MJ, McDonnel J, Van Busschbach JJ *et al.* Quality of life after infrainguinal bypass grafting surgery. Dutch Bypass Oral Anticoagulants or Aspirin (BOA) Study Group. *J Vasc Surg* 1999; 29: 913–919.

11. Humphreys WV, Evans F, Watkin G, Williams T. Critical limb ischaemia in patients over 80 years of age: options in a district general hospital. *Br J Surg* 1995; 82: 1361–1363.

12. Albers M, Fratezi AC, De Luccia N. Walking ability and quality of life as outcome measures in a comparison of arterial reconstruction and leg amputation for the treatment of vascular disease. *Eur J Vasc Endovasc Surg* 1996; 11: 308–314.

13. Pell JP, Donnan PT, Fowkes FG, Ruckley CV. Quality of life following lower limb amputation for peripheral arterial disease. *Eur J Vasc Surg* 1993; 7: 448–451.

14. Holtzman J, Caldwell M, Walvatne C, Kane R. Long-term functional status and quality of life after lower extremity revascularization. *J Vasc Surg* 1999; 29: 395–402.

15. Hobson RW, Lynch TG, Jamil Z *et al.* Results of revascularization and amputation in severe lower extremity ischemia: a five-year clinical experience. *J Vasc Surg* 1985; 2:174–185.

16. Leather RP, Shah DM, Chang BB, Kaufman JL. Resurrection of the *in situ* saphenous vein bypass. 1000 cases later. *Ann Surg* 1988; 208: 435–442.

17. Second European Consensus Document on chronic critical leg ischemia. *Eur J Vasc Surg* 1992; 6 Suppl A: 1–32.

18. Sayers RD, Thompson MM, Hartshorne T, Budd JS, Bell PR. Treatment and outcome of severe lower-limb ischaemia. *Br J Surg* 1994; 81: 521–523.

19. Whittemore AD, Donaldson MC, Mannick JA. Infrainguinal reconstruction for patients with chronic renal insufficiency. *J Vasc Surg* 1993; 17: 32–39.

20. Nehler MR, Moneta GL, Edwards JM *et al.* Surgery for chronic lower extremity ischemia in patients eighty or more years of age: operative results and assessment of postoperative independence. *J Vasc Surg* 1993; 18: 618–624.

21. Hosie KB, Kockelberg R, Newbury-Ecob RA, Callum KG, Nash JR. A retrospective review of the outcome of patients over 70 years of age considered for vascular reconstruction in a district general hospital. *Eur J Vasc Surg* 1990; 4: 313–315.

22. Rosenwaike I. A demographic portrait of the oldest old. *Milbank Mem Fund Q Health Soc* 1985; 63: 187–205.

23. Reyes RL, Leahey EB, Leahey EB Jr. Elderly patients with lower extremity amputations: three-year study in a rehabilitation setting. *Arch Phys Med Rehabil* 1977; 58: 116–123.

24. Cutler BS, Thompson JE, Kleinsasser LJ, Hempel GK. Autologus saphenous vein femoropopliteal bypass: analysis of 298 cases. *Surgery* 1976; 79: 325–331.

25. Reichle FA, Rankin KP, Tyson RR, Finestone AJ, Shuman CR. Long-term results of femoroinfrapopliteal bypass in diabetic patients with severe ischemia of the lower extremity. *Am J Surg* 1979; 137: 653–656.

26. Calle-Pascual AL, Duran A, Diaz A *et al.* Comparison of peripheral arterial reconstruction in diabetic and non-diabetic patients: a prospective clinic-based study. *Diabetes Res Clin Pract* 2001; 53: 129–136.

27. Karacagil S, Almgren B, Bowald S, Bergqvist D. Comparative analysis of patency, limb salvage and survival in diabetic and non-diabetic patients undergoing infrainguinal bypass surgery. *Diabet Med* 1995; 12: 537–541.

28. Leers SA, Reifsnyder T, Delmonte R, Caron M. Realistic expectations for pedal bypass grafts in patients with end-stage renal disease. *J Vasc Surg* 1998; 28: 976–980.

29. Edwards JM, Taylor LM, Jr, Porter JM. Limb salvage in end-stage renal disease (ESRD). Comparison of modern results in patients with and without ESRD. *Arch Surg* 1988; 123: 1164–1168.

30. Baele HR, Piotrowski JJ, Yuhas J, Anderson C, Alexander JJ. Infrainguinal bypass in patients with end-stage renal disease. *Surgery* 1995; 117: 319–324.

31. Chang BB, Paty PS, Shah DM, Kaufman JL, Leather RP. Results of infrainguinal bypass for limb salvage in patients with end-stage renal disease. *Surgery* 1990; 108: 742–746.

32. Meyerson SL, Skelly CL, Curi MA *et al.* Long-term results justify autogenous infrainguinal bypass grafting in patients with end-stage renal failure. *J Vasc Surg* 2001; 34: 27–33.

33. Lantis JC, Conte MS, Belkin M *et al.* Infrainguinal bypass grafting in patients with end-stage renal disease: improving outcomes? *J Vasc Surg* 2001; 33: 1171–1178.

34. Harrington EB, Harrington ME, Schanzer H, Haimov M. End-stage renal disease—is infrainguinal limb revascularization justified? *J Vasc Surg* 1990; 12: 691–695.

35. Harpavat M, Gahtan V, Ierardi R, Kerstein MD, Roberts AB. Does renal failure influence infrainguinal bypass graft outcome? *Am Surg* 1998; 64: 155–159.

36. Blankensteijn JD, Gertler JP, Petersen MJ *et al.* Avoiding infrainguinal bypass wound complications in patients with chronic renal insufficiency: the role of the anatomic plane. *Eur J Vasc Endovasc Surg* 1996; 11: 98–104.

37. Isiklar MH, Kulbaski M, MacDonald MJ, Lumsden AB. Infrainguinal bypass in end-stage renal disease: when is it justified? *Semin Vasc Surg* 1997; 10: 42–48.

38. Cheshire NJ, Wolfe JH, Noone MA, Davies L, Drummond M. The economics of femorocrural reconstruction for critical leg ischemia with and without autologous vein. *J Vasc Surg* 1992; 15: 167–174.

39. Panayiotopoulos YP, Tyrrell MR, Owen SE, Reidy JF, Taylor PR. Outcome and cost analysis after femorocrural and femoropedal grafting for critical limb ischaemia. *Br J Surg* 1997; 84: 207–212.

40. Leather RP, Shah DM, Chang BB, Clement Darling R. The *in situ* saphenous vein arterial bypass by valve incision. In *Vascular and Endovascular Surgical Techniques* 4th edn. Greenhalgh RM (ed). London: WB Saunders, 2001: 347–352.

There is a place for primary amputation for critical ischaemia • **Against the motion** • J D Blankensteijn

There is a place for primary amputation for critical ischaemia

Charing Cross Editorial Comments towards Consensus

Every vascular specialist is inclined to perform an arterial reconstruction by vascular or endovascular means to save a leg if they feel it is possible. Back in the late 1980s at a Charing Cross meeting on limb salvage and amputation for vascular disease we were prompted to review the outcome of 100 consecutive critical ischaemic patients: 89% had successful limb salvage in the sense that major amputation was not required. Of the remaining 11%, only 3% had above-knee amputation and 8% below-knee amputation. It seems an open and closed argument that arterial reconstruction of a vascular or endovascular nature should be undertaken but the problems come when reconstructions are attempted in patients in whom the chances of success are very poor. Such patients include those with severely calcified vessels with distal disease and poor run-off and also those with severe infection, especially those whose veins are inadequate for a long reconstruction. We have read about the claims of subintimal angioplasty elsewhere in this book. Undoubtedly, the argument for the occasional primary amputation is well made and I suspect that every vascular surgeon amongst our group will feel that on occasions a primary amputation is required. The question is how many times this should be performed. The absolutely disastrous situation is when an arterial reconstruction is performed with great pain and reduction in quality of life and then after that an amputation is required possibly at a higher level than would have been previously required and possibly with attendant infection. All vascular surgeons have seen this and this scenario translates into the most awful long-term hospital stay which outweighs much benefit at an attempt at reconstruction. Balance has to be struck and these chapters have gone a long way to identify the vital issues to be considered. Nevertheless it is still the specialist on the spot who has to decide on the optimal treatment at the moment.

Roger M Greenhalgh
Editor

Vein graft duplex surveillance is a waste of time

For the motion
DK Beattie, A Hawdon, AH Davies

Introduction

The increase in the availability of duplex scanning in recent years has been mirrored by an increase in the number of institutions entering those patients who have undergone infrainguinal arterial reconstruction with vein into vein graft surveillance programmes. The rationale behind this is the supposition that duplex scanning will detect haemodynamically significant lesions within the graft or within the inflow and outflow vessels, and that correction of these will improve both graft patency rates and limb salvage. This concept has not, however, been proven.

The delivery of healthcare to populations has undergone considerable change in recent years. This change has been provoked by a number of factors but perhaps most important is the vast increase in the range and complexity of diagnostic and therapeutic procedures available. Increasing pressure on resources means that, for a test or procedure to become accepted, efficacy must be proven. The burden of proof is also more rigid in that it requires not just an improvement in the health parameter being targeted, but a demonstrable effect on the patients' quality of life as measured by disease-specific or generic quality of life tools. Economic evaluation techniques are increasing in importance with cost-benefit, cost-effectiveness and cost-utility analyses the tools by which efficacy will be judged. This is the climate in which screening tests, diagnostic procedures, and interventions, surgical or otherwise, must be evaluated and it is as a consequence of this climate that the science of Health Economics is one of the fastest growing areas in modern health care delivery.

The above is demonstrated nowhere better than in the United Kingdom National Health Service. The current government has put in place a strategy, *The NHS Plan*, that aims to alter the manner in which health care is delivered to the nation. A key element of this plan has been the foundation of the National Institute for Clinical Excellence, a body mandated to analyse and make recommendations with respect to the efficacy of interventions and treatments. The Institute is charged with developing clear sets of clinical guidelines and these will be incorporated into National Service Frameworks that are specialty specific. By this means it is expected that treatment regimens will be standardized across the country *according to the best evidence* available, whilst ensuring that unproven or ineffective diagnostic tests and therapeutic manoeuvres do not become part of routine practice.

Given the above, it is appropriate to ask whether vein graft surveillance has sufficient weight of evidence behind it to withstand close scrutiny. If it does not it has no place currently in a modern health care system unless being applied under the scrutiny of a properly controlled trial. This chapter aims to demonstrate that there remains considerable doubt as to the value of vein graft surveillance. The corollary of this is that it may, indeed, be a waste of time as well as a considerable waste of valuable resources.

Vein graft surveillance may be considered as a screening test

The requirements of duplex ultrasound in graft surveillance are akin to those of a screening test applicable to a whole population. The duplex is looking for a specific problem – detection of the threatened 'at risk' graft in a well-defined population – those who have undergone infrainguinal arterial reconstruction with vein. Table 1 shows some of the criteria for the ideal screening test and it can be readily appreciated that they apply equally well to duplex used in the context of vein graft surveillance.

Table 1.   Requirements of a screening test / requirements of duplex ultrasound in vein graft surveillance

Requirements of the duplex

It should be easy to perform.
It should have few or no recognized side-effects.
It should have proven sensitivity and specificity in detecting the problem.
It should have good inter- and intra-observer reproducibility.
It should be cheap.
It should be readily available.

Requirements of the condition being screened for i.e. the 'at risk' graft

It should be detectable at a point where intervention is possible and will alter outcome.
There should be a demonstrable beneficial effect with respect to defined and accepted end-points.
There should be easily determined and agreed criteria as to what constitutes a positive test.
Intervention deemed appropriate as a result of the test should be of proven efficacy and should be cost-effective. The appropriate resources for such intervention should be available.

Requirements of the population

The population should be easily defined.
The population should find the test acceptable.

Evidence

Does duplex measure up?

In some respects duplex clearly meets the requirements detailed. It is applicable to an easily definable population, is non-invasive with no obvious side-effects and is hence acceptable. These criteria require no further consideration. In all other respects, however, there are serious question marks as to the use of duplex in graft surveillance.

The first issue to be addressed is that concerning the criteria by which benefit should be measured. Most published series suggest that benefit equates with improvements in primary-assisted and secondary patency rates. It is well recognized, however, that graft occlusion does not necessarily result in critical ischaemia or limb loss.[1] It may be argued pragmatically that patency of a bypass merely for the period required to heal any tissue loss may be considered a success. The hard and easily definable end-point of amputation is of far greater practical importance than graft patency. Sadly few series publish these important figures, and many argue strongly in favour of duplex surveillance solely on the basis of patency.[2,3]

The importance of assessing limb salvage was shown in a review by this department published in 1996.[4] We reported a summation analysis on a total of 6649 grafts taken both from published series where duplex surveillance had been employed and those where it had not. The results demonstrated that duplex surveillance had been responsible for an improvement in graft patency rates, but that no improvement in limb salvage had resulted. In performing the review it proved difficult to extract accurate data, primarily due to the variety of techniques that had been employed to confirm patency. This supports the importance of using the definite end-point of limb salvage. However, of 17 series only six reported amputation rates. At the time only one prospective study had been reported, that by Lundell et al.[5] This likewise showed improved graft patency but no alteration in limb salvage.

A more recent randomized trial looked at the end-points of patency and limb salvage in 185 grafts randomized to either duplex surveillance or simple ankle:brachial pressure index measurement.[6] There was no difference between the two groups with respect to either end-point. The difficulty of providing a comprehensive surveillance programme within the confines of a clinical service were, however, noted. The same group presented the results of a larger study a year later with the same conclusions.[7] Figure 1 shows the results of a meta-analysis of these two trials with respect to the effects of graft surveillance on both primary-assisted and secondary patency rates. The US Agency for Health Care Policy and Research classification for the grading of evidence and the strength of recommendations based on such evidence (Table 2) demonstrates how tenuous the current evidence for vein graft surveillance is.[8]

Table 2. The US Agency for Health Care Policy and Research classification for the grading of evidence and recommendations

Evidence

Ia.   Obtained from meta-analysis of randomized controlled trials.
Ib.   Obtained from at least one well-conducted randomized controlled trial.
IIa. Obtained from at least one controlled study without randomization.
IIb. Obtained from at least one other well-designed quasi-experimental study.
III. Obtained from expert committee reports and/or clinical experience of respected authorities.

Recommendation

A.   Requires at least one randomized controlled trial as part of a body of literature of overall good quality and consistency addressing the specific recommendation.
B.   Requires the availability of well conducted clinical studies but no randomized clinical trials on the topic of recommendation.
C.   Requires evidence obtained from expert committee reports and/or clinical experiences of respected authorities. Indicates the absence of directly applicable clinical studies of good quality.

The concept of graft surveillance has been built upon the supposition that a duplex-detected stenosis inevitably means a much-increased risk of graft failure and thus

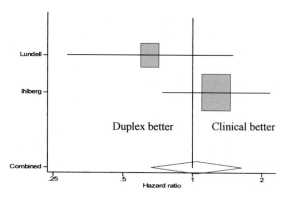

Figure 1a. Fixed effects meta-analysis of primary-assisted patency rates with graft surveillance.

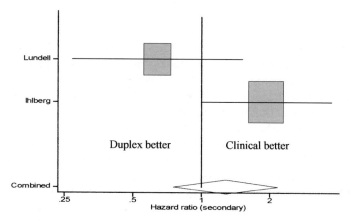

Figure 1b. Fixed effects meta-analysis of secondary patency rates with graft surveillance.

amputation. Detection and correction of such stenoses is hence deemed desirable. This has never been adequately proven, again primarily because most series do not publish amputation rates. There is, however, data to suggest that the opposite is true i.e. that although duplex can certainly detect graft stenosis, it is not able to distinguish those stenoses that are likely to lead to graft failure from those that are not.

In one study[9] only 12% of patients progressed to occlusion whereas it is recognized that up to 30% of grafts develop a stenosis, usually within 1 year. Revision of all duplex-detected stenoses is thus likely to result in multiple unnecessary operations. Furthermore the perceived greater sensitivity of duplex in detecting lesions did not translate into an improved outcome as there was no significant difference in outcome in those stenoses identified only by duplex, without synchronous symptomatology or ankle:brachial pressure change.

A study from Bristol[10] supports the above: 275 grafts were studied. In total 85 grafts subjected to surveillance developed a stenosis, 24 which were not treated. A further 28 of 64 that developed a *de novo* in-flow or out-flow problem were left untreated. At 12 months there were no differences between the cumulative patency rates for treated and untreated grafts. Other studies have left similar doubt. Barnes *et al.*[11] concluded that serial non-invasive studies do not herald postoperative failure of femoropopliteal or femorotibial bypass grafts and Mattos *et al.*[12] concluded that the majority of stenoses stay patent whether treated or not.

A large multicentred randomized trial assessing the benefits of duplex graft surveillance with respect to graft patency, limb salvage, quality of life analysis and cost-benefit is clearly needed before it can be stated confidently that duplex surveillance is not a waste of time. Fortunately such a trial is in progress.[13]

The above evidence demonstrates that duplex graft surveillance is of doubtable value with respect to many of the factors shown in Table 1, particularly the question of a demonstrable beneficial effect with respect to defined and accepted end-points.

Even if it is accepted that correction of a graft stenosis translated into improved limb salvage rates there are problems with respect to the other criteria, however.

The generally accepted duplex criteria for the identification of a haemodynamically significant stenosis are:

1. ABPI fall > 0.2.
2. Peak systolic velocity < 45 cm/s.
3. Increase in peak systolic velocity to > 150 cm/s.
4. Peak systolic velocity ratio across a stenosis > 2.0.

Standardized criteria mean that the reproducibility of duplex data from laboratory to laboratory must be excellent. Ihlberg et al.[14] investigated the interobserver agreement in duplex scanning for vein grafts and found a 'Kappa' value of 0.69. Statistically this equates merely to 'good' agreement and thus significant errors are introduced into what is already an inexact science.

There is debate as to the levels of peak systolic velocity and peak systolic velocity ratios that should be used to deem a graft 'at risk' without compromising either sensitivity or specificity unacceptable. A peak systolic velocity of 150cm/s and a ratio in excess of 2.0 are indicative of a stenosis in excess of 50%, a level at which haemodynamic significance is implied. However, there is evidence that, as long as a graft is surveyed every 3 months, a graft stenosis can be left untreated until the ratio is in excess of 3.0.[15] In one series, 46 grafts with duplex-detected abnormalities as defined by a peak systolic velocity ratio in excess of 3.0 were followed up.[16] Of the 46, just 14 grafts were revised at some point and just three occluded during follow-up.

All three demonstrated a peak systolic velocity ratio in excess of 7.0 before they occluded. Of great significance the same investigators performed a trial comparing the outcome for failing grafts as identified by duplex and where revision was undertaken with similar grafts where, despite the duplex findings, no revision was performed. The outcome with respect to primary and secondary patency rates, and with respect to limb salvage, was the same for the two groups.[17] This suggests that the currently accepted duplex criteria of a failing graft are significantly oversensitive and that the specificity of duplex in the detection of vein grafts that are truly at risk is unacceptable low. Furthermore, these criteria do not take into account factors such as graft diameter and outflow and the location of the distal anastomosis, all of which it is suggested are important.[18]

If the appropriate criteria for a failing graft are in some doubt, then so is the length of time for which a graft surveillance programme should run. The Leicester group studied 112 vein grafts using duplex surveillance.[19] Eight of 38 duplex-detected stenoses occurred more than a year after operation, the implication being that curtailment of duplex surveillance at a year would result in decreased primary-assisted patency rates. A further paper has re-confirmed their belief that duplex graft surveillance should be indefinite.[20] In the trial referred to earlier, Lundell et al.[5] found that there were only differences in patency between grafts randomized to duplex surveillance and those not followed up with duplex by the second year. There is significant evidence that refutes this however. Mills et al.[21] examined 91 grafts that were normal

3 months postoperatively and found that only two subsequently developed new stenoses. Furthermore, all grafts progressing to high-grade stenosis had a duplex-detected abnormality by 6 weeks. This suggests that a normal early postoperative duplex surveillance scan selects a group of patients who do not require and will not benefit from further intensive surveillance. A further study looking prospectively at 300 patients concluded that surveillance may be restricted to 6 months in those who have no abnormality within that period.[22]

A full appraisal of duplex-based graft surveillance requires, as noted above, consideration of not only patency and limb salvage rates, but also of the quality-of-life and economic aspects. Neither has been reported on in a prospective trial as yet and there is little data on quality of life. Some consideration of the economic aspects has been made, however.

The costs of a duplex-based graft surveillance programme are considerable. It has been estimated that to make a surveillance programme cost-effective, limb salvage rates would have to be improved by around 5%.[23]

It has been shown in a number of studies that the costs of primary reconstruction are cheaper than those of primary amputation. Panayiotopoulos *et al.*[24] looked at femorocrural and femoropedal bypass. Cost analysis showed that, in their hands, the median price of a successful bypass was £4320. This compared with a cost of £12 730 for primary amputation and £17 066 for amputation following a failed reconstruction. The primary determinant of cost was length of hospital stay, which was four times longer for amputees than for those who underwent successful reconstruction. It was noted that repeated attempts at revascularization significantly increased costs and the importance of identifying patients who would ultimately benefit most from amputation at an early stage was shown.

Singh *et al.*[25] reported their costs for the operative period and the 12 months beyond. Reconstruction for acute ischaemia had a median cost of £3970, but was increased to £6766 in chronic disease. Primary amputation cost £13 848. The costs of acute ischaemia were lower as the patients required much shorter rehabilitation. The differential between reconstruction in chronic disease and primary amputation was only maintained as long as repeated intervention was not required.

Data from Finland reflects the UK experience.[26] It was found that patients undergoing reconstruction needed frequent reinterventions for graft problems, further symptoms and revision of ischaemic tissue. Mean costs for reconstruction were 240 000 FIM or 70 000 FIM per survival year, including subsequent amputations. Where no amputation was required the corresponding costs were 175 000 and 47 000 FIM. Reconstruction with subsequent amputation was most expensive of all, costing 402 000 FIM per patient and 148 000 per year. Primary amputees cost 313 000 FIM or 150 000 FIM per year. Again the costs of amputation were shown to be considerably in excess of revascularization, where the latter is successful.

It is tempting to extrapolate these figures to the situation where the choice rests between intervention and non-intervention for a duplex-detected stenosis. This is wholly inappropriate, however, given that it has never been adequately shown that such a stenosis leads to inevitable critical ischaemia, nor that limb salvage rates are improved by a policy of intervention.

One recent study has looked at the economic effects of lower extremity bypass graft maintenance.[27] This retrospective study was performed due to the authors increasing concerns as to the volume and the cost of revision procedures deemed necessary consequent upon duplex surveillance; 155 grafts required 86 revisions; 36% of grafts were revised within 1 year. The mean costs of reconstruction and a subsequent 5-year graft maintenance programme were the same as those of primary amputation. Grafts revised for duplex-detected stenoses in comparison with those revised after graft occlusion demonstrated improved 1-year patency, required fewer amputations and were cheaper to treat. This was taken as justification for the considerable expenses associated with graft surveillance. No morbidity or quality of life data were presented with respect to those patients who may have undergone unnecessary revision for duplex-detected stenoses.

Conclusion

Vein graft surveillance programmes following infrainguinal arterial reconstruction with vein are becoming more common. There is little evidence, however, that the efficacy of the surveillance has been proven to the level required and expected in modern day surgery. Many standard techniques of assessment have not yet been applied prospectively to graft surveillance, though trials involving economic and quality of life analyses are on going. Put simply, it has never been shown which of the very large numbers of stenoses that are detected by a duplex programme are responsible for subsequent graft failure and amputation; indeed the literature contains significant data suggesting the opposite. If that is so, then duplex-based graft surveillance may indeed be a waste of time. Given that modern medicine requires adequate proof of the validity of a technique before its use becomes widespread, and given that this proof is not available, then duplex-based vein graft surveillance should currently be considered a waste of time. The situation may indeed be worse than this, however. If duplex surveillance is not effective in improving outcome than it follows that its use condemns many people to revision procedures from which they have no chance of benefiting. The quality-of-life of these patients is likely to be significantly worsened by these unnecessary procedures and, if this is the case, the use of this very expensive surveillance technique becomes untenable.

Summary

- Current opinion demands that techniques or procedures accepted into routine medical practice should be of proven efficacy. Level I evidence of such efficacy should be sought.

- There is no level I evidence available to support vein graft surveillance in terms of limb salvage rates and quality of life.

- Level I evidence with respect to graft patency is contradictory.

- There is poor agreement in the literature as to the duplex criteria that should be used in vein graft surveillance.

- There is poor agreement in the literature as to the optimum duration for vein graft surveillance.

- Until the above are addressed, recommendations for duplex-based vein graft surveillance programmes cannot be included in clinical guidelines or service frameworks following infrainguinal reconstruction with vein.

References

1. Brewster DC, Lasalle AJ, Robinson JG, Strayhorn EC, Darling RC. Femoropoliteal graft failures: Clinical consequences of success of secondary reconstructions. *Arch Surg* 1983; 118: 1043–1047.

2. Moody P, Gould DA, Harris PL. Vein graft surveillance improves patency in femoro-popliteal bypass. *Eur J Vasc Surg* 1990; 4: 117–121.

3. Dunlop P, Hartshorne T, Bolia A, Bell PR, London NJ. The long-term outcome of infrainguinal vein graft surveillance. *Eur J Vasc Endovasc Surg* 1995; 10: 352–355.

4. Golledge J, Beattie DK, Greenhalgh RM, Davies AH. Have the results of infrainguinal bypass improved with the widespread utilisation of postoperative surveillance? *Eur J Vasc Endovasc Surg* 1996; 11: 388–392.

5. Lundell A, Lindblad B, Bergqvist D, Hansen F. Femoropopliteal-crural graft patency is improved by an intensive graft surveillance programme: A prospective randomised study. *J Vasc Surg* 1995; 21: 26–34.

6. Ihlberg L, Luther M, Tierala E, Lapantalo M. The utility of duplex scanning in infrainguinal vein graft surveillance: results from a randomised controlled study. *Eur J Vasc Endovasc Surg* 1998; 16: 19–27.

7. Ihlberg L, Luther M, Alback A, Kantonen I, Lepantalo M. Does a completely accomplished duplex-based surveillance programme prevent vein-graft failure? *Eur J Vasc Endovasc Surg* 1999; 18: 395–400.

8. US Department of Health and Human Services. Agency for health care policy and research. The Agency; Clinical practice guidelines. AHCPR publication No 92-0023 1993: 107.

9. Grigg MJ, Nicolaides AN, Wolfe JH. Femorodistal vein bypass graft stenoses. *Br J Surg* 1988; 75: 737–740.

10. Wilson YG, Davies AH, Currie IC *et al*. Vein graft stenosis; incidence and intervention. *Eur J Vasc Endovasc Surg* 1996; 11: 164–169.

11. Barnes RW, Thompson BW, MacDonald CM *et al*. Serial non-invasive studies do not herald post-operative failure of femoropopliteal or femorotibial bypass grafts. *Ann Surg* 1989; 210: 486–493.

12. Mattos MA, Van Bremmelen PS, Hodgson KJ *et al*. Does correction of stenoses identified with colour duplex scanning improve infrainguinal graft patency? *J Vasc Surg* 1993; 17: 54–66.

13. Kirby PL, Brady AR, Thompson SG, Torgerson D, Davies AH. The vein graft surveillance trial: rationale, design and methods. VGST participants. *Eur J Vasc Endovasc Surg* 1999; 18: 469–474.

14. Ihlberg L, Alback A, Roth WD, Edgren J, Lepantalo M. Interobserver agreement in duplex scanning for vein grafts. *Eur J Vasc Endovasc Surg* 2000; 19: 504–508.

15. Olojugba DH, McCarthy MJ, Naylor AR, Bell PR, London NJ. At what peak velocity ratio should duplex-detected vein graft stenoses be revised? *Eur J Vasc Endovasc Surg* 1998; 15: 258–260.

16. Dougherty MJ, Calligaro KD, DeLaurentis DA. The natural history of 'failing' arterial bypass grafts in a duplex surveillance protocol. *Ann Vasc Surg* 1998; 12: 255–259.

17. Dougherty MJ, Calligaro KD, DeLaurentis DA. Revision of failing lower extremity bypass grafts. *Am J Surg* 1998; 176: 126–130.

18. Treiman GS, Lawrence PF, Bhirangi K, Gazak CE. Effect of outflow level and maximum graft diameter on the velocity parameters of reversed vein bypass grafts. *J Vasc Surg* 1999; 30: 16–25.

19. Mills JL, Harris EJ, Taylor LM, Beckett WC, Porter JM. The importance of routine surveillance of distal bypass grafts with duplex scanning: a study of 379 reversed vein grafts. *J Vasc Surg* 1990; 12: 379–386.

20. McCarthy MJ, Olojugba D, Loftus IM *et al*. Lower limb surveillance following autologous vein bypass should be life long. *Br J Surg* 1998; 85: 1369–1372.

21. Mills JL, Bandyk DF, Gahtan V, Esses G. The origin of infrainguinal vein graft stenosis: a prospective randomised trial based on duplex surveillance. *J Vasc Surg* 1995; 21: 16–25.

22. Idu MM, Buth J, Cuypers P *et al*. Economising vein-graft surveillance programmes. *Eur J Vasc Endovasc Surg* 1998; 15: 432–438.

23. Cheshire NJW, Wolfe JHN. Infrainguinal graft surveillance: a biased overview. *Sem Vasc Surg* 1993; 6: 143–149.

24. Panayiotopoulos YP, Tyrrell MR, Owen SE, Reidy JF, Taylor PR. Outcome and cost analysis after femorocrural and femoropedal grafting for critical limb ischaemia. *Br J Surg* 1997; 84: 207–212.

25. Singh S, Evans L, Datta D, Gaines P, Beard JD. The costs of managing lower limb-threatening ischaemia. *Eur J Vasc Endovasc Surg* 1996; 12: 359–362.

26. Luther M, Lepantalo M. Femorotibial reconstructions for chronic critical leg ischaemia: influence on outcome by diabetes, gender and age. *Eur J Vasc Endovasc Surg* 1997; 13: 569–577.

27. Wixon CL, Mills JL, Westerband A, Hughes JD, Ihnat DM. An economic appraisal of lower extremity bypass graft maintenance. *J Vasc Surg* 2000; 32: 1–12.

Vein graft duplex surveillance is a waste of time

Against the motion

Geoffrey L Gilling-Smith, Thomas Nicholas

Introduction

Duplex scanning is routinely employed to monitor infrainguinal vein graft performance during the first 12–24 months after operation. The justification for such a surveillance programme relies on a number of assumptions:

1. That infrainguinal vein grafts fail often enough and that the consequences of such failure are important enough that it is worth trying to prevent failure.
2. That the cause or causes of vein graft failure can be detected before failure occurs.
3. That duplex scanning is the most reliable and cost-effective method of detecting such causes of failure.
4. That secondary intervention to correct such causes prevents failure and improves the long-term clinical performance of the vein graft.

In order to determine whether or not duplex surveillance of vein grafts is indeed worthwhile, one must examine the validity of these assumptions.

The clinical problem

Numerous clinical reports attest to the limited durability of infrainguinal vein grafts. Primary patency rates are reported to vary between 52 and 67% after 2 years and between 49 and 76% after 4 years.[1,2] Thus up to one-third of vein grafts occlude within 2 years of surgery.

Vein graft failure is rarely a benign event. Thrombotic occlusion of the graft will often result in recurrence of the symptoms for which bypass was originally performed although it is important to note that vein grafts performed to treat critical limb-threatening ischaemia can sometimes occlude without such occlusion resulting in limb loss. This may reflect the development of a collateral circulation (unlikely) or it may indicate that the limb was not in fact as threatened as the surgeon thought. In many cases, however, amputation is not performed because the patient is unfit and/or because rest pain can be managed conservatively.

On the other hand, it is important to differentiate between thrombotic failure (graft occlusion) and clinical or haemodynamic failure. A reduction in blood flow through a narrowed but patent graft can result in recurrence of symptoms without necessarily resulting in thrombosis of the graft (i.e. haemodynamic and clinical failure despite continued technical success).

Causes of vein graft failure

Szilagyi first drew attention to the development of structural abnormalities in vein grafts throughout follow-up. He noted fibrotic strictures, progression of atherosclerosis and/or aneurysmal dilatation in almost one-third of 289 vein grafts followed angiographically for up to 5 years.[3]

In a prospective study of 227 vein grafts followed by serial duplex scanning, Mills et al.[4] subsequently documented haemodynamic or clinical failure in 47 grafts (21%). Failure was most commonly due to focal stenosis at or adjacent to proximal or distal anastomoses (28 cases) with a further 10 cases resulting from progression of inflow or outflow disease. The authors further noted that 70% of failures occurred within 12 months of operation and 80% within 18 months of operation.

Donaldson et al.[5] examined the causes of failure in 92 of 455 *in situ* vein grafts. In 48 cases, failure was attributed to focal peri-anastomotic stenosis, in 29 to focal mid-graft stenosis. Overall, 63% of failures were ascribed to structural abnormalities that had developed in the graft itself while in 37%, failure was attributed to extrinsic causes including progression of inflow and outflow disease.

Thus in a majority of cases, vein graft failure results from the development of focal lesions which reduce blood flow through the graft. Identification and correction of such lesions might be expected to improve blood flow and avert thrombosis.

Detection of the failing graft

Various strategies and techniques have been proposed to monitor vein graft performance.

Clinical review, although important, is of limited value. In one study, Veith et al.[6] noted that 80% of patients presenting with recurrent symptoms had already occluded their grafts. Others have confirmed the unreliability of clinical review alone.

Serial measurement of the ankle brachial index is more sensitive than simple clinical review but has also been shown to be unreliable. In one study, Wolfe et al.[7] noted that a fall in ankle brachial index identified only 50% of angiographically documented stenoses while Barnes et al.[8] noted that the risk of graft occlusion was no greater in patients who developed a fall in ankle brachial index than in those who did not.

Angiography remains the gold standard for detection of both focal graft stenoses and progression of inflow or outflow disease. There is general agreement, however, that this method is too invasive, time-consuming and costly for routine surveillance and attention has focussed, therefore, on non-invasive alternatives.

Duplex scanning is non-invasive, quick and relatively cheap. It can detect and assess the haemodynamic significance of focal stenoses. It can also detect low flow throughout a graft which is suggestive of inflow or outflow problems. The reliability of duplex scanning when compared with angiography is now well established.[9,10]

The natural history of vein graft stenosis

The natural history of haemodynamically significant vein graft stenosis remains largely unknown. There is widespread belief that the majority of vein graft stenoses will, if left untreated, result in graft occlusion. It is also generally held that the results of re-intervention to disobliterate an occluded graft are often disappointing. There is, therefore, an understandable reluctance to simply observe haemodynamically signif-icant graft stenoses. Once detected, they are usually corrected by secondary intervention.

It is, however, probable that some vein graft stenoses regress and/or do not result in graft thrombosis. It is also accepted that re-intervention to correct vein graft steno-sis is not always successful. Indeed, it may be argued that in some cases, attempted correction actually precipitates thrombosis that might not otherwise have occurred. What then is the evidence that intervention is beneficial ?

Does correction of graft stenosis improve outcome?

In an analysis of published reports of vein bypass grafting, Golledge et al.[11] compared the fate of 2680 vein grafts which had been monitored by serial duplex scanning with the fate of 3969 vein grafts that had not. The indications for operation and the level of distal anastomosis did not differ significantly between the two groups. The authors noted a significantly higher incidence of graft thrombosis (27%) in patients who had not undergone duplex surveillance when compared with those who had (15%). There was no statistically significant difference in the rate of limb loss but amputation rates were not, in fact, reported in 11 of the 17 publications reviewed to assess the results of duplex surveillance.

In a retrospective review of 251 vein grafts followed by duplex scanning, Wilson et al.[12] documented 85 angiographically confirmed stenoses in 59 patients; 40 of these stenoses were treated by secondary intervention while 45 were not. Cumulative 12-month patency was 87.5% in the treated group compared with 75% in the untreated group.

To date there has only been a single small prospective randomized study compar-ing combined clinical and duplex surveillance with clinical surveillance alone.[13] In this study, the fate of 45 vein grafts surveilled by duplex scanning was compared with the fate of 43 vein grafts that were not. Both primary assisted and secondary 3-year patency was significantly higher (78% and 82%) in the duplex surveillance group than in the clinical surveillance group (53% and 56%). It is interesting to note that clinical surveillance (including monitoring of ankle brachial index) identified only 13 of 18 failing grafts.

Conclusion

There is a need for larger prospective randomized studies to firmly establish the benefit of duplex surveillance of vein grafts, but it is clear from the available evi-dence that duplex scanning is not a waste of time.

Summary

- Vein graft failure is common and clinically significant.

- Vein graft failure most commonly results from the development of focal fibrotic strictures and from progression of inflow or outflow disease.

- Duplex scanning can reliably detect both focal graft stenoses and evidence of a reduction in graft flow secondary to progression of inflow or outflow disease.

- Duplex scanning has been shown to be more sensitive and reliable than clinical examination and/or serial measurement of the ankle brachial index.

- Duplex scanning is simpler, cheaper and less invasive than angiography.

- There is evidence that the incidence of vein graft thrombosis is reduced by secondary intervention to correct haemodynamically significant lesions noted on surveillance.

References

1. Veith FJ, Gupta SK, Ascer E *et al.* Six year prospective multicentre randomised comparison of autologous saphenous vein and expanded polytetrafluoroethylene grafts in infrainguinal arterial reconstructions. *J Vasc Surg* 1986; 3: 104–114.
2. Lawson JA, Tangelder MJD, Algra A, Eikelboom BC, on behalf of the Dutch BOA Study Group. The myth of the *in situ* graft: Superiority in infrainguinal bypass surgery? *Eur J Vasc Endovasc Surg* 1999; 18: 149–157.
3. Szilagyi DE, Elliott JP, Hageman JH, Smith RF, Dall'olmo CA. Biological fate of autogenous vein implants as arterial substitutes. *Annl Surg* 1973; 178: 232–245.
4. Mills JL, Fujitani RM, Taylor SM. The characteristics and anatomic distribution of lesions that cause reversed vein graft failure: a five year prospective study. *J Vasc Surg* 1993; 17: 195–206.
5. Donaldson MC, Mannick JA, Whittemore AD. Causes of primary graft failure after *in situ* saphenous vein bypass grafting. *J Vasc Surg* 1992; 15: 113–120.
6. Veith FJ, Weiser RK, Gupta SK. Diagnosis and management of failing lower extremity arterial reconstructions prior to graft occlusion. *J Cardiovasc Surg* 1984; 25: 381–384.
7. Wolfe JHN, Thomas ML, Jamieson CW *et al.* Early diagnosis of femoro-distal graft stenoses. *Br J Surg* 1987; 74: 268–270.
8. Barnes RW, Thompson BW, MacDonald CM. Serail non-invasive studies do not herald post operative failure of femoro-popliteal or femoro-tibial bypass grafts. *Annl Surg* 1989; 210: 486–494.
9. Taylor PR, Tyrrell MR, Crofton M. Colour flow imaging in the detection of femoro-distal graft and native artery stenosis: improved criteria. *Eur J Vasc Surg* 1992; 6: 232–236.
10. Davies AH, Magee TR, Tennant SGW *et al.* Criteria for identification of the at-risk infra-inguinal bypass graft. *Eur J Vasc Surg* 1994; 8: 315–319.
11. Golledge J, Beattie DK, Greenhalgh RM, Davies AH. Have the results of infrainguinal bypass improved with the widespread utilisation of postoperative surveillance? *Eur J Vasc Endovasc Surg* 1996; 11: 388–392.
12. Wilson YG, Davies AH, Currie IC *et al.* Vein graft stenosis: incidence and intervention. *Eur J Vasc Endovasc Surg* 1996; 11: 164–169.
13. Lundell A, Lindblad B, Bergqvist D, Hansen F. Femoropopliteal-crural graft patency is improved by an intensive surveillance program: a prospective randomised study. *J Vasc Surg* 1995; 21: 26–34.

Vein graft duplex surveillance is a waste of time

Charing Cross Editorial Comments towards Consensus

A decade ago vein graft surveillance was all the rage. Everyone was remiss unless they were doing it. Every duplex scanner was employed for accessing vein graft surveillance looking for stenoses and this produced a problem. What should one do next? Should it be scheduled for angioplasty? Should a stent be used? Would an operation be better? What was the evidence that any intervention was beneficial? What measures would one consider to be important to justify vein graft surveillance? Alun Davies is to be credited with having raised the alarm on vein graft surveillance and having pointed out to us that we need to look at the evidence for doing it. A random controlled trial is underway. For the moment all the question marks against vein graft surveillance are rehearsed and a sceptic is pitted against an enthusiast. At the time of writing it is simply not a subject that has been resolved but it would be fair to say that the onus has now swung to those who wish to justify vein graft surveillance as a mandatory investigation to the same extent as those who question it.

Roger M Greenhalgh
Editor

Phlebectomy is the treatment of choice for varicose veins

For the motion
R Kolvenbach, L Pinter, M Kirch

Introduction

The treatment of varicose veins provides a good example for the role of economics in venous therapy. Varicose veins are common and patients are referred to either a phlebologist, a dermatologist a general or a vascular surgeon. The threshold for intervention is not agreed and varies widely, with considerable implications for resources. For vein surgery to compete with other less invasive interventions, economic and clinical outcome assessment of new surgical techniques will be increasingly important. Many patients are told that a radical surgical treatment could worsen their symptoms and that they should choose a more conservative therapy as an alternative.

Evidence

The use of more conservative treatment protocols has been the centre of controversy from two groups of advocates. On one side are phlebologists who use sclerotherapy as a major form of treatment of varicose veins of all sizes and aetiology. On the other side are surgeons who are operating a patient with an incurable disease. Dodd stated 'the worst aspects of injection therapy are seen when varicose vein patients are herded into injection clinics without appropriate follow-up'.[1] Hobbs carried out a random trial at St Mary´s Hospital in London comparing surgery vs sclerotherapy.[2] During a 6-year follow-up study fewer than 10% of the injected legs had no remnant or recurrent varicosities vs 84% in the surgical group. There is no controversy about injection therapy having a beneficial role when treating small (< 3–4 mm) side-branches or reticular varicosities. Yet an increasing number of patients is admitted for surgery in whom sclerotherapy of the saphenofemoral junction or of one of the large veins of the proximal thigh has been attempted. This includes the long saphenous vein, the accessory medial saphenous vein (posteromedial thigh vein), or the accessory lateral saphenous vein (anterolateral thigh vein). Assuming that varicosities (> 4 mm) in this part of the proximal leg are best treated surgically we tried to evaluate the clinical and cosmetic outcome of patients after previous sclerotherapy in this region of the leg.

In addition to the clinical data we looked at the answers of a patient questionnaire trying to assess the benefit of a treatment as perceived by the patient. Quality of life after varicose vein surgery is an important aspect when evaluating new techniques and cosmetic results.[3]

Operative technique

The main principle behind a successful therapy includes the correct identification of the site of valvular incompetence and the subsequent control of this site by either surgery or sclerotherapy.

In our study we concentrated on class C2 and C3 patients according to the CEAP classification.[4,5] C2 are patients with varicose vein clusters and C3 are patients with varicose veins and oedema.

The basic surgical principles are:

1. Flush ligation of the saphenofemoral junction including ligation of all major tributaries, particularly the accessory saphenous veins.
2. Microsurgical excision of local varicosities
3. Limited inversion stripping of the greater saphenous vein.

In addition to these principles we have added in our institution a fourth paradigm:

4. Intraoperative quality control!

Microsurgical techniques include 1 mm incisions and extraction of varicose branches with special hooks (Varaday hooks, Storz, Tuttlingen FRG).[6] The incisions do not require any sutures. A refluxing varicose greater saphenous vein is stripped. When the duplex examination of the greater saphenous vein shows reflux of the proximal segment only without clinically visible varicose changes flush ligation without stripping is performed. Limited inversion stripping is performed no further distally than to the medial part of the knee to avoid saphenous nerve injury and to spare intact vein segments.[7] More recently we started removing large varicose vein clusters with the TriVex technique to safe time and to reduce the number of incisions. This novel technique can only be used for side-branches.

Intraoperative quality control to assess the completeness of the procedure is performed using transillumination with the TriVex cannula (Fig. 1).

The TriVex procedure is combined with Tumescent anaesthesia.[8] Tumescent anaesthesia is achieved with infusions of 1000 ml of 0.9% normal saline with 50 ml of 1%

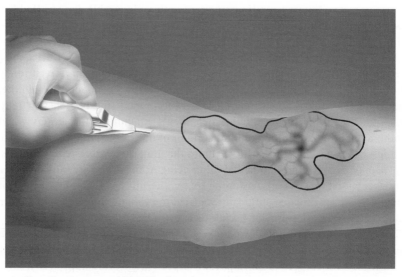

Figure 1. Transillumination and identification of venous clusters.

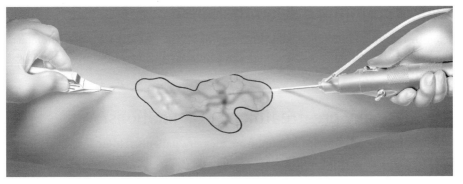

Figure 2. Transilluminator and resection device placed opposite to each other. Vein clusters were marked preoperatively.

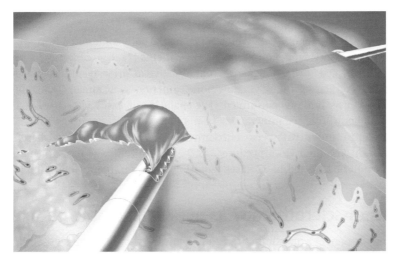

Figure 3. The vein is morcellated and suctioned in through the resector.

lidocaine with 2 ml of epinephrine added (Fig. 2). The TriVex system vein resector is a rotating, tubular inner cannula encased in a stationary outer sheath dissector. Through a working tip the vein is suctioned in, morcellated, and removed (Fig. 3). In our experience this device is most effective when used in combination with hook phlebectomy to extract the morcellated venous remnants. The resector–suction device also serves to evacuate any haematoma from the extracted side-branches or the subcutaneous saphenous vein canal.

Results

During a 20-month period 1000 patients were referred to us for varicose vein surgery. Among these were 146 cases (14.6%) where sclerotherapy of the proximal greater saphenous vein, the accessory saphenous vein or other major tributaries of the saphenofemoral junction had been performed; 117 patients (117/1000) were admitted with recurrent varicosities. This group (11.7%) served as a control cohort to compare the outcome of surgery with sclerotherapy.

Who is performing sclerotherapy?

Sclerotherapy of the inguinal and thigh region was performed by a dermatologist/phlebologist in 121 (82.8%) cases and by general practitioners with a special interest in phlebology in the remaining 25 patients.

Are there any pre-treatment examinations?

Checking the doctors bill or recalling from memory patients told us that a pre-treatment duplex examination was performed in 37 cases (25.3%) only .

Intermediate results of sclerotherapy

When performing a preoperative duplex examination in the group of 146 patients who were referred to us for surgery after failed sclerotherapy, we could detect a refluxing greater saphenous vein which was only partially obliterated in combination with patent accessory saphenous veins in 113 patients (77.3%). Since injection treatment was performed during a mean interval of 3.2 years prior to surgery it is justified to infer that reflux of the saphenofemoral junction was already existent when sclerotherapy was initially performed. The majority of cases (129 patients) had a median number of five sclerotherapy sessions.

In the control group with recurrent varicosities the median interval between the first operation and the redo procedure was 9.2 years. Reflux of the saphenofemoral junction could be detected in 37 cases requiring re-exploration of the groin (31.6%).

Results of sclerotherapy as perceived by the patient

Analysing the patient's questionnaire 123 patients (84.2%) complained that they were not informed about possible side-effects, alternative treatments and the lack of durability of the procedure. In 77 cases (52.7%) the patient was told that any kind of surgery could be detrimental for him. In 69 cases the patients (47.2%) complained about the costs, and the duration of the treatment.

As a side-effect of sclerotherapy, hyperpigmentation, thrombosed veins or cutaneous discolouration was seen in 29 cases (19.8%) and considered by most patients as a cosmetically unsatisfactory result.

Discussion

We can conclude that in C2 and C3 patients with saphenofemoral reflux sclerotherapy of the saphenous vein or one of its major tributaries does not present an alternative compared with surgery using microsurgical techniques and intraoperative quality control.

Only a minority of our patients had a pre-interventional duplex examination although most of the patients were treated by phlebologists.

Sclerotherapy of the long saphenous vein during a 3-year period prior to surgery was inefficient with a recurrence rate of almost 80%. Injection treatment could eventually not avoid the surgical procedure. The treatment interval was prolonged combined with increased costs.

The costs for a surgical outpatient treatment were calculated including the costs for theatre staff, anaesthesia, surgeon and one assistant, suture material, drapes and disposable strippers as well as the material required for a TriVex operation.

The median costs for an operative outpatient treatment were 796.4 EURO (approx. £497.75). When TriVex was used we had to add 204.5 EURO (approx. £127.81). The median costs for the preoperative sclerotherapy and phlebological treatment were 409 EURO (approx. £255.62) for each patient. If these costs are added to a finally required operative treatment then injection therapy for saphenofemoral reflux and major varicose side-branches is not cost-effective. This calculation will change even more unfavourably when more expensive agents for injection therapy are used.

Surgery is cost-effective as a radical procedure, even when using relatively expensive adjuncts, when it is offered as a day-care operation.

Sclerotherapy is supposed to be a less invasive alternative to any surgical technique, which should even make surgery redundant in most instances.[9] Our own experience and the results published so far indicate that the recurrence rate is too high to permit a cost-effective approach which can satisfy the majority of patients.

If symptom control and recurrence rates are the endpoints, conservative treatment options deserve assessment against modern surgical techniques. The time has come to subject the therapy for varicose veins to the same rigours of economic assessments that other health care sectors are already receiving – namely, the comparative assessment of costs and benefits.[10,11]

When respecting the results of preoperative venous duplex tests, and when using microsurgical techniques, excellent functional and cosmetic results can be obtained in varicose vein surgery. The operative approach is significantly more durable and cost-effective than any kind of injection therapy.

Summary

- Clinical trials performed so far show that conservative and injection therapy in patients with advanced chronic venous insufficiency is associated with a high recurrence rate.

- Sclerotherapy of the greater saphenous vein is useless and not cost-effective.

- Varicose vein surgery using microsurgical techniques can be performed safely with significantly better intermediate term results.

- Intraoperative quality control can improve the outcome of surgical procedures.

References

1. Dodd H, Cockett FB. *Pathology and Surgery of the Veins of the Lower Limb* 2nd edn. Edinburgh: Churchill Livingston, 1976: 106.
2. Hobbs JT. The management of varicose veins. *Surg Ann* 1980; 12: 169.
3. Smith JJ, Garratt AM, Guest M, Greenhalgh RM, Davies AH. Evaluating and improving health-related quality of life in patients with varicose veins. *J Vasc Surg* 1999; 30: 710–719.
4. Rutherford RB, Padberg FT, Comerota AJ *et al*. Venous severity scoring: An adjunct to venous outcome assessment. *J Vasc Surg* 2000; 31: 1307–1312.
5. Porter JM, Moneta GL *et al*. Consensus comittee on chronic venous disease. Reporting standards in venous disease: an update. *J Vasc Surg* 1995; 21: 635–645.

6. Varaday Z. Microsurgical venous extraction. *Vasomed* 1990; 3: 23–25.
7. Wilson S, Prye S, Scott R Inversion stripping of the long saphenous vein. *Phleblogy* 1997; 12: 91–95.
8. Yanke CW, Bernstein G, Bullock S. Safety of tumescent liposuction in 15,336 patients. *Dermatol Surg* 1995; 21: 459–462.
9. Sigg K. Treatment of varicose veins by injection sclerotherapy: a method practiced in Switzerland. In *The Treatment of Venous Disorders*. Hobbs JT (ed). Philadelphia: JB Lippincott, 1977: 113.
10. JE Brazier, Johnson AG Economics of surgery. *Lancet* 2001; 358: 1077–1081.
11. Bishop Ch, Fronek HS, Fronek A, Dilley RB, Bernstein EF Real-time color duplex scanning after sclerotherapy of the greater saphenous vein. *J Vasc Surg* 1991; 14: 505–510.

Phlebectomy is the treatment of choice for varicose veins

Against the motion
Charles N McCollum, Francis Dix

Introduction

Approximately 15–20% of the adult population have varicose veins with an annual incidence in adults of 2.5%.[1] This equates to 4–5 million patients with varicose veins in the UK of whom 600 000 approach their General Practitioner each year for advice on treatment, yet only 60 000 operations for varicose veins are performed by the National Health Service (NHS) with perhaps another 15 000 operations performed privately.[2] Not surprisingly, surgeons and health authorities have been attracted to alternative and relatively simple approaches to treatment such as injection sclerotherapy or phlebectomy. This chapter will show that these suboptimal approaches to treatment have resulted in high recurrence rates and subsequently greater demands on health services.

Varicose vein surgery has been done badly for many years with unacceptable recurrence rates and many patients requiring re-operation. Patients rightly expect an improvement in symptoms, limb function and appearance which is only temporary for most with recurrence rates ranging from 7 to 65%,[3–5] despite difficulties in the adequate classification of what constitutes recurrence. In a study of 1014 consecutive varicose vein operations undertaken in the Lothian region in the early 1990s, 20% were performed for recurrent disease.[6,7] It is generally accepted that recurrence now represents over 30% of varicose vein practice in England with more challenging surgery associated with more frequent complications. The cost for health authorities is considerable, as operations for recurrence are more expensive than the original surgery and could have been avoided had an accurate diagnosis and appropriate surgery been offered in the first instance. In an audit of practice at Surgicare (a specialist independent surgical provider) in 1992–1994, 40% of patients were referred for recurrent varicose veins.

Causes of varicose veins

The pathophysiology remains contentious but incompetence of the superficial venous valves appears to be the initiating event. The resulting high retrograde flow leads to turbulence and variable sheer stresses on the vein walls resulting in tortuous dilatation (Fig. 1).

The figures from our NHS practice suggest that this incompetence may be through the long saphenous vein (62%), the short saphenous vein (16%), through perforators (2%) or a combination of these (20%).

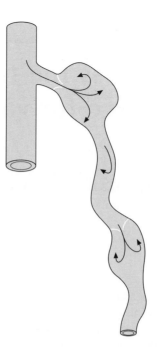

Figure 1. Incompetence of the superficial venous valves leads to turbulent retrograde flow, variable sheer stresses on the vein wall and tortuous dilatation.

Diagnosis of varicose veins

Appropriate surgery can only be performed if venous incompetence is correctly investigated by an ultrasound technique. Hand-held Doppler should be routine in the outpatient clinic.

Duplex imaging may be required for more complex cases such as those with recurrence or incompetence in the popliteal fossa.

Hand-held Doppler ultrasound

The patient should be adequately assessed in the outpatient department using hand-held Doppler to identify sites of reflux. The technique is important and should be standardized: the patient is examined standing on a step and with the examined leg slightly bent at the knee with the calf relaxed. Body weight is supported on the opposite leg. The saphenofemoral junction is located by identifying the femoral artery and moving the probe medially to lie over the femoral vein. An 8MHz Doppler probe is used for most cases but a 5MHz probe can be used in the obese and for assessing reflux in the deep veins. With manual squeeze and release of the calf, antegrade and retrograde flow in the superficial veins can be heard and timed. Moving the probe inferomedially from the common femoral vein locates the long saphenous vein. This should be examined at the groin, mid-thigh level and at the knee. The popliteal fossa is then examined for any source of incompetence. The short saphenous vein is usually found overlying or just lateral to the signal from the popliteal artery. Gentle pressure on an incompetent short saphenous vein using the Doppler probe will usually prevent reflux which is difficult to control in deep veins. The level of the saphenopopliteal junction can be estimated by moving the probe proximally along the vein until the reflux signal becomes loud as the short saphenous vein passes through the deep fascia; the signal becomes soft, almost inaudible just above the junction with the polpliteal vein.

The assessment of sites of venous reflux and the duration of reflux can be performed just as accurately and more cost-effectively by a trained vascular nurse specialist in a nurse-led varicose vein clinic. We compared the varicose vein nurse specialist using hand-held Doppler, with duplex imaging by an experienced vascular laboratory technician in the diagnosis of reflux in primary varicose veins. Following 9 months of training, our varicose vein nurse-specialist achieved 99% concordance with duplex imaging. Colour duplex imaging is essential for complex cases, popliteal recurrence or when there is any doubt on hand-held Doppler examination.

Surgical technique

Precise and appropriate surgery depends on accurate preoperative diagnosis and marking using hand-held Doppler or duplex imaging. The incision, while usually small, must allow adequate access to all tributaries especially in operations for recurrent varicose veins. In the groin the femoral vein should be explored 5cm proximally and 2cm distally to the saphenofemoral junction so that all potential sites of incompetence are divided (Fig. 2). All the tributaries should be ligated as far from the saphenofemoral junction as possible to avoid recurrence by neovascularization. The saphenofemoral junction should be ligated flush with the femoral vein and the long saphenous vein everted using a rod stripper to the knee avoiding the risk of saphenous nerve injury. Exploring the groin for recurrent varicose veins, the femoral vein is best approached from its lateral aspect by exposing the femoral artery first. The long saphenous vein is often still present in the thigh where it is easier to identify just above the knee. This can be brought to the surface through a 1 cm incision and everted using a rod stripper passed proximally to the groin wound.

In short saphenous vein incompetence, the saphenopopliteal junction should be clearly located and marked preoperatively. The skin incision should be transverse but

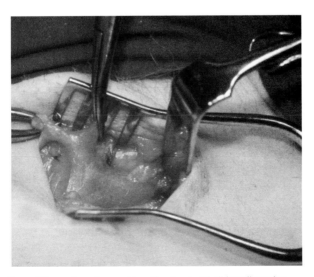

Figure 2. Dissection of the saphenofemoral junction to reveal all its tributaries.

adequate access to the saphenofemoral junction is best achieved by a vertical incision in the popliteal fascia. The saphenofemoral junction must be clearly identified and followed as it passes around the lateral politeal nerve to join the popliteal vein. The sural nerve should be identified and preserved. Whether the short saphenous vein should be removed remains uncertain but we remove at least the proximal 5–10 cm. Avulsions are performed using small transverse stab incisions and a phlebectomy hook.

Causes of recurrence

Inadequate diagnosis is perhaps the main cause of recurrence as it leads to inappropriate surgery. In patients with calf varicose veins, saphenofemoral ligation ignoring saphenopopliteal incompetence will inevitably lead to rapid recurrence.

Inadequate surgery is also a frequent cause of recurrence. All tributaries in the groin must be divided and the saphenofemoral junction ligated flush with the femoral vein. Misidentification of the anterior vein of thigh as the long saphenous vein will leave an incompetent long saphenous vein *in situ* and cause rapid recurrence. A prospective audit by Lees of 50 limbs undergoing superficial venous surgery assessed by duplex scanning showed that trainees were responsible for 14 of 15 cases of persisting incompetence in the groin or popliteal fossa presumably due to inadequate saphenofemoral dissection.[8] The conclusion from this is that improved training, technique and supervision are necessary, particularly as the groin is the commonest site of failure in most recurrences.

Failure to strip an incompetent long saphenous vein may also lead to recurrence, either through proximal or mid-thigh perforating veins or by incompetence developing through neovascularization in the groin wound. In a prospective study using duplex imaging, neoreflux appeared in 9 of 46 limbs (20%) at only 6 weeks postoperatively.[9] Long saphenous vein reflux may also occur with a competent saphenofemoral junction and in this situation saphenofemoral junction ligation alone would clearly achieve little.[10,11] It is important to ablate the most proximal point of reflux and remove an incompetent long saphenous vein when present.

Neovascularization, the growth of thin-walled incompetent veins in healing tissue, is an important cause of recurrence and is difficult to prevent.[12,13] Originally proposed by Glass, and generally regarded as an extension of wound healing during angiogenesis, it has been suggested that covering the ligated saphenofemoral junction with mersilene mesh or a polytetrafluoroethylene patch may prevent neovascularization.[14,15] There is little convincing evidence that these approaches are better than careful saphenofemoral junction division with removal of the incompetent long saphenous vein.

Results of appropriate varicose vein surgery

Guided surgical management by precise preoperative ultrasound diagnosis and standardized operative techniques have been used at Surgicare for 10 years. Of the first 250 consecutive operations, 197 (79%) were for primary varicose veins (including patients who had previous sclerotherapy) and 53 (21%) were for recurrent disease. All underwent continuous wave Doppler assessment and photoplethysmography in the outpatient department and were marked preoperatively by the operating surgeon using hand-held Doppler. Surgery was performed by two surgeons working to the same detailed protocol. All patients were sent a questionnaire at least 1 year after surgery. Any responses suggesting recurrence were recalled for repeat investigation. Responses were obtained from 208. Recurrence was defined as incompetence in any dilated superficial vein or at the saphenofemoral junction/saphenopopliteal junction, whether or not there were visible varicosities or symptoms.

There were five recurrences (2.3%) at the saphenofemoral junction in patients operated on for primary long saphenous vein varicosities and five recurrences (9.5%) at the saphenofemoral junction in patients undergoing surgery for recurrent disease. Incompetent perforators were found in 47 limbs where no other source of incompetence was identified. New site incompetence was detected in five saphenofemoral junctions (5%) and six saphenopopliteal junctions (2%) after 2 years.

This study demonstrates that the rate of recurrence after accurate investigation and precise surgery can be good leading to long-term patient satisfaction. Patients can expect little pain following varicose vein surgery with an early return to work or normal full activity (mean of 16 days postoperatively) .

Should the long saphenous vein be removed?

Table 1 shows the clinical trial evidence on the role of long saphenous vein stripping. A range of procedures were performed in these various studies with different criteria for recurrence. Jakobsen *et al.* randomized 320 limbs to stripping or not stripping of the long saphenous vein, clearly demonstrating fewer recurrences when the long saphenous vein was stripped.[16] The incidence of paraesthesia in the saphenous nerve distribution when the long saphenous vein was stripped to the ankle was high.[17] Later studies included both a measure of the clinical outcome and an objective measure such as photoplethysmography combined with duplex imaging.[13,18-21] In each of these studies, the frequency of reflux was approximately halved by removing the long saphenous vein in the thigh. Clinical outcome was also generally improved, with lower clinical recurrence rates in those patients where the long saphenous vein was removed.

Novel techniques for long saphenous ablation

More recently we have seen the introduction of new techniques to obliterate the incompetent long saphenous vein. Minimally invasive techniques are being developed in an attempt to reduce discomfort and recovery time whilst improving the cosmetic outcome. These include endoluminal laser and microwave techniques which ablate the long saphenous vein by thermal injury.[22] Although short-term 'closure rates' are good it is unclear whether these techniques adequately ablate tributaries in the groin. They are slow and painful requiring extensive local anaesthesia or in some cases general anaesthesia. Long-term randomized studies are required to compare these novel techniques with the standards achieved by good surgery .

Table 1. Trials of saphenofemoral ligation with and without long saphenous vein (LSV) stripping.

Author	Limbs	Mean follow-up (months)	Diagnostic tests	LSV strip		LSV not stripped			Comments
				Limbs	Recurrence (%)	Limbs	Recurrence (%)	p value	
Jakobsen [16] 1979	320	36	Clinical	158	16 (10)	162	56 (35)	p < 0.05	Strip from ankle to groin
Munn [17] 1981	114	36	Clinical	57	21 (37)	57	34 (60)	p < 0.01	
Neglen [18] 1993	137	60	Clinical	74	30 (40)	63	53 (84)	p < 0.05	
Sarin [19] 1994	89	21	Clinical, duplex, photoplethysmogram	43	clinical 15 (35) reflux 21 (49)	46	clinical 38 (83) reflux 38 (83)	p < 0.05	Includes trivial recurrences
Rutgers [20] 1994	142	36	Clinical, Doppler	69	clinical 27 (39) reflux 10 (14)	73	clinical 44 (60) reflux 34 (47)	p < 0.05	
Jones [13] 1996	113	31	Clinical, duplex	53	13 (25)	60	26 (43)	p < 0.04	
Dwerryhouse [21] 1999	110	60	Clinical, duplex	52	11 (21) reflux 15 (29)	58	8 (14) reflux 41 (71)	p < 0.59	Reoperations more frequent where LSV not removed

p Values represent the difference in recurrence between stripping the long saphenous vein and not stripping.
All are randomized controlled trials (Neglen trial only partly randomized).

Polidocanol microfoam sclerotherapy has the advantage of simplicity as the microfoam is easily visualized on duplex imaging and its injection can therefore be precisely controlled. Polidocanol is an established sclerosant which interferes with cell surface lipids and promotes intense spasm and thrombosis. The foam has the additional advantage that it displaces blood as it fills the venous lumen greatly reducing subsequent thrombophlebitis. Dr Cabrera demonstrated that this technique may be used on large veins such as the incompetent long saphenous vein.[23] With Mr Harper in Aberdeen we conducted a pilot study in primary varicose veins due to major long saphenous incompetence with reflux times of under 6 seconds and a long saphenous vein diameter of >7 mm. Forty-one patients (median age of 43, range 25–64 years, 23 women and 18 men) were assessed clinically, by duplex and digital photography preoperatively and at 1, 2, 6, 12 and 52 weeks following foam sclerotherapy. Following local anaesthesia, a cannula was introduced into the long saphenous vein in the mid-thigh under duplex guidance. With the leg elevated, Polidocanol foam was then injected and its passage proximally along the long saphenous vein imaged by duplex until it reached the saphenofemoral junction. This junction was then compressed while further foam was injected, refluxing down the incompetent long saphenous vein to fill calf varices. The leg was rested in the elevated position for 5–10 minutes before a class II full length elastic stocking was applied. The patient was then immediately mobilized and allowed to go home. The elastic stocking was worn day and night for the first week and then throughout the day for a further 3 weeks.

At 3 months after sclerotherapy duplex imaging revealed that 66% of patients had complete occlusion of the long saphenous vein and saphenofemoral junction, 14% had an occluded saphenofemoral junction alone and 20% had recanalized (Fig. 3). The 1-year follow-up data for the 21 patients from our department are very encouraging; 18 patients (86%) had sustained occlusion of the long saphenous vein (Fig. 4). The procedure was almost pain-free, only 14 patients (34%) took any form of analgesia, usually a non-steroidal anti-inflammatory and only seven (17%) patients continued analgesia after the first postoperative day. Two patients had asymptomatic short segment occlusions of the posterior tibial vein demonstrated on subsequent duplex imaging; there were no other complications. A randomized clinical trial comparing polidocanol foam sclerotherapy with standard surgical techniques for long saphenous varicose veins is now underway. This novel approach has the advantage that the long saphenous vein can be ablated up to the saphenofemoral junction without inhibiting the subsequent use of microfoam sclerotherapy or surgery should this be indicated.

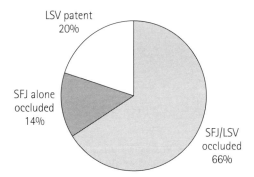

Figure 3. Occlusion rates by Polidocanol microfoam sclerotherapy of the long saphenous vein (LSV) and saphenofemoral junction (SFJ) assessed by duplex imaging at 3 months (n=41).

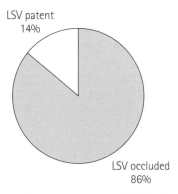

LSV patent
14%

LSV occluded
86%

Figure 4. The occlusion rates of the long saphenous vein (LSV) by Polidocanol microfoam sclerotherapy from our unit assessed by duplex imaging at 1 year (n=21).

Conclusion

Phlebectomy alone is inadequate in the treatment of varicose veins. Recurrence will be frequent unless the proximal source of incompetence is also ablated. The principles of treatment include :

1. Obliteration of the highest point of reflux.
2. Ablation of the incompetent trunk vein.
3. Removal or sclerosis of other varices.

At present this is best achieved by flush saphenofemoral or saphenopopliteal ligation with rod eversion of the long saphenous vein and multiple avulsions .

Summary

- Recurrence rates after varicose vein surgery are unacceptably high due to inaccurate preoperative diagnosis, inadequate surgery and neovascularization.

- Varicose vein surgery requires accurate diagnosis by ultrasound and precise surgery to sites of incompetence.

- Failure to remove an incompetent long saphenous vein in the thigh doubles the risk of recurrence over 2–5 years.

- Phlebectomy alone is insufficient and almost inevitably leads to recurrence.

- For the future, less invasive methods of long saphenous ablation may prove acceptable.

References

1. Brand FN, Dannenberg AL, Abbott RD, Kannel WB. The epidemiology of varicose veins: The Framingham study. *Am J Prev Med*, 1988; 4: 96–101.
2. Bradbury A, Evans CJ, Allan P *et al.* The relationship between lower limb symptoms and superficial and deep venous reflux on duplex ultrasonography: The Edinburgh vein study. *J Vasc Surg*, 2000; 32: 921–931.

3. Negus D. Recurrent varicose veins: a national problem. *Br J Surg* 1993; **80**: 823–824.

4. Rivlin S. The surgical cure of primary varicose veins. *Br J Surg* 1975; **62**: 913–917.

5. Royle JP. Recurrent varicose veins. *World J Surg* 1986; **10**: 944–953.

6. Bradbury AW, Stonebridge PA, Ruckley CV, Beggs I. Recurrent varicose veins: correlation between preoperative clinical and hand-held Doppler ultrasonographic examination,and findings at surgery. *Br J Surg* 1993; **80**: 849–851.

7. Davies GC. The Lothian surgical audit. *Medical Audit News* 1991; **1**: 26–27.

8. Lees T, Singh S, Beard J, Spencer P, Rigby C. Prospective audit of surgery for varicose veins. *Br J Surg* 1997; **84**: 44–46.

9. Turton E, Scott D, Richards S *et al*. Duplex-derived Evidence of reflux after varicose vein surgery: neoreflux or neovascularisation? *Eur J Vasc Endovasc Surg* 1999; **17**: 230–233.

10. Abu-Own A, Scurr JH, Coleridge Smith PD.Saphenous vein reflux without incompetence at the saphenofemoral junction. *Br J Surg* 1994; **81**: 1452–1454.

11. McMullin GM, Coleridge Smith PD, Scurr JH. Objective assessment of high ligation without stripping the long saphenous vein. *Br J Surg* 1991; **78**: 1139–1142.

12. Nyamekye I, Shephard NA, Davies B, Heather BP, Earnshaw JJ. Clinicopathological evidence that neovascularisation is a cause of recurrent varicose veins. *Eur J Vasc Endovasc Surg* 1998; **15**: 412–415.

13. Jones L, Braithwaite BD, Selwyn D, Cooke S, Earnshaw JJ. Neovascularisation is the principal cause of varicose vein recurrence: results of a randomised trial of stripping the long saphenous vein. *Eur J Vasc Endovasc Surg* 1996; **12**: 442–445.

14. Glass GM. Prevention of recurrent saphenofemoral incompetence after surgery for varicose veins. *Br J Surg* 1989; **76**: 1210.

15. Earnshaw JJ, Davies B, Harradine K, Heather BP. Preliminary results of PTFE patch saphenoplasty to prevent neovascularisation leading to recurrent varicose veins. *Phlebology* 1998; **13**: 10–13.

16. Jakobsen BH. The value of different forms of treatment for varicose veins. *Br J Surg* 1979; **66**: 182–184.

17. Munn SR, Morton JB, Macbeth WA, McLeish AR. To strip or not to strip the long saphenous vein? A varicose veins trial. *Br J Surg* 1981; **68**: 426–428.

18. Neglen P, Einarsson E, Eklof B. The functional longterm value of different types of treatment for saphenous vein incompetence. *J Cardiovasc Surg* 1993; **34**: 295–301.

19. Sarin S, Scurr JH, Coleridge Smith PD. Stripping of the long saphenous vein in the treatment of primary varicose veins. *Br J Surg* 1994; **81**: 1455–1458.

20. Rutgers PH, Kitslaar PJ. Randomised trial of stripping versus high ligation combined with sclerotherapy in the treatment of the incompetent greater saphenous vein. *Am J Surg* 1994; **168**: 311–315.

21. Dwerryhouse S, Davies B, Harradine K, Earnshaw J. Stripping of the long saphenous vein reduces the rate of reoperation for recurrent varicose veins: five-year results of a randomised trial. *J Vasc Surg* 1999; **29**: 589–592.

22. Navarro L, Min RJ, Bone C. Endovenous laser : a new minimally invasive method of treatment for varicose veins – preliminary observations using an 810nm diode laser. *Dermatol Surg* 2001; **27**: 117–122.

23. Cabrera Garrido JR *et al*. Elargissement des limites de la sclérothérapie. Nouveaux produits sclérosants. *J Phlébologie* 1995; **50**: 181–188.

Phlebectomy is the treatment of choice for varicose veins

Charing Cross Editorial Comments towards Consensus

You would have thought that this matter would be settled by now. It has raged on for 40 years or more. An era of injection sclerosant therapy by George Fegan of Dublin threatened to blow varicose vein surgery away but it is still with us. Now we hear of the hot wire and injection of solid particles once again to establish that surgery is not the gold standard. Trials are underway to convince us which is the best way to do it. At the time of writing to say the least there is uncertainty.

Roger M Greenhalgh
Editor

Surgery heals venous ulcers

For the motion
Rachel E Bell, Peter R Taylor

Introduction

The advent of imaging techniques, particularly duplex scanning, has allowed the role of superficial vein reflux in the genesis of varicose ulcers to be identified. Isolated superficial vein incompetence can be detected in over half of all venous ulcers.[1-3] High healing rates of up to 91% can be achieved with saphenous vein surgery alone in this group of patients.[4] It follows that the majority of patients with venous ulceration can be healed with surgery. Surgery can also help to heal venous ulceration which is secondary to a combination of primary valvular incompetence in the deep system, superficial and perforator incompetence. However, the role of surgery in the post-phlebitic limb is controversial.

Imaging

Duplex and venography have been used to accurately assess the various components of the venous system in patients with venous ulceration. The results of these series are summarized in Table 1.

Table 1. Sites of venous reflux in venous ulceration.

Series	Year	Reflux (%)		
		Superficial	Deep	Combined
Hanrahan et al[5]	1991	36	6	43
Darke and Penfold[4]	1992	39	21	36
Shami et al[1]	1993	53	15	32
Van Rij et al[2]	1994	72	9	19
Labropoulos et al[6]	1994	38	6	53
Scriven et al[3]	1997	63	1	35
Ghauri et al[7]	1998	44	6	49

This shows that superficial vein reflux alone is responsible for the majority of patients developing venous ulceration in most series. Combined deep and superficial reflux comprise the next largest group while deep venous problems alone are rare. Those with perforator incompetence alone form the smallest subgroup (4–8.4%).[4,5] Several studies have shown the benefit of open or subfascial endoscopic perforator surgery (SEPS) in these patients.[8,9]

Patients with deep venous disease have either primary valvular incompetence or the post-phlebitic limb which results from a combination of venous outflow obstruction and reflux. Good results have been reported with valve reconstruction in patients with primary valvular incompetence, however, the post-phlebitic limb is notoriously difficult to treat surgically.[10,11]

Evidence

Surgery for superficial venous incompetence

The benefit of saphenous vein surgery in patients with venous ulceration attributable to isolated superficial vein incompetence has been shown by several authors.[4,12,13] Darke *et al.* showed that 91% of ulcers caused by superficial and perforator incompetence could be healed by saphenous surgery alone at a median follow-up of 3.5 years.[4,14] However, 33% of patients in this study used some form of compression therapy after surgery, making it difficult to state categorically that surgery was responsible for healing in all cases. Short saphenous vein surgery in patients with lateral venous ulcers resulted in 100% being healed at 12 weeks.[12] However, all patients in this study were put into three-layer compression postoperatively. Another series was specifically designed to determine whether saphenous vein surgery alone could heal venous ulcers due to superficial incompetence.[13] The 1-year healing rate for small, medium and large ulcers was 94, 74 and 60% respectively. Further study of those who failed to heal suggested that there was an additional impairment of calf muscle pump function.

In patients with both saphenous reflux and incompetent perforatoring veins, 80% of the perforator veins regain their competence after superficial surgery alone.[15] This finding is in agreement with other studies and supports the theory that venous ulceration may result from calf muscle pump overload rather than superficial venous incompetence alone.[4,16]

One important beneficial effect of surgery would be to minimize the risk of recurrent venous ulceration. It has been convincingly shown that patients with normal deep veins who have surgery for superficial vein incompetence have a significantly lower recurrence rate of venous ulceration (9%) than patients treated with compression therapy alone (50%).[7] This important finding also has a significant bearing on the cost-effectiveness of the treatment. Clearly, a patient who has surgery which is curative will benefit more and cost less than a patient wearing compression hosiery for life.

In conclusion, therefore, there can be no doubt that saphenous vein surgery can heal venous ulcers and prevent recurrence in the majority of patients who have isolated superficial venous incompetence.

Surgery for combined superficial and deep venous reflux

Surgery in patients who have combined deep and superficial venous reflux is more controversial but has been shown to improve ulcer healing. There is a higher success rate for patients with primary valvular incompetence than for those presenting with the post-phlebitic limb.

It has been shown that saphenous vein surgery alone does not correct perforator incompetence in the presence of deep venous reflux.[15] Therefore this group of patients could benefit from additional perforator surgery. Saphenous vein surgery alone performed in patients with multi-system reflux achieved healing in 21/52 (40%) of patients.[17] Of the 31(60%) patients who failed to heal, 19 went on to have open perforator surgery and 10/19 healed post-surgery. Therefore a total of 40/52 (80%) healed their ulcer with surgery. This is similar to another series which reported a 70% healing rate after superficial and perforator surgery.[18]

There have also been reports of improved haemodynamics in addition to ulcer healing following superficial and perforator surgery. Clinical and haemodynamic improvement was demonstrated in 11 patients following superficial and perforator ablation.[19] However, all these patients had primary valvular incompetence.

From this evidence it appears that patients with primary valvular incompetence are more likely to benefit from superficial and perforator surgery than patients with the post-phlebitic limb. Patients with any element of deep venous obstruction do not do well with venous surgery and are better managed with compression bandaging and skin grafting to achieve healing.

Surgery for perforator incompetence

Since Linton and Cockett there has been a great controversy surrounding the contribution of calf perforator veins to venous ulceration.[20,21] Cockett's seminal paper describing the 'ankle blow-out syndrome' was based mainly on subjective analysis.[22] Burnand *et al.* showed that perforator surgery alone resulted in a high ulcer recurrence rate (55%) particularly in patients with the post-phlebitic limb.[23] The same group also demonstrated that there was no improvement in venous function following perforator ligation.[24] There is some evidence that superficial vein surgery combined with subfascial ligation of incompetent perforating veins and the use of elastic stockings for deep venous incompetence can attain good results with up to 92% of venous ulcers remaining healed at 6 years.[25] However, surgery for perforating veins fell out of favour because of poor results and the high incidence of wound complications (>50%). Since the development of SEPS, the enthusiasm for perforator surgery has been rekindled.

Some claim 100% healing rates following SEPS; however, more than half of the patients in this study had concomitant superficial saphenous surgery, and very few patients had the post-phlebitic limb.[26] Another small study showed healing rates of 85% after SEPS with no recurrence at 1 year.[9] The North American SEPS study group showed a cumulative ulcer-healing rate of 88% at 1 year.[8] However, 28% of ulcers had recurred at 2 years and the recurrence rate was noted to be higher in patients with the post-phlebitic limb (46%) than in those with primary valvular incompetence (20%).

Perforator surgery does have a role in the management of venous ulceration in the presence of multi-system reflux but only in combination with superficial venous surgery. Perforator surgery alone is only suitable for the small group of patients where incompetent perforators are the only identifiable venous abnormality. There is no evidence to suggest that perforator surgery alone is better than medical treatment or saphenous surgery alone.

Surgery for deep venous incompetence

Excellent results have been reported for deep venous surgery in patients with primary valvular incompetence.[10,11] The results are not as good for patients with post-thrombotic problems." One series reported a 10-year ulcer-free survival rate of 73% in patients with primary valvular incompetence compared with 43% in post-thrombotic cases." Another reported a 74% ulcer-free survival at 10 years.[10] In this series, no significant difference was demonstrated between patients with primary valvular incompetence and post-phlebitic limb. This may be explained by the use of multiple valve reconstructions in the post-thrombotic cases.

Both studies showed that valvuloplasty was more durable than valve transposition. To date there is a dearth of randomized trials comparing best medical treatment with deep venous surgery in the treatment of venous ulceration.

Conclusions

There is a large amount of evidence that surgery heals venous ulcers. Duplex scanning is very useful in detecting abnormalities in the superficial, deep and perforating venous systems of the leg. The majority of patients with a venous ulcer have correctable superficial vein reflux. Surgical intervention in the small number of patients with isolated incompetent perforators is also justified. Deep vein reconstruction may help patients with primary valvular incompetence. Patients with deep venous obstruction and those with incompetent deep veins as a consequence of the post-phlebitic limb do not respond well to venous surgery, but may still benefit from non-venous surgery for excision and skin grafting of ulcers that are difficult to heal.

Summary

- The majority of venous ulcers attributable to superficial and perforator reflux alone will heal following saphenous surgery alone.

- In patients with a combination of superficial and deep incompetence there is a role for saphenous and perforator surgery in patients with primary valvular incompetence.

- The results of venous surgery in patients with post-phlebitic limbs are poor.

- Prospective randomized studies are needed to define the role of perforator surgery and deep venous construction in patients with chronic venous insufficiency.

References

1. Shami SK, Sarin S, Cheatle TR *et al.* Venous ulcers and the superficial venous system. *J Vasc Surg* 1993; **17**: 487–490.
2. van Rij AM, Solomon C, Christie R. Anatomic and physiologic characteristics of venous ulceration. *J Vasc Surg* 1994; **20**: 759–764.
3. Scriven JM, Hartshorne T, Bell PRF *et al.* Single-visit venous ulcer assessment clinic: the first year. *Br J Surg* 1997; **84**: 334–336.
4. Darke SG, Penfold C. Venous ulceration and saphenous ligation. *Eur J Vasc Surg* 1992; **6**: 4–9.
5. Hanrahan LM, Araki CT, Rodriguez AA. Distribution of valvular incompetence in patients with venous stasis ulceration. *J Vasc Surg* 1991; **13**: 805–812.
6. Labropoulos N, Leon M, Nicolaides AN *et al.* Superficial venous insufficiency: Correlation of anatomic extent of reflux with clinical symptoms and signs. *J Vasc Surg* 1994; **20**: 953–8.

7. Ghauri AS, Nyamekye A, Grabs AJ *et al.* Influence of a specialised leg ulcer service and venous surgery on the outcome of venous leg ulcers. *Eur J Vasc Endovasc Surg* 1998; **16**: 238–244.

8. Gloviczki P, Bergan JJ, Rhodes JM *et al.* Midterm results of endoscopic perforator vein interruption for chronic venous insufficiency: lessons learned from the North American Study Group. *J Vasc Surg* 1999; **29**: 489–502.

9. Pierik EG, van Urk H, Wittens CH *et al.* Efficacy of subfascial endoscopy in eradicating perforating veins of the lower leg and its relation with venous ulcer healing. *J Vasc Surg* 1997; **26**: 255–259.

10. Raju S, Fredericks RK, Neglen PN *et al.* Durability of venous valve reconstruction techniques for "primary" and postthrombotic reflux. *J Vasc Surg* 1996; **23**: 357–367.

11. Masuda EM, Kistner RL. Long-term results of venous valve reconstruction: A four-to twenty-one-year follow-up. *J Vasc Surg* 1994; **19**: 391-403.

12. Bass A, Chayen D, Weinmann EE. Lateral venous ulcer and short saphenous vein insufficiency. *J Vasc Surg* 1997; **25**:654–657.

13. Bello M, Scriven M, Hartshorne T *et al.* Role of saphenous surgery in the treatment of venous ulceration. *Br J Surg* 1999; **86**: 755–759.

14. Sethia KK and Darke SG. Long saphenous incompetence as a cause of venous ulceration. *Br J Surg* 1984; **71**: 754–755.

15. Stuart WP, Adam DJ, Allan PL *et al.* Saphenous surgery does not correct perforator incompetence in the presence of deep venous reflux. *J Vasc Surg* 1998; **28**: 834–838.

16. Scriven JM, Hartshorne T, Thrush AJ et al. Role of saphenous surgery in the treatment of venous ulceration. *Br J Surg* 1998; **85**: 781–784.

17. Darke SG. Can we tailor surgery to the venous abnormality? In: *Venous Disease, Epidemiology Management and Delivery of Care.* Ruckley CV, Fowkes FGR, Bradbury AW (eds). London: Springer 1998: 139–42.

18. Akesson H. Long-term clinical results following correction of incompetent superficial and perforating veins in patients with deep venous incompetence and ulcers. *Phlebology* 1993; **81**: 29–131.

19. Padberg FT, Pappas PJ, Araki CT *et al.* Haemodynamic and clinical improvement after superficial vein ablation in primary combined venous insufficiency with ulceration. *J Vasc Surg* 1996; **24**: 711–718.

20. Linton RR. The communicating veins of the lower leg and operative techniques for their ligation. *Ann Surg* 1938; **107**: 582–593.

21. Dodd H, Cockett FB. *The Pathology and Surgery of the Veins of the Lower Limb* 2nd edn. Edinburgh: Churchill Livingstone, 1976.

22. Cockett FB, Elgan-Jones DE. The ankle-blow-out syndrome. *Lancet* 1953; **1**: 17–53.

23. Burnand K, Thomas ML, O'Donnell T *et al.* Relationship between post-phlebitic changes in the deep veins and the results of surgical treatment of venous leg ulcers. *Lancet* 1976; **1**: 936–938.

24. Stacey MC, Burnand KG, Layer GT *et al.* Calf pump function in patients with healed venous ulcers is not improved by surgery to the communicating veins or by elastic stockings. *Br J Surg* 1988; **75**: 436–439.

25. Negus D and Friegood A. The effective management of venous ulceration. *Br J Surg* 1983; **70**: 623–627.

26. Rhodes JM, Gloviczki P, Canton L *et al.* Endoscopic perforator division with ablation of superficial reflux improves venous haemodynamics. *J Vasc Surg* 1998; **28**: 839–847.

Surgery heals venous ulcers

Against the motion
RM Greenhalgh

Introduction

Chronic venous ulcers are a major problem with 1% of the population suffering from them. The prevalence ranges from 1% for all adults[1] to more than 3.6% for people over 65 years of age.[2] Venous ulceration occurs when venous blood of high pressure gravitates to the ankles. The ulcers are sometimes referred to as gravitational ulcers. In simple terms the process of competitive inhibition occurs at the ankle when the venous pressure is so high at the ankle level that the arterial circulation is compromised, ulceration follows. The distribution of the ulceration is generally either predominantly on the medial aspect of the so-called 'gaiter' area or on the lateral aspect. Traditionally it has been reckoned that if more contribution comes from the long saphenous vein, the medial situation is more likely and when more contribution comes from the short saphenous system the lateral ulceration is more likely. However, the findings are never absolute. If venous ulcer is caused essentially by high pressure of venous blood around the ankle level, then certainly there is known to be a multiplicity of venous problems which can lead to such high pressure of venous blood.[3] High pressure of venous blood may be simply due to underlying varicose veins which account for 20–50% of venous leg ulcers[4, 5] or rise from incompetence of the valves of the deep veins. The latter may be due to previous deep vein thrombosis or primary valve failure.[6]

Various mechanisms for venous ulceration have been suggested including the stagnant blood theory of Homans[7] and the 'Fibrin cuff' hypothesis of Browse and Burnand.[8] Also the 'white cell trapping' hypothesis has been suggested.[9]

Despite these theories of mechanism, it has been shown that compression therapy heals venous ulceration and has become the mainstay of treatment. The use of compression therapy has resulted in vastly improved healing rates of venous ulcers.[10,11,12]

In the United Kingdom £400 million per annum is spent managing patients with venous ulceration.[13] Compression bandaging is effective in some 60% of patients.

Evidence

A number of systematic reviews on venous ulcer treatment have been undertaken. A systematic review covering compression therapy as treatment and strategies to reduce venous ulcer recurrence concluded that the use of high compression therapy improves healing.[10]

Only one randomized trial has been identified for the efficacy of surgery.[14] It is a very small trial and inconclusive. Recurrence following compression treatment ranges from 7 to 69% at 1 year and can be reduced by compression hosiery.[15,16,17]

Superficial venous incompetence contributes to the aetiology of venous ulcers and it is therefore suprising that a recent review using a comprehensive search strategy identified only one randomized controlled trial comparing the effects of venous surgery with no surgery on the outcome of leg ulcer healing.[18] This randomized controlled trial involved 47 patients. There was no difference in the proportion of ulcers healed at 1 year or the rate of ulcer healing. The trial was extremely small.

Therefore, the basic facts are that it can be fairly assumed that venous ulceration is caused by high pressure of venous blood at the ankles and that healing of venous ulcers can be achieved by reducing this high pressure of venous blood. This is successfully achieved by bedrest, elevation and compression bandaging such as the four-layer bandage technique. It is remarkable that surgery has never been proved to be beneficial in the healing rate of venous ulcers.

On the contrary there seems to be good evidence that it is likely that surgery will affect beneficially the recurrence rate of venous ulceration after healing. Undoubtedly once a ulcer is healed the patient will be asked to wear compression stockings and some will and some will not. Those who do not will have exactly the same risk of developing venous ulceration again as they had in the first place. If the venous abnormalities have been corrected surgically then it is possible and more likely that venous ulceration will not occur again.

A multicentre ulcer surgery against bandaging (USABLE) trial is currently underway supported by the Medical Research Council in Britain. Patients receive compression bandaging until healing, then stockings. Half of the patients are randomized to receive vein surgery in addition. Ulcer healing and recurrence of ulceration are the main endpoints.

Summary

- Venous ulceration is caused by high pressure venous blood around the ankles.

- Elastic compression techniques with bandages have been shown to hasten healing of venous ulcers.

- Hosiery and compression techniques reduce recurrence of venous ulcers.

- There is no evidence that surgery hastens the healing of venous ulcers.

- Surgery probably reduces the recurrence rate of venous ulcers.

References

1. Dale JJ, Callam MJ, Ruckley CV, Harper DR, Berrey PN. Chronic ulcer of the leg: a study of prevalence in a Scottish community. *Health Bull* 1983; 41: 310–314.

2. Bobek K, Cajzl L, Cepelak V, Slaisova V *et al*. Etude de la frequence des maladies phlebologiques et de l'influence de quelques facteurs etiologiques. *Phlebologie* 1996; 19: 217–230.

3. Nicholaides AN, Zukowski A, Lewis R, Kyprianou P, Malouf GM. Venous pressure measurements in venous problems. In *Surgery of the Veins*. JJ Bergan, JST Yao (eds). Orlando: Grune and Stratton, 1985: 111–118.

4. Dodd H, Cockett FB. *The Pathology and Surgery of the Veins of the Lower Limb*. Edinburgh: Churchill Livingston, 1976.

5. Hoare MC, Nicholaides AN, Miles CR *et al*. The role of primary varicose veins in venous ulceration. *Surgery* 1982 **92**: 450–453.

6. Kistner RL. Primary venous valve incompetence of the leg. *Am J Surg* 1980; **140**: 218–224.

7. Homans J. The aetiology and treatment of varicose ulcers of the leg. *Surg Gynaecol Obstet* 1917; 24: 300–311.

8. Browse NL, Burnand KG. The cause of venous ulceration. *Lancet* 1982; 2: 243–245.

9. Coleridge Smith PD, Thomas P, Scurr JH, Dormandy JA. Causes of venous ulceration: a new hypothesis. *BMJ* 1988; **296**: 1726–1727.

10. Effective Health Care Bulletin. Compression therapy for venous leg ulcers. EHCB 3, no4. 1997.

11. Partsch H, Ruckley CV, Fowkes FGR, Bradbury AW (eds). Compression therapy: is it worthwhile? In. *Venous Disease*. Berlin: Springer-Verlag, 1999: 117–125.

12. Fletcher A, Cullum N, Sheldon TA. A systematic review of compression treatment for venous leg ulcers. *BMJ* 1997; **315**: 576–580.

13. Wilson E. Prevention and treatment of venous leg ulcers. *Health Trends* 1989; **21**: 97.

14. Stacey M, Burnand K, Layer G *et al*. Calf pump function in patients with healed venous ulcers is not improved by surgery to the communicating veins or by elastic stockings. *Br J Surg* 1988; **75**: 436–439.

15. Duby T, Hoffman D, Cameron J *et al*. A randomised trial in the treatment of venous leg ulcers comparing short stretch bandages, four layer bandage system and long stretch-paste bandage system. Wounds – A compendium of clinical research and practice 1993; **5**: 276–279.

16. Morrell CJ, Walters SJ, Dixon S *et al*. Cost effectiveness of community leg ulcer clinics: randomised controlled trial. *BMJ* 1998; **6**: 1487–1491.

17. Lagatolla NRF, Burnand KG, Eastham D. A comparison of perforating vein ligation, stanzol and stockings in the prevention of recurrent venous ulceration. *Phlebology* 1985; **10**: 79–85.

18. Warburg FE, Danielsen L, Madsen SM *et al*. Vein surgery with or without skin grafting versus conservative treatment for leg ulcers. *Acta Dermatol Venereol* 1994; **74**: 307–309.

Surgery heals venous ulcers

Charing Cross Editorial Comments towards Consensus

As the reason for venous ulcer is known to be high pressure venous blood often caused by demonstrable incompetence of the superficial veins, the common view is that surgery should be performed wherever possible to cure the ulcer. In an earlier era there was a search for perforating veins to be ligated to correct the so-called 'blow-out' veins described by Cockett. It is now known that stagnation ulceration can be caused by a multiplicity of venous abnormalities and there is a great temptation to think that surgery, to correct the underlying problem, should heal venous ulcers more rapidly. The evidence has been slow to emerge and Peter Taylor has given his evidence in support of surgery of various types.

However, there is less controversy about the value of surgery to prevent recurrence of ulceration. So whereas it has also been argued that there is simply not strong enough evidence to support the concept that surgery is effective in causing more rapid healing of venous ulcers there is less opposition to the suspected value of surgery to maintain ulcer healing. The debate will certainly lead to heated exchange and even possibly consensus in some areas, but there needs to be hard data and we hope it will come from the USABLE trial.

Roger M Greenhalgh
Editor

Below-knee venous thrombosis merits treatment

For the motion

Jean-Georges Kretz, Nabil Chakfe,
Simon Rinckenbach, Othman Hassani,
Jocelyn Celerien

Introduction

Preventive treatment for thrombophlebitis has been widely accepted since the publication by Kakkar *et al.*[1] and is actually part of a postoperative routine treatment. Duplex scanning is actually the most common method for diagnosis of venous thrombosis of the lower extremity.

Conflicting opinions have been published concerning calf vein thrombosis but we are still convinced that calf vein thrombosis is not a minor problem. Most often calf vein thrombosis is found as the starting point of more proximal deep venous thrombosis. Calf vein thrombosis may be complicated by pulmonary emboli and has also a strong potential for late complications such as post-thrombotic syndrome.

Therefore calf vein thrombosis has to be considered in the same way as any other location of deep venous thrombosis and has to be treated as well. The last point to be discussed is how calf vein thrombosis should be treated and for how long?

Evidence

Frequency of below-knee venous thrombosis

Kakkar *et al.* in 1969 suggested that the majority of deep venous thrombosis originated in the calf veins especially in the soleal sinuses and clotting begins most frequently in calf veins.[1] The first group of papers to suggest that deep vein thrombosis usually begins in the calf were mostly using I_{125} or labelled fibrinogen and phlebography to assess their statements.[2-6] Browse in 1974, using phlebography, reported a 43% incidence of calf vein thrombosis in 430 cases of phlebitis.[6] In 35% calf vein thrombus was contiguous to more proximal thrombosis and in 14% calf vein thrombosis coexisted with another location of thrombosis but without contiguity.

Calf vein thrombi often propagate more proximally. The frequency of upward propagation was estimated as 20% by Kakkar[1] and 30% by Nicolaides.[5]

Most recently non-invasive diagnosis of deep vein thrombosis has been proposed and nowadays duplex ultrasound is the most common method to assess deep venous thrombosis.[7-10] Mattos[7] reviewed 540 symptomatic patients with suspected deep vein thrombosis. He found that all three paired calf veins were visualized in 94% of cases. Calf vein thrombosis was present in 69% of the limbs with deep vein thrombosis. Clots were confined in the calf in 33%. The most locations were the peroneal (81%) and the posterior tibial vein (69%).

These data were confirmed by Labropoulos[8] in 1999 in a series of 5250 patients refered for suspected deep venous thrombosis. He reported an isolated calf vein thrombosis incidence of 4.8% (282 limbs). In this group he demonstrated that thrombus involved most frequently (40%) muscular veins that are not usually investigated in routine screenings using duplex ultrasound. Therefore he recommended routine examination of soleal and gastrocnemial veins.

Diagnosis of calf vein thrombosis

In the past, diagnosis of deep venous thrombosis was mostly assessed by invasive methods such as venous angiogram or fibrinogen uptake test. Ultrasonography is now used as a routine examination to screen the patients suspected of deep venous thrombosis or in patients suspected of pulmonary emboli.

Duplex ultrasound was rapidly accepted as the method of choice for non-invasive diagnosis of deep venous thrombosis. As showed by Lensing in 1989,[11] in a comparative study between B mode ultrasonography and venogram, the sensitivity of ultrasounds in proximal deep venous thrombosis was 100% with a 99% specificity. But it was not sensitive in detection of calf vein thrombi.

Further developments in ultrasonography were proposed and accuracy of deep venous thrombosis diagnosis progressively became more performant. The reasons for this evolution appear in the literature (Table 1). In fact the most effective progress was in the quality control of the technique of the duplex examination. Most of the published series only used limited exploration of the inguinal and popliteal areas and very few used compression and routinely detected calf veins and deep muscular vein thrombosis.

Table 1. Prevalence of deep venous thrombosis (DVT) detected by duplex.

Authors	DVT % by duplex	Type of exploration
Fowl[12]	11 (45/412)	Crural popliteal
Perrier[13]	11 (48/444)	Inguinal and popliteal
Turkstra[14]	15 (52/357)	Inguinal and popliteal
Barrelier[15]	30.4 (107/352)	IVC to the ankles
Van Rossum[9]		
Meta analysis of 12 studies	18	

Diagnosis of calf vein thrombosis requires appropriate duplex examination. All the veins of both legs have to be explored especially muscular veins such as solear and gastrocnemial veins[7] and since peroneal and posterior tibial veins are most frequently involved they should routinely be scrutinized.[8]

Below-knee thrombosis and pulmonary emboli

We have very few data on pulmonary emboli in non-treated isolated calf vein thrombosis. In his meta-analysis, Philbrick[16] was able to collect data from five studies. Two of them suggested that the risk of pulmonary migration was low but their follow-up seems to be weak since they only examined their patients once at 3 months.[3,17] Others like Kakkar[1] confirm that propagation from the calf veins to the proximal veins occurs in 23% but pulmonary emboli occured only in those patients with proximal propagation. So if propagation definitely can occur, reported cases with pulmonary emboli in isolated calf vein thrombosis were not obviously demonstrated in this study.

Passmann reported a 35% incidence of pulmonary embolism in isolated calf vein thrombosis.[18]

In 1999, Kazmers published more convincing data in a study on the incidence of propagation and pulmonary emboli in isolated calf vein thrombosis.[19] The incidence of proximal progression was 25% with an incidence of 36% of pulmonary emboli and 27% mortality in the group with proximal progression of the thrombus.

Guias in 1999 also reported an incidence of 15% pulmonary emboli in isolated calf vein thrombosis.[20]

So, it appears clearly that pulmonary emboli can complicate isolated vein thrombosis below the knee especially in case of proximal propagation of the thrombus originally located in the calf veins.[21]

Below-knee thrombosis and post-phlebitis syndrome

Does isolated calf vein thrombosis have potential to cause complications in the long-term with post-phlebitis syndrome?

Philbrick in 1988[16] gave some answer to this question. He studied nine published series on long-term complications of calf vein thrombosis. One study followed non-treated patients, two followed patients with only initial anticoagulants and seven studies followed patients treated initially and in the long-term with anticoagulants. Follow-up varied from 6 months to 10 years. Most of these studies were given a rather weak evidence rate. Post-thrombotic venous disease was found in 21–79% of the cases, but in the two studies where both legs were examined, bilateral venous disease was found even if the contralateral leg was initially not involved.

More recently, Ziegler[22] studied post-thrombotic syndrome in patients treated for deep venous thrombosis 10 to 20 years ago. They demonstrate that calf vein thrombosis is one of the four significant factors predicting clinically relevant post-thrombotic syndrome within 10 to 20 years of deep venous thrombosis.

In fact even if there is no prospective study available some data suggest that isolated calf vein thrombosis may cause complications in the later follow-up with post-thrombotic syndrome.

Treatment of isolated below-knee deep venous thrombosis

In our opinion there is no question whether to treat or not to treat isolated below-knee deep venous thrombosis. Because of its frequency as an isolated phenomenom, because of its potential to propagate more proximally in 25–30%, because of its potential risk of pulmonary embolism which is not zero and because of its tendency to evolve in the later follow-up to post-thrombotic syndrome, isolated below-knee deep venous thrombosis is all but not benign and should definitely be treated medically.

These data have been accepted in UK vascular practice since 74% of the vascular consultants in UK[23] report that calf veins are specifically sought during routine investigation for deep venous thrombosis. In the case of thrombosis of calf veins, a majority of them will be treated classically using heparin first followed by oral anticoagulants.

Calf vein thrombosis should be treated initially using either heparin or low molecular weight heparin for a 5-day period followed by a switch to oral anticoagulants. One issue to be discussed is how long should we treat?

Recently a randomized trial compared a short oral anticoagulant course (6 weeks) with a long course (12 weeks) in isolated calf vein thrombosis.[24] The outcome events were recurrence, major, minor or lethal bleeding complications. Conclusions were that a 6-week treatment for isolated calf vein thrombosis is sufficient in the absence of permanent recurrence risk factors. In the case of specific risk factors for recurrence, further trials are requested.

Summary

- Calf vein thrombosis is frequent in deep venous thrombosis and is most often located in muscular veins.

- Proximal propagation of calf vein thrombosis is observed within 20–30% of deep venous thrombosis.

- Accuracy of duplex in calf vein thrombosis diagnosis is good.

- When proximal propagation occurs, pulmonary emboli are frequent.

- There is no predictive factor available for proximal propagation or pulmonary emboli.

- Isolated calf vein thrombosis may lead to post-thrombotic syndrome in the later follow-up.

- Isolated calf vein thrombosis has to be treated for at least 6 weeks.

References

1. Kakkar VV, Howe CT, Flanc C, Clarke MB. The natural history of post-operative deep vein thrombosis. *Lancet* 1969; **2**: 230–232.
2. Nicolaides AN, Kakkar VV, Field ES, Renney JT. The origin of deep vein thrombosis: a venographic study. *Br J Radiol* 1971; **44**: 653–663.
3. Hunter WC, Krygier JJ, Kennedy JC *et al.* Etiology and prevention of thrombosis of the deep veins: a study of 400 cases. *Surgery* 1945; **17**: 178.
4. Moreno-Cabral R, Kistner RL, Nordyke RA. Importance of calf vein thrombosis. *Surgery* 1976; **80**: 735–742.
5. Nicolaides AN, Desai S, Dupont PA *et al.* Small doses of subcutaneous sodium heparin in preventing deep venous thrombosis after major surgery. *Lancet* 1972; **2**: 890.
6. Browse NL, Thomas ML. Source of non-lethal pulmonary emboli. *Lancet* 1974; **1**: 258.
7. Mattos MA, Melendres G, Sumner DS *et al.* Prevalence and distribution of calf vein thrombosis in patients with symptomatic deep venous thrombosis: a color-flow duplex study. *J Vasc Surg* 1996; **24**: 738–744.
8. Labropoulos N, Webb KM, Kang SS *et al.* Patterns and distribution of isolated calf vein thrombosis. *J Vasc Surg* 1999; **30**: 787–793.

9. Van Rossum AB, Van Houwelingen HC, Kieft GJ, Pattynama PM. Prevalence of deep vein thrombosis in suspected and proven pulmonary embolism: a meta analysis. *Br J Radiol* 1998; **71**: 1260–1265.

10. Ouriel K, Green RM, Greenberg RK, Clair DG. The anatomy of deep venous thrombosis of the lower extremity. *J Vasc Surg* 2000; **31**: 895–900.

11. Lensing AW, Prandoni P, Brandjes D *et al.* Detection of deep vein thrombosis by real time B mode ultrasonography. *N Engl J Med* 1989; **320**: 342–345.

12. Fowl RJ, Stothman GB, Bleblea J *et al.* Inappropriate use of venous duplex scans: an analysis of indications and results. *J Vasc Surg* 1996; **23**: 881–886.

13. Perrier A, Desmarais S, Miron MJ *et al.* Non-invasive diagnosis of venous thromboembolism in outpatients. *Lancet* 1999; **353**: 190–195.

14. Turkstra F, Kuijer PM, Van Beek EJ *et al.* Diagnosis utility of ultrasonography of leg veins in patients suspected of having pulmonary embolism. *Ann Intern Med* 1997; **126**: 775–781.

15. Barrelier MT, Lezin B, Landy S , Le Hello C. Prévalence de la thrombose veineuse diagnostiquée par échographie-doppler des membres inférieurs dans la suspiscion d'embolie pulmonaire. *J Mal Vasc* 2001; **26**: 23–30.

16. Philbrick JT, Becker DM. Calf vein thrombosis: a wolf in sheep's clothing? *Arch Int Med* 1988; **148**: 2131–2138.

17. Moser KM, Le Moine JR Is embolic risk conditionned by location of deep venous thrombosis? *Ann Intern Med* 1981; **94**: 439–444.

18. Passman MA, Moneta GL, Taylor LM *et al.* Pulmonary embolism is associated with the combination of isolated calf vein thrombosis and respiratory symptoms. *J Vasc Surg* 1997; **25**: 39–45.

19. Kazmers A, Groehn H, Meeker C. Acute calf vein thrombosis: outcomes and implications. *Am Surg* 1999; **65**: 1124–1127.

20. Guias B, Simoni G, Oger E *et al.* Calf muscle venous thrombosis and pulmonary embolism. *J Mal Vasc* 1999; **24**: 132–134.

21. Lohr JM, Kerr TM, Lutter KS *et al.* Lower extremity calf thrombosis: to treat or not to treat? *J Vasc Surg* 1991; **14**: 618–623.

22. Ziegler S, Schillinger M, Maca TH, Minar E. Post-thrombotic syndrome after primary event of deep venous thrombosis 10 to 20 years ago. *Thromb Res* 2001; **15**: 23–33.

23. Turton EPL, Coughlin PA, Berridge DC, Mercer KG. A survey of deep venous thrombosis management by consultant vascular surgeons in the United Kingdom and Ireland. *Eur J Vasc Endovasc Surg* 2001; **21**: 558–563.

24. Pinede L, Ninet J, Duhaut P *et al.* Comparison of 3 and 6 months of oral anticoagulant therapy after a first episode of proximal deep vein thrombosis or pulmonary embolism and comparison of 6 and 12 weeks of therapy after isolated calf deep vein thrombosis. *Circulation* 2001; **103**: 2453–2460.

Below-knee venous thrombosis merits treatment

Against the motion
W Bruce Campbell

Introduction

Deep vein thrombosis usually begins in veins below the knee – particularly the venous sinuses within soleus. If thrombus propagates to involves the above-knee popliteal, femoral, or iliac veins, then there is a risk that a portion may detach, causing pulmonary embolism which may be fatal. In the longer term persistent obstruction to veins or damage to their valves may result in leg swelling, skin damage and pain. Anticoagulant treatment for above-knee deep vein thrombosis is well accepted clinical practice, but treatment of calf vein thrombosis remains controversial: at an international venous meeting in 1996 a poll of the 150 delegates showed almost equal numbers for and against the practice of anticoagulation for calf vein thrombosis.[1]

The proposition that isolated calf vein thrombosis merits treatment by anticoagulants would rely upon evidence that anticoagulation influences one or more of the following:

1. the short-term effects of calf vein thrombosis,
2. the risk of propagation or pulmonary embolism,
3. the risk of recurrence of deep vein thrombosis,
4. the risk of long-term venous dysfunction and symptoms (post-phlebitic syndrome).

A review of all English language papers 14 years ago (1942–1987)[2] concluded that there was no convincing evidence that calf vein thrombosis led to chronic venous insufficiency or that anticoagulation conferred any benefit. Since that time, however, serial examination of the lower limb veins has become much easier and more commonplace with the use of duplex ultrasound, and a numbers of recent papers have described cohorts of patients in whom isolated calf vein thrombosis has been found on duplex scanning. There are no prospective or randomized studies of anticoagulation for treatment of isolated calf vein thrombosis, but sufficient data exist to show that routine use of anticoagulants is not indicated.

The natural history and short-term effects of calf vein thrombosis

Studies done 30 years ago using ^{125}I-labelled fibrinogen showed that calf vein thrombosis was common in the postoperative period, affecting 30% of patients.[3] Of 40 patients with deep vein thrombosis in the thigh or calf, Kakkar et al.[3] observed that 14 had had raised ^{125}I counts for less than 72 hours, and venography showed only localized deep vein thrombosis less than 5 cm long in the tibial or soleal veins. This clear evidence that calf vein thrombosis frequently remains minor and undergoes rapid lysis is supported by more recent work: Masuda et al.[1] studied 54 limbs with isolated calf vein thrombosis using serial duplex scans and showed complete resolution of thrombi by 3 months in 88% (half the patients had received no anticoagulants). In addition, studies which used 'normal control subjects' have found evidence of reflux in the calf veins in 6–19% of controls.[1,4] This suggests that minor calf vein thrombosis may be a common asymptomatic phenomenon, which resolves unnoticed. Even when patients present with symptoms of possible deep vein thrombosis, it is common practice to scan only veins above the knee,[5] and if duplex scanning of calf veins is done minor calf vein thrombosis is easy to miss.[6,7] All this suggests that many cases of calf vein thrombosis remain undetected and untreated without any clinical sequelae.

Propagation of isolated calf vein thrombosis

The observed incidence of propagation of calf vein thrombosis varies from 0–25% in different studies, with most reporting propagation rates around 15%.[1,6,8–10] Anticoagulation seems to have no significant effect on the risk of propagation, based on the raw data from retrospective studies. Indeed, anticoagulated patients showed a greater tendency to propagation of calf vein thrombosis than those did not receive anticoagulants in two studies.[6,9] Solis et al.[6] reported propagation in 3 of 13 (23%) anticoaglated patients after hip and knee surgery, compared with 2 of 25 (8%) who were not treated. Kazmers et al.[9] performed serial duplex scans on 71 patients, and showed propagation to proximal deep vein thrombosis in 25% of those receiving anticoagulants at the time of the initial scan, compared with 6% of those not receiving anticoagulants. Clearly the referring clinicians had already made a judgement about the need for anticoagulants based on a variety of clinical features, but nevertheless these data show that very few patients propagate their calf vein thrombosis without anticoagulant treatment, while propagation is a common phenomenon despite anticoagulation.

Two separate studies have each documented proximal propagation of calf vein thrombosis despite anticoagulant treatment – in 15% of 50 patients studied by O'Shaughnessy et al. (85% anticoagulated),[10] and 18% of 28 fully heparinized patients reported by Langerstadt et al.[11] By contrast, propagation occurred in only 2 of 26 (8%) limbs with calf vein thrombosis which were not treated by anticoagulants in the study by Masuda et al.[1] These observations provide an argument for serial duplex scanning of patients with calf vein thrombosis to detect proximal progression, but not for routine use of anticoagulants.

Isolated calf vein thrombosis and pulmonary embolism

A number of studies have reported an association between the finding of calf vein thrombosis and pulmonary embolism. For example, Kazmers et al.[9] documented a high probability result for pulmonary embolism in 10 of 18 ventilation/perfusion scans, among a cohort of 118 patients with calf vein thrombosis; Masuda et al.[1] described an initial presentation with pulmonary symptoms and highly suggestive scans in 8 of 54 patients who then had only calf vein thrombosis on duplex examination; and Guias et al.[12] documented an association between calf vein thrombosis and pulmonary embolism in 16 of 106 patients (15%). In all these patients presenting with pulmonary symptoms, however, it is possible that the fragments of deep vein thrombosis which had embolized to the lungs detached from more proximal veins (the commonly accepted reason for pulmonary embolism) and that the calf vein thrombosis then observed on duplex scans was all that remained of the original lower limb deep vein thrombosis.

Few studies have sought an association between calf vein thrombosis, pulmonary embolism and anticoagulants, but Meissner et al.[8] observed pulmonary embolism in just one patient (treated with anticoagulants) among 58 calf vein thrombosis patients; while Moser et al.[13] observed none in a follow-up study of 21 patients who did not receive anticoagulants.

There is no doubt that occasional patients progress from an initial presentation with calf vein thrombosis to suffer pulmonary embolism, but those cases which have been clearly described have had other major risk factors suggesting the need for anti-coagulants. Specific examples are patients with cancer[10,14] and those with a past history of venous thromboembolism.[1] Such patients ought to be considered for anti-coagulation: they constitute a different group to those with isolated calf vein thrombosis in the absence of other major risk factors.

The recurrence rate of calf vein thrombosis

There is no evidence that anticoagulants affect the rate of recurrence after calf vein thrombosis. Indeed, the one recent study which addressed this issue provides a particular example of inadequate methodology and inappropriate extrapolation of data. Astermark et al.[15] reviewed a cohort of 126 patients shown to have calf vein thrombosis on venograms, who had nearly all been treated with 6 weeks of anticoagulation, in accordance with their unit policy. Four (3%) had recurrent thromboembolism within 3 months, and 11 (9%) within 2 years. There was no serial imaging of the leg veins; no organized follow-up was done; and there was no control group. On this basis the authors concluded that their policy to treat calf vein thrombosis with 6 weeks of anticoagulants was justified, but their data provided no scientific basis for this conclusion.

The findings of recent long-term follow-up studies after calf vein thrombosis are shown in Table 1 below.

Points to note from these studies are

1. Long-term symptoms are quite uncommon, mostly mild, and seldom attributable to venous disease.
2. Function in the calf veins is frequently abnormal in control subjects.
3. Taken together, these studies show little difference between calf vein thrombosis patients followed up in the long-term and controls.
4. Calf vein segments found to be occluded years after calf vein thrombosis are usually in vein segments which were not affected by the original thrombosis.

All these observations testify to the relatively benign prognosis of calf vein thrombosis in the long-term.

Table 1. The risk of long-term venous dysfunction or symptoms (post-phlebitic syndrome).

Authors and year	No. of patients	Method of follow-up	Duration of follow-up	Findings
Meissner et al. 1997[8] *72% anticoagulated*	29	Clinical Duplex	1 year	Symptoms in 23% Reflux in 24% No residual thrombus in any case
Haenen et al. 1998[16] *100% anticoagulated*	16	Clinical Duplex	10 years	83% thrombosed segments patent No difference between initially thombosed and non-thrombosed segments for reflux (7% vs 5%) and non-compressibility (10% vs 5%)
Masuda et al. 1998[1] *51% anticoagulated*	23 CVT Controls – 26 for duplex – 10 for APG	Clinical Duplex APG	1–6 years (median 3)	Limb pain in one-third, but none typically venous. Reflux (>0.5s) in 9% initially thrombosed veins. Any reflux in 39% CVT group vs 19% controls (n.s.) APG abnormal in 26% CVT patients vs 30% controls
McLafferty et al. 1998[4] *51% anticoagulated*	37 CVT 17 controls	Clinical Duplex PPG	2–6 years (median 3.4)	Abnormal valve closure in 26% CVT legs (but mostly NOT segments initially thrombosed) PPG abnormal in 23% CVT vs 9% controls

APG: Air plethysmography.
PPG: Photoplethysmography.
CVT: Calf vein thrombosis.

Summary

- Minor calf vein thrombosis is common and usually resolves spontaneously.

- The incidence of proximal propagation is low; propagation can occur in anticoagulated patients; and anticoagulants have not been shown to reduce the risk.

- Pulmonary embolism in the presence of calf vein thrombosis is likely to be due to more proximal deep vein thrombosis which has already embolized.

- There is no evidence that anticoagulants reduce the recurrence rate of calf vein thrombosis.

- Post-phlebitic syndrome is rare after calf vein thrombosis.

- Long-term follow-up studies show few differences between calf vein thrombosis patients and controls.

- There is an argument for serial duplex scanning of isolated calf vein thrombosis, but not for the routine use of anticoagulants.

References

1. Masuda EM, Kessler DM, Kistner RL, Eklof B, Sato DT. The natural history of calf vein thrombosis: lysis of thrombi and development of reflux. *J Vasc Surg* 1998; 28: 67–74.
2. Philbrick JT, Becker DM. Calf vein thrombosis. A wolf in sheep's clothing? *Arch Intern Med* 1988; 148: 2131–2138.
3. Kakkar VV, Howe CT, Flanc C, Clarke MB. Natural history of postoperative deep-vein thrombosis. *Lancet* 1969; 2: 230–232.
4. McLafferty RB, Moneta GL, Brant BM *et al*. Late clinical and hemodynamic sequelae of isolated calf vein thrombosis. *J Vasc Surg* 1998; 27: 50–57.
5. Gottleib RH, Widjaja J, Mehra S, Robinetta WB. Clinically important pulmonary pulmonary emboli: does calf vein US alter outcomes? *Radiology* 1999; 211: 25–29.
6. Solis MM, Ranval TJ, Nix ML *et al*. Is anticoagulation indicated for asymptomatic postoperative calf vein thrombosis? *J Vasc Surg* 1992; 16: 414–419.
7. Labropoulos N, Webb KM, Kang SS *et al*. Patterns and distribution of isolated calf deep vein thrombosis. *J Vasc Surg* 1999; 30: 787–793.
8. Meissner MH, Caps MT, Bergelin RO, Manzo RA, Strandness DE. Early outcome after isolated calf vein thrombosis. *J Vasc Surg* 1992; 26: 749–756.
9. Kazmers A, Groehn H, Meeker C. Acute calf vein thrombosis: outcomes and implications. *Am Surg* 1999; 65: 1124–1128.
10. O'Shaughnessey AM, Fitzgerald DE. The value of duplex ultrasound in the follow-up of acute calf vein thrombosis. *Int Angiol* 1997; 16: 142–146.
11. Langerstadt CI, Olsson CG, Fagher BO *et al*. Need for long-term anticoagulant treatment in symptomatic calf-vein thrombosis *J Vasc Surg* 1985; 2: 515–518.
12. Guias B, Simoni G, Oger E *et al*. Thrombose veineuse musculaire du mollet et embolie pulmonaire. *J Malad Vasc (Paris)* 1999; 24: 132–134.
13. Moser KM, LeMoine JR. Is embolic risk conditioned by location of deep vein thrombosis? *Ann Intern Med* 1981; 94: 439–444.
14. Bartter T, Hollingsworth HM, Irwin RS *et al*. Pulmonary embolism from a venous thrombus located below the knee. *Arch Intern Med* 1987; 147: 373–375.
15. Astermark J, Bjorgell O, Linden E *et al*. Low recurrence rate after deep calf-vein thrombosis with 6 weeks of oral anticoagulation. *J Intern Med* 1998; 244: 79–82.
16. Haenen JH, Janssen MCH, van Langen H *et al*. Duplex ultrasound in the hemodynamic evaluation of the late sequelae of deep vein thrombosis. *J Vasc Surg* 1998; 27: 472–478.

Below-knee venous thrombosis merits treatment

Charing Cross Editorial Comments towards Consensus

This is an old chestnut. When is a deep venous thrombosis safe to leave? If it is really tiny it could be argued that even if it moves it could not be fatal. If it is adherent to the vein wall it could be argued that it isn't going to shift and therefore is not a danger. These arguments have been heard but they say nothing of the expectation of propagating thrombus and the reason why the first thrombosis occurred. Others say any deep vein thrombosis once diagnosed should be treated with anticoagulants for 6 months.

One of the problems is that accurate diagnosis of early venous thrombosis has not been with us for long, and in addition venography was not performed at every hospital with great care; plus duplex scan is at its worst in the calf vessels. I think it would be a fair conclusion to say that there are safe deep venous thrombi which can be left without anticoagulants but it is mighty hard to decide at any time to leave one alone and not to use anticoagulants once a diagnosis of deep vein thrombosis has been made accurately.

Roger M Greenhalgh
Editor